# Praise for Toni Weschler's *Taking Charge of Your Fertility*

*❦ From Clients of Toni Weschler's Fertility Awareness Seminars:*

"I had noticed certain changes in my cycle for years, but I never knew what it all meant until Toni Weschler's Fertility Awareness seminar. It was the missing link. Initially, I felt liberated, privileged to have this knowledge and to really know the most personal, basic things I should know about myself. Am I pregnant? Am I fertile? When will I get my period? After the initial joy, I felt some anger. Why hadn't someone told me earlier?"     —Therese Frare

"Toni Weschler's Fertility Awareness seminars changed my life, and her book is long overdue. Women everywhere should have the opportunity to learn what I learned in her class—that I can be in control of my body, that I can read my body's own signs that reveal when I'm fertile and when I'm not, and so much more. Learning all this and when I'm about to menstruate with astonishing accuracy was a true revelation. I have used Fertility Awareness as a method of birth control now for six years. Not only has it been completely reliable for preventing pregnancy, but when my husband and I decided we wanted a baby, we were able to conceive on our very first try."     —Heather Worthley

"We had been trying to become pregnant for about a year. Two months after we completed Toni Weschler's Fertility Awareness seminar, we conceived. I truly believe this was due to the knowledge we received from the class. We discovered that my 'fertile window' was very brief compared to many women. We were both fascinated by the information about the human body and how it works, most of which we didn't know or had been misinformed about prior to taking her class."     —Mark and Judy Jorgensen

*❦ From Health Professionals:*

"Toni Weschler is stupendous. Her book addresses hardcore facts and functions to each and every person's individual variations in their body and body fluids. Toni's knowledge, depth, sincerity, and appreciation for couples trying to conceive is most heartwarming. The small details that her book goes into are not possible in the course of a daily busy office routine."

—Michael Greer, M.D.,
Obstetrician/Gynecologist

"From my eighteen years of experience teaching college students about women's bodies and their hormonal cycles, I can say without hesitation that *Taking Charge of Your Fertility* is desperately needed and desired by a large number of women. My students have made it clear that they want to know more about their bodies and their cycles. They want detailed information that is truthful and comprehensible. Toni Weschler had provided it."

—Nancy Kenney, Associate Professor,
University of Washington

"This is a much-needed resource for women as well as health-care professionals. Until this book's emergence on the scene, I was aware of no other publication that deals with this topic in a very helpful and accurate way. It will be exciting to have this book available to all women. Although women claim to desire control over their own bodies, it seems there is increasing pressure on them to succumb to technology and commercial invasiveness when it comes to birth control and pregnancy. How wonderful to know that control can be returned to where it belongs."

—Molly Pessl, R.N., B.S.N.

# TAKING CHARGE OF YOUR FERTILITY

*The Definitive Guide to Natural Birth Control and Pregnancy Achievement*

## TONI WESCHLER, M.P.H.

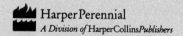
HarperPerennial
*A Division of HarperCollinsPublishers*

If you would like to be put on a mailing list for a possible newsletter or video on Fertility Awareness, please send your name and address to FACTS (Fertility Awareness Counseling and Training Seminars). In addition, any comments or suggestions for future editions of this book would be greatly appreciated:

FACTS
P.O. Box 31111
Seattle, WA 98103

Requests of Ms. Weschler for assistance with curriculum development and public speaking engagements should be accompanied by a self-addressed stamped envelope.

For individual questions about Fertility Awareness, please refer to Appendix M for various FAM/NFP resources. You may also want to check the Internet to see if a Fertility Awareness Bulletin Board has been established.

Grateful acknowledgment is made for permission to reprint the following:

Cartoons: page 45, copyright © Los Angeles Times Syndicate; page 67, copyright © Viv Quillin, "The Opposite Sex"; page 112, OFF THE LEASH reprinted by permission of UFS, Inc.; page 150, copyright © 1982, 1991 by Lynn Johnston Productions Inc. and Lynn Johnston. Reprinted from *David, We're Pregnant!* with permission of its publisher, Meadowbrook Press; page 186, copyright © David Horsey, *Seattle Post-Intelligencer,* page 215, copyright © 1988, Los Angeles Times Syndicate. Reprinted by permission; and PMS Attacks by Steve Phillips, Copyright © 1988 by Steve Phillips. Used by permission of Ten Speed Press, P.O. Box 7123, Berkeley, CA.

Adaptation of the graph on effective rates from *Contraceptive Technology* on page 313: *Contraceptive Technology,* Hatcher, R. A., Trussell, J., Stewart, F., Stewart, G. K., Kowal, P., Guest, F., Cates, W., Policar, M.S. Irvington Publishers, 1994.

Color insert: pages 1–2 of insert, photographs by Frankie Collins; page 3, photographs by Lennart Nilsson, *A Child Is Born,* Dell Publishing Company; page 4, ovulation photographs by Erlandsen/Magney: *Color Atlas of Histology,* 1992; page 5, hormone graph by Kate Sweeney; page 6, photograph of egg in fallopian tube by Lennart Nilsson, *A Child Is Born,* Dell Publishing Company, and photographs of cervical fluid and baby by Bruce Bobman.

HarperCollins books may be purchased for educational, business, or sales promotional use. For information please write: Special Markets Department, HarperCollins Publishers, Inc., 10 East 53rd Street, New York, NY 10022.

FIRST EDITION

*Medical Illustrations by Kate Sweeney & Christine Shafner*

Library of Congress Cataloging-in-Publication Data
Weschler, Toni, 1955–
   Taking charge of your fertility : the definitive guide to natural birth control and pregnancy achievement / Toni Weschler.—1st ed.
     p.  cm.
   Includes bibliographical references and index.
   ISBN 0-06-095053-6
   1. Natural family planning.  I. Title.
RG136.5.W47  1995
613.9'4—dc20                        95-13496

99  DT/RRD  20 19

*In loving memory of my mother,*
*Franzi Toch Weschler,*
*whose strength always amazed me*

# Contents

# Acknowledgments

They say women are blessed with the ability to forget the pain of childbirth so they will be able to have more than one child. I often wonder whether the same principle applies to the pain of writing a book. Had another author warned me about what a monumental task it would be, I'm not sure I would have been so intent on pursuing the dream. But I suppose writers are deluded, or perhaps their memories are simply fried from their own projects! Either way, I've come away from this endeavor having experienced the gamut of human emotion, from total frustration and misery to incredible joy and pride. Along the way, as the following list will attest, I've had the privilege of being supported by numerous people to whom I owe a debt of gratitude:

To the many health practitioners and professionals who were my advocates when this book was but a concept in my head: Andrea Brass, Suzannah Cooper Doyle, CFE, Michael Greer, M.D., Vivien Webb Hanson, M.D., Joan Helmich, Patricia Kato, M.D., Nancy Kenney, Ph.D., Chris Leininger, M.D., Zora Pesio, M.S.N., Molly Pessl, B.S.N., Suzanne Poppema, M.D., Deb Van Derhei, and Aradia Women's Health Center.

To the excellent naturopathic doctor, Rebecca Wynsome, N.D., whom I would like to single out for being especially helpful in this project and providing invaluable professional expertise.

To numerous clients who offered so much encouragement, especially Cathy, Heather, Jane, Tera, Therese, Gwen and Joe, Jan and Mike, Judy and Mark, Karen and Bruce, Sandy and Steve, and Valerie and Larry.

To the research assistants I had over the years from the University of Washington, in particular to Wendy Blair and Robin Cutler, for their excellent detective work.

To my brother Lawrence Weschler, whose remarkable literary achievements gave me the inspiration to write this book. And to my brother Robert Weschler, for his many insightful contributions.

To my agent, Joy Harris, and her assistants, Leslie and Paul, for guiding me through the ominous publishing maze. To my first editor, Jenna Hull, for her sweet encouragement and direction. And to my second editor, Janet Goldstein, as well as her team at HarperCollins including Betsy Thorpe, Pam LaBarbiera, and Linda Dingler for their wizardry in pulling it all together at the eleventh hour.

To the individuals who were kind enough to wade through my initial drafts of the manuscript, including Diana Brement, Emilie Coulter, Barbara Feldman, Susan Specht Fleagle, Stephanie Irving, Miriam Labbok, M.D., and Janet Yoder.

To my medical illustrator, Kate Sweeney, and her assistant, Christine Shafner, whose beautiful artwork has helped make this book so visually appealing.

To my photographer, Frankie Collins, who was instrumental in so many ways, especially for her constant generosity and the ease with which she made herself available to take pictures of the cervix and cervical fluid at the oddest hours.

To my cervix model, Deanna Hope, who was so proud of her contribution to the enlightenment of women that she wanted to be mentioned by name (if this book is read by as many women as I hope it will be, then I imagine her cervix will be the most appreciated ever).

To the many clients I've had over the years who continue to swell my "Thank You" file with their letters of gratitude for the ways in which I have apparently enriched their lives. It is this type of appreciation that buoys me when I occasionally feel disheartened by a medical community that has yet to fully grasp the scientific validity and practicality of the Fertility Awareness Method.

To my wonderful associate, Melanie Warren, who was also my first research assistant and the standard by which I judged all others. I am forever indebted to her for freeing me to focus on this endeavor. Her sense of humor and shared passion for this field contributed to this project in ways she'll never know.

To my cherished friends who helped me maintain a sense of perspective when I kept wondering whether I would ever have a life again, especially to Aud, Susan, Cath, and of course Roger, whose presence helped give me the sanity and stability to get through it all.

Finally, and most important, to my younger brother Raymond Weschler, without whom this book could never have been written. He was an indispensable editor, researcher, and organizer, as well as an endless source of wit and moral support throughout this project. The fact is that we talked about sharing authorship credit, but he insisted that the book came from my passion and experiences, not his, and ultimately it was written with my voice. Perhaps, but truth be told, Raymond was my co-writer. I am eternally grateful to him for all that he's done, although more than any of that, I thank him for simply being the best brother that any sister could have.

# Introduction

I still cringe when I recall my college years and what ironically led me to pursue the field of fertility education. I cannot count the number of times I ran off to the gynecologist with what I thought was a vaginal infection. Most women will agree that no matter how many times they've had a pelvic exam, the experience is still unpleasant and sometimes even traumatic. Yet I remember returning seemingly every month, with the same apparent problem. As usual, I'd be sent home with a patronizing, "Well, Toni, there's really nothing there." So I would leave, feeling like a hypochondriac, only to meekly return when I had what appeared to be the signs of yet another infection.

Along with my frustration at this recurring problem were the inevitable side effects of the various methods of birth control I tried. If I wasn't dealing with weight gain and headaches caused by the Pill, I was enduring urinary tract infections from the diaphragm or irritation from the sponge. Yet, every time I asked the gynecologist for a natural, *effective* alternative to the dismal selection of birth control methods available, I was informed that the only "natural" method was Rhythm, and everyone knew that the Rhythm Method simply didn't work. So back to square one I would go, seeming to have infections all the time and without an acceptable method of birth control.

It wasn't until years later when I took a class in Fertility Awareness that I realized I was absolutely healthy all that time. What I had been perceiving as infections was in fact normal cervical fluid, one of the healthy signs of fertility which all women experience as they approach ovulation. But since discussing one's vaginal secretions is hardly your typical topic of social chitchat, I had no idea that my experiences were normal, universal, and perhaps most important, cyclical.

Because of misleading and inadequate health education, women are rarely taught how to distinguish between normal signs of fertile cervical fluid produced every cycle and the signs of a vaginal infection. Other than the unnecessary expense, inconvenience, and anxiety that women experience, what are the consequences of such a basic omission in upbringing and education? I think that such ignorance can lead to lowered self-esteem and confusion about sexuality.

My negative gynecological experiences gradually led to an interest in women's health that evolved into a real passion. It was that passion which led me to interview for a position as a health educator at a women's clinic—a disastrous experience, which in hindsight provided the final catalyst in my decision to pursue fertility education as a career.

While sitting in the waiting room anticipating my interview with the clinic director, my eyes wandered, glancing over the all-too-familiar paraphernalia of all women's clinics: the posters warning against spreading sexually transmitted diseases, the charts comparing methods of birth control (with their inherent side effects and risks in tiny print), and the plastic models of the female reproductive system.

I remember being suddenly struck with the futility of my situation. Here I was, applying to be a health educator in a women's clinic, with absolutely no training in the field. While fidgeting, I noticed a brochure about classes on the Fertility Awareness Method that were available at the clinic.

I could not believe that this supposedly reputable clinic seemed to be teaching the discredited Rhythm Method. I was in a dilemma. The cover of the brochure mentioned natural birth control, but I knew of no natural contraceptive methods that weren't synonymous with Rhythm. Should I risk losing this coveted position by expressing my dismay, or should I keep my mouth shut and get the job?

In the end, I would have felt dishonest if I had said nothing. My heart skipped a beat when the clinic director called my name. The pressure was on. The director was cordial, but I barely gave her a moment to introduce herself before I blurted out: "I don't understand why you teach Rhythm here. Everybody knows it doesn't work!"

"Oh really? We teach *what?*" she inquired with obvious surprise. "Don't you teach the Rhythm Method?" I muttered shyly. "I noticed your brochure here about the Fertility Awareness Method. Isn't that the same thing?" She looked a bit irritated and responded, "Actually, Toni, no. It's not the Rhythm Method, and frankly, your lack of knowledge about such an important facet of women's health wouldn't bode well at our clinic."

Needless to say, I didn't get the job. But that embarrassing experience years ago helped transform my perspective about women's health care. After swallowing my pride, I took the clinic's class on Fertility Awareness and was amazed. What I learned is that not only was it possible for me to take control of my cycles, but I no longer needed to feel uncertain about various secretions, pains, and symptoms. I could finally understand the subtle changes I experienced every month. I could place my menstrual cycle in the context of my overall health—both physiological and psychological. And no more unnecessary trips to the gynecologist.

By taking just a couple of minutes a day, I am able to utilize a highly effective method of natural birth control in which I can accurately determine those days of my cycle when I am potentially fertile. And if I want to get pregnant, I can avoid the guessing game so many couples play by learning precisely when to time intercourse. I can also identify for myself problems that could potentially impede pregnancy achievement. And the fact is, so can you.

Probably the best thing to come out of my years using the Fertility Awareness Method is the privilege I feel in being so knowledgeable about such a fundamental part of being a woman. I no longer question when I will get my period. I always know. I know what to expect physically and emotionally at different times in my cycle. I've also gained confidence in a way that is reflected in other areas of my life.

Your menstrual cycle is not something that should be shrouded in mystery. By the end of this book, I hope you will also experience the liberation of feeling in control of your body. Beyond its practical value in giving you the tools to avoid or achieve pregnancy naturally, this information about your cycle and body will empower you with numerous facets of self-knowledge that you rightly deserve.

# PART ONE

# BREAKING FERTILE GROUND: TOWARD A NEW WAY OF THINKING

# Fertility Awareness:
# What You Should Know and
# Why You Probably Don't

ow often have you heard that a menstrual cycle should be 28 days and that ovulation usually occurs on Day 14? This is a myth, pure and simple. And yet it is so accepted that it's sadly responsible for countless unplanned pregnancies. Furthermore, it has prevented many couples who have desired a pregnancy from attaining one. Much of this fallacy is a legacy of the dangerously inaccurate Rhythm Method, which falsely assumes that individual women have cycle lengths that, if not precisely 28 days, are reliably consistent over time. The result is that Rhythm is nothing more than a flawed statistical prediction using a mathematical formula based on the average of *past* cycles to predict *future* fertility.

In reality, cycles vary tremendously among women and often within each woman herself, though most cycle lengths are 24 to 36 days. The myth of Day 14 can affect individuals in the most astounding ways:

*Ilene and Mick were virgins when they got married on May 21. They wanted to start a family soon after their wedding, so they had their joint medical insurance start on May 15. When they discovered that Ilene had gotten pregnant on their honeymoon, they were pleasantly surprised that it happened so fast. Imagine their shock when the insurance company refused to cover the pregnancy and delivery, claiming that since her last period started on April 19, she must have gotten pregnant about three weeks before the wedding.*

*"That's impossible," she insisted, "we were both virgins until our wedding day." She tried to explain to them that her cycles had become quite long and irregular since she started jogging and dieting in order to be a "picturesque bride."*

*The insurance company wouldn't hear of it. They adhered to the frequently used pregnancy wheel, the calculating device that doctors rely on to determine the woman's due date. It is based on the assumption that ovulation always occurs on Day 14. As Ilene lamented, "We were sunk. How does one prove virginity in a courtroom? And why should it be anyone else's business?"*

*Needless to say, the Day-14 myth had very expensive consequences for Ilene and Mick. The only consolation they took from their experience was the fact that their son was born just when they expected, three weeks after the insurance company's due date! He was, in the words of Ilene "worth all the trouble anyway."*

Luckily, with advances in our understanding of human reproduction, we now have a highly accurate and effective method of identifying the woman's fertile phase: The Fertility Awareness Method (FAM). Fertility Awareness is simply a means of understanding human reproduction. It is based on the observation and charting of scientifically proven fertility signs that determine whether or not a woman is fertile on any given day. The three primary fertility signs are waking temperature, cervical fluid, and cervical position (the last one being an optional sign that simply corroborates the first two). FAM is an empowering method of natural birth control or pregnancy achievement, and is an excellent tool for assessing gynecological problems and understanding your body.

## 🐚 WHY THE FERTILITY AWARENESS METHOD IS NOT BETTER KNOWN

As you saw in the introduction, probably the greatest resistance to the acceptance of FAM has been its dubious misassociation with the Rhythm Method. Unfortunately, just the phrases "Natural Birth Control" or "Fertility Awareness" inevitably conjure up jokes along the lines of "What do you call Rhythm Method users?"—"Parents." Given the prevalence of this type of joke and the confusion of Rhythm with Fertility Awareness, is it any wonder that FAM is so misunderstood?

Furthermore, because the Rhythm Method is still practiced by people morally opposed to artificial methods of birth control, FAM tends to be falsely perceived as used only by such individuals. But in fact women from all over the world have been drawn to FAM simply because it is free of the chemicals associated with hormonal methods such as the Pill. Just as important, it allows them to minimize the time they need to use the devices that make other methods unpleasant, impractical, or unspontaneous. Many of these people tend to be oriented toward leading a natural and health-conscious life in other ways besides taking control of their fertility and reproduction.

It is true that many religious people have discovered the benefits of Fertility Awareness, though they may technically practice Natural Family Planning (NFP). The primary distinction between FAM and NFP is that those who use NFP choose to abstain rather than use barrier methods of contraception during the woman's fertile phase. But regardless of the differing values that often divide users of FAM and NFP, all are drawn by the desire for a natural method of effective contraception.*

## FAM's Conspicuous Absence from Medical School

If FAM has so many benefits as a method of birth control (and as an aid to pregnancy achievement, as you will later read), why, then, is it not better known? One of the most critical and mystifying reasons that people have rarely heard of it is that doctors are seldom taught a comprehensive version of this scientific method in medical school. It is amazing to think that women who practice the Fertility Awareness Method are often more knowledgeable about their own fertility than gynecologists who are trained to be experts in female physiology!

> *Years ago when I taught at a women's clinic, the entire staff except one doctor took my seminar to use FAM as a method of contraception. One day, the one who had never attended pulled me aside and whispered, "Toni, I'll be honest with you. I don't refer my patients to your classes." "Oh, really, why is that?" I casually asked, trying not to act surprised. "I got pregnant using your method and haven't trusted it since," she replied. "You're kidding? What rules did you use?" I inquired. "What do you mean, what rules?" she asked. "You know, did you observe the rules for both waking temperature and cervical fluid or just one of them?" She looked at me totally confused, as if she had no clue about what I had just asked. It was then that I realized just how widespread ignorance of Fertility Awareness was in the medical community. Even among doctors, I thought, Fertility Awareness still meant Rhythm, or perhaps a flower child's intuition.*

* Appendix D extensively discusses contraceptive efficacy rates.

What is especially remarkable about the glaring omission of Fertility Awareness education from medical school curricula is the fact that the method's effectiveness is based on purely biological principles, all discussed in greater detail in Chapter 4. They include the functions of estrogen, progesterone, luteinizing hormone, and the corpus luteum, all of which have been scientifically proven.

Because Fertility Awareness is useful not only for birth control and pregnancy achievement but for promoting gynecological health in general, it is even more surprising that this information is not part of a complete medical education. Indeed, FAM can be a vital aid to doctors and their patients in diagnosing a number of conditions, including:

1. anovulation (lack of ovulation)
2. late ovulation
3. short luteal phases (the second phase of the cycle)
4. infertile cervical fluid
5. hormonal imbalances
6. insufficient progesterone levels
7. occurrence of miscarriages

Another advantage of charting the three fertility signs is that it facilitates diagnosis of gynecological problems. Women who chart are so aware of what is normal for themselves that they can help their clinician determine irregularities based on their own cycles. Examples of potential gynecological problems that can be more easily diagnosed through daily charting include:

1. irregular or abnormal bleeding
2. vaginal infections
3. urinary tract infections
4. cervical anomalies
5. breast lumps
6. premenstrual syndrome
7. miscalculated date of conception

By not being taught FAM, doctors are denied an excellent tool with which to better diagnose and counsel their female patients. Moreover, this lack of knowledge on the part of doctors often results in patients being unnecessarily subjected to invasive, painful, and frequently expensive tests to diagnose an apparent menstrual problem. If women were taught how to chart for their fertility-related health, they would not need to visit their doctor nearly as often and substantial numbers of useless medical procedures could be avoided.

As the list on page 6 should make clear, charting would reveal a myriad of potential impediments to pregnancy, ranging from the woman not ovulating to her simply not producing the cervical fluid necessary for conception. It may even show that this woman is consistently getting pregnant, but having repeated miscarriages of which neither she nor her doctor had been aware. And for those seeking to prevent pregnancy, charting would eliminate the anxiety so many feel as they run off to the store or their gynecologist for expensive and inconvenient pregnancy tests. Women who chart know if they are pregnant just by observing their waking temperatures, and thus they can eliminate that recurrent doubt while awaiting the arrival of a "late period."

## Politics, Profit, and Natural Contraception

Another reason this method is not better known or promoted for birth control is that it is not profitable for either physicians or the major pharmaceutical companies such as those that produce the Pill or IUD. In other words, beyond the initial investment in a book or class and a thermometer, there is little further cost to the woman or couple using FAM. Compare this to the cost of the Pill, which can range from $2,000 to $4,000 for a 10-year supply.*

Given the profitability of other contraceptives, is it any wonder that FAM is not promoted more enthusiastically by the medical community? It's no secret that great sums of money are spent in order to present the Pill as a contraceptive panacea, but what is often overlooked is the bias with which various pharmaceutical companies distort the effectiveness and validity of other birth control methods, particularly Fertility Awareness.

Corporate literature that summarizes the various contraceptives for public consumption is consistently filled with blatant inaccuracies, such as one pamphlet entitled "Contraception: The Choice Is Yours," which claims that "Natural Family Planning is based on the fact that fertilization is most likely to occur just before, during, and just after ovulation." This would almost make sense, except for the tiny detail that fertilization cannot take place without an egg present, so it would be no small feat for fertilization to take place before the egg is released!

Of course, more important than any individual misrepresentation is the overall way FAM and NFP are portrayed. This particular pamphlet was typical

---

* Of course, you will still incur the cost of barriers for the fertile phase if you choose not to abstain while using Fertility Awareness.

in that its "Natural Family Planning" heading was followed by a clarification in parentheses, which as you could guess, simply said "The Rhythm Method."

## The Language of "Palatability"

Finally, the last reason FAM is not better known is that it suffers from the misfortune of being a method that many, especially in the media, refer to as "unpalatable." Why is this?

> *We have a doctor on the Seattle news who does medical stories every week. I had approached him about the possibility of doing a feature about the Fertility Awareness Method a number of times over the years, but he was always noncommittal while still acknowledging that he sincerely believed the method was effective. I could never grasp why he felt it wouldn't be suitable for the news until he finally admitted that he felt the subject was simply "unpalatable" for the general public.*
>
> *Perhaps his concern was about the term used for one of the three fertility signs: "cervical mucus." Maybe if it were referred to as "cervical fluid" he would find it suitable for the evening news. No sooner had I written him with that suggestion, when he called to tell me he thought that change in vocabulary was just the modification necessary to make FAM acceptable for the news. Within a few weeks, he did a story about Fertility Awareness.*

It took that experience to make me realize how powerful language can be in the acceptance of FAM. Since that news feature years ago, I have found that people are infinitely more attentive to and interested in FAM when cervical mucus is referred to by the more neutral term cervical *fluid*. Perhaps the increased acceptability of that terminology is less puzzling when you consider that the woman's *cervical* fluid is analogous to the man's *seminal* fluid. One would never refer to seminal fluid as seminal mucus, and yet the purpose of the fluid in both the man and woman is comparable: to nourish and provide a medium in which the sperm can travel.

Of course, the media is an extension of our culture, which tends to promote a sanitized, unrealistic view of human physical processes. The purpose of FAM, however, is to enlighten people with a clear and empowering knowledge of their bodies' functioning. Thus, if coining a term such as "cervical fluid" makes that task easier, so much the better.

## ꙮ WHY SOME DOCTORS FAMILIAR WITH THE FERTILITY AWARENESS METHOD DO NOT INFORM THEIR PATIENTS

Many doctors know that FAM is a scientifically validated, natural method of effective birth control, pregnancy achievement, and health awareness, but they may still cite various reasons why they don't recommend it to their patients. Some say that women cannot be bothered to learn it because it's complicated and difficult to use, requires high intelligence in order to apply, and takes too much time to learn and practice. But for the vast majority of women, I believe that these assertions are simply not valid.

It is unfortunate that many doctors believe and help disseminate the erroneous assumption that FAM is complicated and difficult to use. Actually, it is generally simple and easy, once you learn its basic principles. (Many will be able to learn those principles in this book. Others will need to take a class, where a certified instructor can typically teach a comprehensive course in a couple of evening sessions.) The method is no different from many skills in life, such as learning to drive a car. It may seem intimidating at first, until a little practice gives you the confidence you need.

Some doctors may genuinely believe that women are not smart enough to understand and assimilate the information taught in FAM classes. While I find this perspective discouraging, I understand why they believe this. It is true that the type of people attracted to FAM tend to be quite educated. However, I think this is more a function of the way in which people have initially learned about it, and not the inherent intelligence required to use it. It often takes a very motivated individual to seek out information about a subject which, until now, has typically been reserved for the few who are resourceful enough to research the topic.

I personally have taught FAM to over 1,000 clients, and can assure you that virtually all women can internalize the method and its biological foundation within a few hours. I also suspect few of them are particularly burdened by the couple of minutes a day it takes to apply.

### In Defense of Doctors

The above is not meant to be a diatribe against the medical community. In an industry that is becoming increasingly high tech, many doctors may be truly skeptical, precisely because FAM is so *nontech*. Indeed, they may believe that they are not active enough in their patients' care if they do not prescribe drugs or perform procedures.

But most important, clinicians don't realistically have the time to thoroughly explain the method in a typical office visit, and thus few women ever learn it. Ultimately, there is a perpetual circle of ignorance, for even those physicians who are especially supportive of women taking control of their own reproductive health cannot be as effective as they would like to be. Indeed, the benefits of FAM cannot become commonplace in the doctor-patient relationship until more women do *their* part by charting their cycles.

# Taking Control of Your Reproductive Health

*D*uring every cycle, a woman's body prepares for a potential pregnancy, much to the frustration of those who prefer not to become pregnant. But a woman is actually fertile only a few days per cycle, around ovulation (when the egg is released). The only practical, noninvasive way to reliably identify that fertile time is through observing the woman's waking temperature and cervical fluid, as well as the optional sign of cervical position. By charting these primary fertility signs, a woman can tell on a day-to-day basis whether or not she is capable of getting pregnant on any given day. Because the actual day of ovulation can vary from cycle to cycle, the determination of those few days around ovulation becomes critical; therein lies the value of the Fertility Awareness Method.

## $\mathcal{L}$ THE POLITICS OF NATURAL BIRTH CONTROL

> *We want far better reasons for having children than not knowing how to prevent them.*
>
> —DORA RUSSELL

Why are so many women frustrated with the state of contraception today? Why is the vast majority of birth control designed for women to use even though it is men who are fertile every single day? Wouldn't it make more sense for birth control to be developed for the gender that is the most fertile? Consider the following table:

## METHODS OF BIRTH CONTROL AVAILABLE TODAY
(listed in approximate order of most invasive)

**For Women**
Tubal ligation
Norplant
Depo-Provera
Pill
IUD (intrauterine device)
Diaphragm
Cervical cap
Sponge
Female condom
Suppositories
Spermicides
Natural methods

**For Men**
Vasectomy
Condom
Withdrawal

Given that women are only fertile a few days per cycle, it's ironic that they're the ones who risk the vast array of side effects and physical ramifications of birth control. These include increased risk of blood clots, strokes, breast cancer, irregular spotting, severe pelvic inflammatory disease or uterine perforation, heavy and crampy periods, urinary tract infections, cervical inflammation, and allergic reactions to spermicides and latex, to name a few. And for what? To protect themselves from a man, who produces millions of sperm per minute!

Imagine the reaction of most males to the following announcement:

## A NEW INTRAPENAL CONTRACEPTIVE

*The newest development in male contraception was unveiled recently at the American Women's Surgical Symposium. Dr. Sophia Merkin announced the preliminary findings of a study conducted on 763 unsuspecting male graduate students at a large midwest university. In her report, Dr. Merkin stated that the new contraceptive—the IPD—was a breakthrough in male contraception. It will be marketed under the trade name "umbrelly."*

*The IPD (intrapenal device) resembles a tiny folded umbrella which is inserted through the head of the penis into the scrotum with a plungerlike instrument. Occasionally there is perforation of the scrotum, but this is disregarded since it is known that the male has few nerve endings in this area of his body. The underside of the umbrella contains a spermicidal jelly, hence the name "umbrelly."*

*Experiments on a thousand white whales from the continental shelf (whose sexual apparatus is said to be closest to man's) proved the umbrelly 100 percent effective in preventing production of sperm, and eminently satisfactory to the female whale since it doesn't interfere with her rutting pleasure.*

*Dr. Merkin declared the umbrelly to be statistically safe for the human male. She reported that of the 763 grad students tested with the device, only two died of scrotal infection, three developed cancer of the testicles, and 13 were too depressed to have an erection. She stated that the common complaints ranged from cramping and bleeding to acute abdominal pain. She emphasized that these symptoms were merely indications that the man's body had not yet adjusted to the device. Hopefully, the symptoms would disappear within a year.*

*One complication caused by the IPD was the incidence of massive scrotal infection necessitating the surgical removal of the testicles. "But this is a rare occurrence," said Merkin, "too rare to be statistically important." She and the other distinguished members of the Women's College of Surgeons agreed that the benefits far outweighed the risk to any individual man.*

*—© 1974 Written by Belita H. Cowan. Reprinted with permission.*

*Illustration by Frankie Collins.*

While the above is only a parody, in reality, the notorious Dalkon Shield IUD rendered many women infertile by causing severe pelvic inflammatory disease. It is but one example of the type of medical nightmares to which many women have been subjected; history reveals countless ways in which women's bodies and those of their potential offspring have been exposed to dangerous drugs and procedures.

From the tragedies caused by thalidomide and DES in the 1950s to the more recent controversies over the side effects of Norplant and Depo-Provera, we've seen an endless stream of revelations that call into question the level of safety that female patients are assured. Beyond the often dubious nature of the drugs we've been prescribed, both contraceptive and otherwise, we've witnessed the anguish surrounding the use of breast implants. In addition, we're now aware of the wide overuse of such "necessary" medical procedures as C-sections and hysterectomies, adding even more confusion to the average woman's relationship with her medical practitioners.

Whether men would submit to all the "inconveniences" is not really the issue. Given all that women have been through, it's only natural that they would desire to take control of their own medical and reproductive needs with the most effective, least intrusive means possible.

## Why Unplanned Pregnancies Occur

> *I remember . . . a friend described her first experience with a contraceptive device, which shot out a bathroom window into the college quadrangle. She never retrieved it. I wouldn't have, either.*
>
> —ANNA QUINDLEN

To understand the politics of natural birth control, we must examine the concept of unplanned pregnancies. Why do unplanned pregnancies occur? * There are four primary reasons:

1. People do not use birth control because they are "swept away with the moment."
2. People do not use birth control because of ignorance.
3. People do not use birth control because they feel no method is acceptable.
4. People use birth control, but the method fails.

How does the Fertility Awareness Method fit into the above scheme? Let us examine each situation individually:

### People Do Not Use Birth Control Because They are Swept Away with the Moment.

All barrier methods leave people vulnerable to the type of passion that reduces them to a momentary lapse in judgment. Who among us has not

---

* By unplanned pregnancies, I am not referring here to the unfortunate practice of many unmarried teenage girls who engage in an intentional pattern of unprotected sex, either out of indifference to the consequences or because they actually want to have babies. This issue, the subject of intensive sociological analysis and public policy debate, is beyond the scope of this book.

thought at one time or another, "Oh, I'm sure we're fine." However, if a woman knows when she is fertile, it eliminates guessing. Being unlucky is no longer an excuse.

### People Do Not Use Birth Control Because of Ignorance.

Many more people would be more inclined to use birth control if they understood the likelihood of pregnancy occurring at specific times in the cycle. There are so many myths perpetuated about human fertility that it's no wonder there are so many unplanned pregnancies. The classic one responsible for probably the most unplanned pregnancies is that ovulation occurs on Day 14. In actuality, ovulation *may* occur on Day 14; it may also occur on Day 10, Day 18, or Day 37. In other words, ovulation is not the consistent event it is presumed to be. But the fallacy of Day 14 is so prevalent that even clinicians perpetuate it.

If a couple thinks a woman can only get pregnant on Day 14, they may feel safe having unprotected intercourse up to Day 13 and again from Day 15 on. Some couples may even feel that they are being conservative if they put a buffer zone of several days on either side of Day 14. But if the woman ovulates on Day 20, for example, no amount of abstinence between Days 11 and 17 will prevent an unplanned pregnancy! The dangerous fiction of Day 14 is but one example in which people simply do not understand human reproduction.

What about the faulty assumption that women cannot get pregnant from intercourse during their periods? (See page 331.) Another common belief is that sperm can only live up to 3 days. (In reality, sperm can survive up to 5 days, *if* fertile quality cervical fluid is present.) Combine this belief with that of ovulation always occurring on Day 14, and undesired results are almost inevitable.

These are just some of the more common misperceptions that people have about basic human biology. Suffice it to say, many unplanned pregnancies occur because people believe such fallacies. Obviously, education is key in dealing with this problem.

### People Do Not Use Birth Control Because They Feel No Method Is Acceptable.

It is hardly surprising that most people find today's contraceptive choices far from ideal. Aside from sterilization, our options include such alternatives as a method that infuses the woman's body with hormones (the Pill), puts women at risk of potential breast cancer or osteoporosis (Depo-Provera), involves inserting six matchstick-size silicone tubes under the skin of the arm (Norplant), maintains the uterus in a constant state of inflammation, causing painful periods (the IUD), fills the woman's vagina with a latex dome that leaks gooey spermicide for at least 24 hours after intercourse (the diaphragm), can be uncomfortable and cause cervical anomalies (the cervical cap), is notorious for causing vaginal infections (the sponge), completely covers the woman's clitoris (the female condom), and places a rubber sheath between the two individuals (the male condom).

Is it any wonder that unplanned pregnancies occur, given the choice of methods people perceive as their only options? With FAM, couples can experience the freedom of effective contraception without devices, chemicals, or side effects for most of the cycle.

### People Use Birth Control, But the Method Fails.

One of the most inflammatory opinions certain people hold is that if a couple has an unplanned pregnancy, it is their fault because they were being careless by not using birth control. Often this is simply not true. According to the Alan Guttmacher Institute, a leading think tank for population research, of the nation's 3.5 million annual unplanned pregnancies, at least 50% result from the failure of various birth control methods. Many of those failures could have been avoided if couples understood the woman's menstrual cycle better.

This fact is particularly interesting given that so many of the barrier methods advertise such impressive "effectiveness rates," often around 95% or higher. These statistics are inherently misleading, primarily because they are based on the faulty assumption that women can get pregnant throughout their cycles, when, in fact, a woman can only get pregnant for about one-fourth of a typical cycle. If a method is going to fail, it is only going to fail during the short fertile phase when her body is even capable of getting pregnant. Given this information, people should know *when* in the cycle a contraceptive has the potential to fail. They can then make an educated decision as to whether they want to abstain or double up on methods of birth control during that very risky phase to reinforce effectiveness of the methods. For example, if a couple normally used the diaphragm and knew that the woman was especially fertile on a particular day, they would be able to increase its effectiveness by using extra spermicide.

## Women, Men, and Contraceptive Responsibility

A common theme in women's conversations is the frustration they often feel when saddled with the full burden of birth control. Once people understand that women are only fertile for a fraction of the time men are, they are especially struck with the inequity of it all. So it is particularly interesting to examine the ways in which women have been disproportionately exposed to side effects throughout their cycle. For example, there are many who will concede that while the Pill was originally designed to sexually emancipate women, what also transpired was burdening the woman with the sole responsibility of birth control.

*Susan and Joe were a very loving couple who grappled with the issue of inequality. Susan had been on the Pill for years even though she often suffered nausea and migraine headaches. So when she suggested they take a class in the Fertility Awareness Method, Joe was more than willing. Three years later they joke about the fact that, even today, every time the alarm rings, he gets up, puts the thermometer in her mouth, brushes his teeth, comes back and removes the thermometer, records it on her chart, and shakes it down. Susan, for her part, remains half asleep, snuggled in bed. No more nausea. No more headaches.*

Unlike most other methods, FAM affords men the opportunity to lovingly and actively share in the responsibility of contraception. In fact, the method is so conducive to male involvement that many couples claim that FAM has strengthened their relationship.

## ✑ THE POLITICS OF PREGNANCY ACHIEVEMENT

*I'll never forget when my client Terry called. She had been trying to get pregnant for over a year before taking my seminar. It was two weeks following the class, and there was a slight hint of panic in her voice as she asked me whether she and her husband should make love that night. They were worried because she thought she had a serious vaginal infection that might affect their chances of conceiving. Just as she began describing what was "coming out of her," I heard someone pick up the other extension. It was her husband James on the other end. "You cannot believe what is leaking out of Terry right now."*

*"Wait a second, you guys. Let me ask you several questions. Is it clear?"*

*"Yes."*

*"Is it slippery?"*

*"Definitely."*

*"Is it stretchy?"*

*"Toni, it's 10 inches!"*

*"Well then, what are you doing talking to me?" I joked, "Get off the phone and take advantage of it!"*

*Before making love that night, Terry and James took a dozen photos of her fertile cervical fluid. Nine months later, their little son was born.*

It is unclear whether the incidence of infertility is actually increasing or people are simply seeking treatment in higher numbers today. Either way, the news is not good. It touches about one in six couples; however, what is often *referred* to as infertility may not necessarily *be* infertility.

The standard definition of infertility is not becoming pregnant after one year of unprotected intercourse. Nevertheless, there are many couples whose infertility problem is so minor that Fertility Awareness alone would facilitate pregnancy. This is not to imply that all infertility can be treated through education. Nor is it to imply that those who are having a fertility problem are uneducated or ignorant. But the medical community itself often inadvertently perpetuates myths that prevent couples from attaining pregnancy.

The classic myth, already discussed in Chapter 1, is that ovulation occurs on Day 14. To use this as an example: A couple may spend a year trying to time intercourse around Day 14, only to discover that in their particular case, the woman didn't usually ovulate until about Day 20. If the couple gets pregnant after learning this information about her particular cycle, would one say that they were infertile up until that point? Clearly they were not. But the emotional and financial consequences are often so great that it's as if they really were.

## Why People Are Often Misled to Believe They Are Infertile

Before discussing the impact on a couple of being inappropriately labeled "infertile," let us examine why people are often misled in the first place.

**1. Infertility is assumed if pregnancy has not occurred after a year.**

If a couple has been unable to get pregnant after a year of unprotected intercourse, the standard wisdom is to assume there is probably a fertility problem, when in reality there may be no medical problem whatsoever.

## 2. Irregular cycles are assumed to be potentially problematic.

The concept that normal cycles are 28 days and ovulation occurs on Day 14 is so entrenched in the medical profession that when a woman's cycles vary from that standard, the variation is often presumed to be a potential concern. "Irregular" cycles are seen as problematic in part because gynecologists need to time fertility procedures around when the egg is released. But if a couple is taught how to identify approaching ovulation to time intercourse appropriately, then it is irrelevant whether it occurs on Day 14, 19, or 25.

*One of my clients was a woman who first called me in a very depressed state because it had been over a year since she and her husband had started trying to get pregnant. She mentioned that she thought the reason she may not be getting pregnant was because her cycles were not a "normal" length. I learned that they were about 35 days, an absolutely normal period of time, but certainly longer than the prototype 28 days. She went on to say that her husband got so frustrated with their apparent infertility that they would have intercourse only up to Day 14, then stop until the next cycle. No wonder they weren't getting pregnant! If a woman has long cycles, by definition she ovulates later than Day 14. Within a month of taking my fertility seminar, the couple got pregnant.*

## 3. Doctors often overlook the most obvious solutions.

Doctors are trained to identify disease and illness, often by diagnosing and treating with the use of high-tech procedures. The result is that the most obvious solutions are often overlooked. A good example of this is the relationship between frequency of intercourse and pregnancy. A couple may have sex twice a week for a year and wonder why they have not gotten pregnant. A doctor may proceed with a fertility workup (including invasive and painful tests) on the assumption that the couple may have a fertility problem, without considering the most rudimentary question, namely, whether the couple is having intercourse *at the right time* in the woman's cycle. It is quite possible to have intercourse twice a week for a year and still be missing the fertile phase each cycle, especially if the woman has only a day or so of fertile cervical fluid, or the man's sperm count is marginal. This is not a fertility problem but an education problem.

This overlooking of fundamental principles is exemplified by Abraham Kaplan's theory, the Law of the Instrument:

Give a small boy a hammer,
and he will find that everything
he encounters needs pounding.

Doctors have a vested interest in using the tools that they have perfected through years of study. It should come as no surprise, then, that infertility specialists initially apply the high-tech tools of the trade. This is very helpful for scores of couples dealing with actual infertility. However, there are many couples for whom the use of these tests and procedures is simply excessive. *Before any high-tech tests or treatments are employed, the man should have a semen analysis. In addition, the couple should chart the woman's fertility signs both to identify when she is the most fertile, and to determine any possible impediments to pregnancy achievement.*

**4. Doctors tend to focus on basal temperatures rather than cervical fluid.**

Doctors will usually focus on basal body temperatures to the exclusion of the most important fertility sign for timing intercourse effectively: cervical fluid. In fact, physicians may unintentionally create a fertility problem by advising their patients to time intercourse for either the drop or rise in temperature. This advice is not only misleading, it can actually impede pregnancy achievement! Cervical fluid is the key to timing intercourse for becoming pregnant, yet many infertility doctors simply assume that women wouldn't want to take the few seconds a day necessary to chart. Informed women should decide that for themselves.

*One of the most glaring examples of a doctor reinforcing the notion of depending on past temperatures to indicate future fertility took place at, of all places, a conference of the infertility organization RESOLVE. The doctor's keynote address was about all the myths surrounding fertility. She was making the correct point that basal body temperatures only indicate fertility after it is too late, after ovulation has already occurred. While sitting in the audience, I remember thinking how gratifying it was to finally hear a physician stress the point that temperatures are invalid for predicting fertility. Imagine my surprise, then, when she continued: "Therefore, to predict impending fertility, you must look back at your previous temperature shifts to predict your upcoming fertile time."*

*I was stunned. Here she was, sustaining the idea of looking at past cycles to predict future fertility, without so much as mentioning the most important fertility sign for pregnancy achievement: the cervical fluid. The irony of the moment would have been amusing if it wasn't such blatantly bad advice, and addressed to such a vulnerable group of people.*

The reason that temperatures don't help determine the best time to achieve pregnancy is *because by the time the temperature shifts up, the egg is typically already dead and gone.* However, the temperature is still very useful in determining several facts about the woman's cycle, including: (1) whether she is ovulating at all, (2) whether the second phase of the cycle (from ovulation until her period) is long enough for the egg to implant in the uterus, and (3) whether she has achieved a pregnancy that particular cycle (see Chapter 11).

**5. Many fertility tests are often timed inappropriately (or simply needlessly performed).**

If infertility is suspected, doctors will often perform a postcoital test to determine if the man's sperm are swimming freely in the woman's cervical fluid. With this test, the couple has intercourse, then the woman goes to the doctor's office within several hours. A few drops of the semen are removed from her vagina and examined under a microscope to determine if sperm are alive and moving in the fluid. The purpose is basically to determine two facts: whether the woman's cervical fluid is conducive to sperm viability, and whether her partner's own sperm will survive in it.

One of the most common mistakes made is the procedure's timing. Many doctors continue to perform it around Day 14 of the woman's cycle, regardless of when she actually ovulates. Unless the woman does ovulate close to that day, the test is usually invalid and leads many couples to believe they have a fertility problem when they do not.

*I will never forget a lecture I gave to a group of nurse practitioners experienced in infertility treatment. As I explained that the test is useless if performed at the wrong time in a woman's cycle (for numerous women Day 14 is simply too early), I could feel the anger build. Finally, one nurse blurted out sarcastically: "And just who do you expect us to refer our patients to for postcoitals where they will be willing to test them based on the woman's cycle rather than the availability of the staff?" All I could think of at that point was that I was not there to tell them what they wanted to hear, but rather what works.*

There are certain medical events over which we simply have no control. Childbirth does not occur merely between the hours of 9 to 5, Monday through Friday. Certainly trauma is treated when it occurs, not just when the clinic is open. To the extent possible, a woman's ovulation should be no different.

A test is only useful if it is both reliable and valid. In the case of the postcoital test, the only information to be obtained from performing it on Day 14 on a woman who ovulates on Day 20, for example, is to prove that Fertility Awareness can also be effectively used as a method of birth control! Sperm die within a few hours of intercourse when a woman is not in her fertile phase, and that phase is only the few days surrounding ovulation. If performed at any other time, the test is useless.

Another frequently mistimed test is the endometrial biopsy, which involves removing a small segment of the uterine lining close to the estimated time of menstruation. This is done in order to determine if the woman is ovulating and producing a suitable lining for implantation. But again, practitioners will often simply assume a Day-14 ovulation, whether this really occurred or not, and thus the procedure's accuracy and relevance are questionable. (Had ovulation actually taken place on Day 21, one should *expect* both endometrial development and the next period to be a week behind.) Clearly, women undergoing these procedures deserve useful information, which is only possible if they are appropriately timed.

It should also be mentioned here that some tests are performed well before it is appropriate to do so, especially given how painful and intrusive they can be. For example, the hysterosalpingogram (HSG) is a dye test used to determine if the woman's fallopian tubes are open. During the procedure a doctor inserts a type of gas inside the abdomen to distend the stomach. As the gas passes under the diaphragm, it can cause a sharp pain in the shoulder area. It is actually quite revealing, but given its discomfort and cost, it should only be performed after it has been determined that potential ovulatory and cervical fluid problems have been ruled out. And needless to say, it is completely useless if in fact the fertility problem is determined to be due to miscarriages. Charting would have revealed all of these problems.

**6. Women are often needlessly prescribed the ovulatory drug Clomid (clomiphene citrate).**

If a couple is presumed to be infertile the woman is often put on an ovulatory drug called Clomid, whether or not she is actually ovulating.

This is especially unfortunate since some studies suggest that Clomid may increase the risk of ovarian cancer. The purpose of the drug is to stimulate egg development in the ovaries. What the couple is usually not told is that it has two paradoxical side effects. One is that it can dry up the cervical fluid which is vital for sperm transport through the cervix. The other is that it can cause the second phase of the cycle to be abnormally short, preventing an egg from being able to implant in the uterus. So while this potent drug is given to increase a woman's fertility, it can ironically act to prevent a pregnancy. (Sometimes, the only way to remedy the former problem is through intrauterine insemination, where the sperm is deposited directly in the uterus, bypassing the cervix altogether.) I have had many clients achieve a pregnancy specifically after discontinuing Clomid.

This is not to suggest that Clomid does not have a role in infertility treatment. Certainly many women do get pregnant by using it, and indeed, it may be possible to alleviate some of the side effects. However, the use of Clomid should be an informed decision, rather than a routine first step. Women should ask their doctors why they think a prescription would be beneficial in their particular case, especially if they already know from charting that they are ovulating normally.

**7. The commonly used ovulation predictor kits can be misleading.**

With the advent of the ovulation predictor kits which are so readily available in drug stores now, many women are led to believe they have a fertility problem if the kits do not show the expected color surge indicating ovulation is about to occur. But even if the kits *do* show a color surge, it does not necessarily mean the woman is fertile. The reasons they can be misleading are all discussed in Chapter 11.

**8. Women are often led to believe they are not getting pregnant, when they are actually having miscarriages.**

There is a huge difference in terms of the fertility of a woman who has never achieved a pregnancy and one who gets pregnant, but then miscarries. I do not mean to imply that women who continually miscarry do not have a fertility problem. However, the diagnostic steps taken for the two women should be drastically different.

The problem with miscarriages is that they can be difficult to diagnose since they often happen so early in the woman's cycle. They may be mistaken for nothing more than a menstrual period. But a woman trained in Fertility Awareness knows that she needs a history of at least 10 days from ovulation to menstruation for implantation to later occur, and that 18 consecutive high temperatures after ovulation almost always indicates a pregnancy. She would therefore be able to determine with a high degree of accuracy whether or not she was indeed pregnant before she bled. But since most women are not taught how to take control of their cycles, they are unable to interpret what is occurring in their bodies. Thus, they may needlessly subject themselves to painful and invasive diagnostic procedures to rule out an infertility problem that may not exist.

> *My client Julie thought she might finally be pregnant because she had taken my class and knew that 18 high temperatures most likely indicated a pregnancy. Upon hearing from her, I suggested she come in to the clinic to get a blood test to confirm her pregnancy. Sure enough, she was pregnant. In fact, she had conceived so early in her cycle (about Day 11) that by the time 18 high temps had been recorded, she was only on Day 29, not a day that most women typically associate with pregnancy. But she knew she was pregnant earlier than most women would typically know because she had educated herself through Fertility Awareness. Unfortunately, within a few days of her positive pregnancy test, she had a miscarriage. While it was sad that she had the miscarriage, the fact that she conceived was nevertheless very helpful in terms of what it told her about her fertility at that time:*
>
> > *a. She was ovulating.*
> > *b. Her fallopian tubes were open.*
> > *c. Her cervical fluid was suitable for sperm penetration.*
> > *d. Her partner's sperm count was fine.*
>
> *What Julie learned from this experience is that she had undoubtedly been having other miscarriages while trying to get pregnant, but would never have known had she not learned how to identify pregnancy through charting. FAM taught her that her problem seemed to be related to a shortened phase of progesterone in the second part of her cycle (the luteal phase). Rather than start the infertility workup from square one, with all of the inherently intrusive tests, she was able to show her charts to her doctor, and immediately address the problem. Several months later, after being treated for a short luteal phase, she got pregnant and carried her baby daughter to term.*

## The Infertility Diagnosis: Staying in Control

As you can see, there are a number of reasons people are led to believe they are infertile when they actually may not be. The physical and emotional ramifications of this misdiagnosis are far reaching and hard to overstate. The cost of infertility diagnosis and treatment is not covered by most insurance companies. Many couples struggling with infertility feel that it is grossly unfair to have years of their insurance fees cover the maternity care of other couples, only to have their own infertility treatment not included. The cost of even a minimal infertility workup can be thousands of dollars, while a comprehensive workup including treatment can amount to tens of thousands of dollars, usually out-of-pocket. What is especially disheartening is that these exorbitant costs are so often totally unnecessary.

While men are impacted to a certain extent, the woman is usually the partner most affected by the whole process. Because a woman's fertility is so integrally related to her menstrual cycle, she must visit the doctor several times a cycle to determine potential fertility problems. Since doctors' offices are rarely open at night or on weekends, many must make arrangements to miss work numerous times, or in some cases quit their jobs to pursue fertility diagnosis and treatment.

As you've read, many of the diagnostic tests are quite uncomfortable or even painful. Even worse, they are often mistimed and simply not needed. But by charting their three primary fertility signs, women can inform their doctors of numerous facts about their fertility which can quickly narrow the range of possible diagnoses. In so doing, they can help exclude those procedures that would serve no purpose, and help to most appropriately time those tests which could reveal valuable information.

Indeed, imagine how much more confident a woman would feel if she could say to her physician:

> Hi, Doctor Smith. Yes, I am basically fine, thank you. But I do have a couple of concerns I wanted to discuss with you. I practice Fertility Awareness and have noticed that my luteal phase is a little short. We plan to get pregnant this spring and would like to try to lengthen it to avoid risking a miscarriage. What would you suggest?

In other words, women and couples can become *active* participants in their health care. By charting, couples facing fertility issues will reduce their feelings of vulnerability, and most important, increase their chances of pregnancy, whether medical intervention is required or not.

### Knowing When: Identifying the Date If Conception Occurs

Interestingly enough, clinicians may even lead couples who have *gotten* pregnant to believe there is a problem when there is not. Once again, it all reverts back to the erroneous assumption that women usually have 28-day cycles and ovulate on Day 14.

> *Dana was a 25-year-old woman who had recently come off the Pill, so her cycles had not yet returned to normal. Because she and her husband wanted to get pregnant, they practiced Fertility Awareness to determine her fertile phase. After she became pregnant, her doctor asked her the date of her last menstrual period to apply the standard pregnancy wheel. Dana mentioned that the pregnancy wheel would be inaccurate in her particular case, since it assumes ovulation on Day 14. She explained that she practiced FAM and knew that she didn't ovulate until about Day 37, so it would inaccurately predict her due date a full 3 weeks earlier than it really should be.*
>
> *You can imagine Dana's surprise when the doctor not only did not give credence to her charts, but actually expressed great concern when his pelvic exam revealed that the fetus was "extremely small for dates." Had this woman not been practicing Fertility Awareness, she would have been distressed to be told by the doctor that there was something wrong with her fetus, all because he was basing her cycles on the average woman's day of ovulation, rather than her own. As if that wasn't enough, he actually red-flagged her chart with a "medical alert" tag, indicating that her pregnancy was high risk and needed to be followed carefully.*

While the use of ultrasound would eliminate this confusion, there are still a great many women who would prefer to avoid such high-tech pregnancies, and thus pregnancy wheel estimations should be approached with caution. Indeed, such miscalculations can and have led to the induced labor of many a premature baby.

## ❧ FERTILITY AWARENESS FOR DETECTING GYNECOLOGICAL PROBLEMS AND UNDERSTANDING THE HEALTHY BODY

How often have you felt a sudden sharp pain in your side, noticed spotting at odd times, or even felt a breast lump that caused you to panic? While all of these experiences may seem confusing, they can be normal occurrences *if they take place at the appropriate time in your cycle.*

The benefits of charting extend far beyond knowing when a woman can and cannot get pregnant. There are many gynecological conditions that can be identified through observing your fertility signs. Women who chart can determine whether they are experiencing normal occurrences or true gynecological problems such as vaginal or urinary tract infections and cervical anomalies. Those who chart are so aware of what is normal for themselves that they can help their clinician determine irregularities based on their *individual* symptoms rather than the average woman's symptoms.

This has tremendous advantages, as seen in the classic example of a woman who may have occasional midcycle spotting, which is usually harmless and often referred to as ovulatory bleeding. But because spotting can be an indication of other potentially serious problems (such as cervical cancer), doctors often feel obligated to pursue unnecessary testing and examinations, needlessly worrying and inconveniencing their patients. A woman who charts would know when this type of bleeding is normal, and thus not seek medical attention unless she really needed it.

Of course, certain unpleasant medical procedures will always be necessary. Most women would say that an annual pelvic exam is hardly one of their favorite activities. The average woman would probably rather be scrubbing a toilet than lying on the exam table, her legs in stirrups, trying to maintain a semblance of dignity. Especially when the doctor walks in, smiling and acting like there's nothing the least bit awkward about her lying there stark naked under a 2-by-2-inch hospital gown.

And what is the first thing that physicians say when they sit down at the foot of the exam table? "Scoot down, please." It's hardly a coincidence that doctors must always request that of their patients. After all, how many women of their own volition would choose to have their derriere hanging off the table if they didn't have to?

Now granted, no amount of fertility consciousness will free you from this unpleasant experience. But taking responsibility for your own health care will at least give you some integrity and a sense of control often lost in a typical office visit. Charting the menstrual cycle allows a woman and her health care practitioner to work together as a team, with the patient contributing to her own well-being.

In addition, FAM will put you so in tune with the normal occurrences of your cycle that it will greatly reduce the number of times you feel a need to consult with your doctor in the first place. For example, how many times have you gone to your gynecologist complaining of an infection only to be assured you were fine? Unfortunately, information about women's fertility signs is not typically taught in school; therefore, many girls and young women grow up thinking they are unhealthy or even dirty. What they really are is simply uninformed.

## So That's What It Is!

There is nothing more confusing than sitting in the library studying for physics one night when you feel a sudden, slippery, wet sensation (you know that physics has never excited you *that* much). What's going on? You run to the bathroom, thinking you may be bleeding, but you find no discoloration on your underwear. In reality, you are no doubt experiencing what is commonly referred to as "eggwhite" cervical fluid, an extremely slippery and fertile secretion that is released as you approach ovulation. As you will learn, such secretions are healthy and normal.

> *The first time Barbara ever noticed fertile cervical fluid as a young teenager, she was horrified. She couldn't imagine what was hanging from her vagina when she went to urinate. The only thing she could think to do in order to remove it was wad up balls of toilet paper and hurl them at this seemingly foreign blob. Barbara is now a FAM instructor.*

Many women today refuse to remain ignorant. They are beginning to actively participate in all facets of their health care, enhancing their understanding of their fertility in the process. FAM gives women these opportunities. Most women are thrilled with the sense of control they feel after spending just a couple of minutes a day charting their cycle, cherishing the privilege of finally understanding their bodies.

## Fertility Awareness as Basic Education

I fully admit that Fertility Awareness is not the best choice of birth control for all women. Indeed, given the reality of AIDS and other sexually transmitted diseases (STDs), FAM as contraception is only recommended for monogamous couples with the maturity and discipline to follow the method correctly. However, even if a woman never uses it for contraceptive purposes, this book will clearly show that the biological principles that form the foundation for FAM should be seen as part of every woman's basic education. If this came to pass, women would be far less dependent on doctors for fundamental answers that should be a part of their own knowledge and understanding.

> *Audrey, one of my clients, had been charting her cycles for several years when she volunteered to be a control for an ultrasound study in abnormal ovulation. Over 5 months, her ovaries were monitored to determine if she was releasing an egg. Every time she went in, she would announce very confidentially that she was about to ovulate, and as usual, the technician would raise her eyebrows in surprise. "Oh really?" she would say. She would then check the monitor and say, "Oh, it looks like you're about to ovulate." "I know, that's what I just told you." And sure enough, the following day, Audrey would indeed ovulate.*
>
> *When she would return the next day, she would say, "By the way, I think you'll find that I've already ovulated." "Oh really?" the technician would say, scratching her head. She would then check the monitor and say, "Oh, it looks like you already ovulated." "I know, that's what I just told you," Audrey would reply, feeling a real sense of confidence about her ability to interpret her fertility signs.*

It is worth noting that the renowned scientist Dr. Carl Djerassi, often honored as the father of the Pill, acknowledges that women should be privy to such basic biological occurrences. "Eventually," he has written, "many a woman in our affluent society may conclude that the determination of when and whether she is ovulating should be a routine item of personal health information to which she is entitled as a matter of course."

# PART TWO

# REDISCOVERING YOUR CYCLE AND YOUR BODY

# CHAPTER 3

# There's More to Your Reproductive Anatomy Than Your Vagina

*W*hat woman doesn't remember awkwardly gathering with other sixth-grade girls to learn about the mysteries of their bodies, and the fascinating world of sanitary napkins they were soon to embark upon? The funny thing is, when all was said and done, most of us came away from the uninspired instruction with hardly a clue as to what was really about to happen to us. We proceeded to grow up with the menstrual cycle still cloaked in mystery, the subject of numerous myths.

We were all led to believe that the main event of every cycle was menstruation, and the primary lesson was proper tampon and sanitary pad etiquette. I can still remember giggling in the corner with my friends as we whispered the joke that was pathetically transformed from one of Stevie Wonder's most popular songs: "What's alright, uptight, and outta sight?" Tampons of course. We were *so* adult now. We sixth-graders could joke about these sorts of things— things the fifth-graders surely would just not get. We were so cool.

So it should come as no surprise that after spending hours in the "feminine hygiene" aisle of the drug store, most of us find that we still know basically nothing about our bodies, but can tell you pretty much anything you ever wanted to know about mini-versus maxipads, napkins with wings versus those with superduper adhesive strips, extrawide versus extralong panty shields, and superabsorbent versus regular tampons.

This is where Fertility Awareness comes in. It is about so much more than merely understanding female hygiene and menstruation. At its core is a philosophy of taking control of, understanding, and demystifying the menstrual cycle and all its effects on you. This is because sexuality, fertility, childbirth, and menopause are all facets of being female, and charting is the edifying window into these aspects of a woman's life. The self-knowledge available from Fertility Awareness is a valuable resource for all kinds of personal decision-making. Perhaps most important, it encourages women to value and trust knowledge provided by their own bodies.

Gynecologists are experts in women's physiology, so it should come as no surprise that most women turn to doctors rather than themselves to interpret their bodies. Reliance on physicians would be understandable if the knowledge doctors possessed about women's cycles was incomprehensible to the general public. But this is basic fertility, not brain surgery. In reality this information is quite simple, and not the mystery so many people believe it is.

In order to understand your cycle, though, you should first have a general knowledge of human reproductive biology. The following pages should familiarize you with both female and male anatomy.

## ❧ INTERNAL FEMALE REPRODUCTIVE ANATOMY

Do you realize that a part of every single one of us resided inside our maternal *grandmother's* uterus, even before our own mothers were born? Unlike male fetuses which contain no sperm, female fetuses already contain all the eggs that the newborn child will ever have. What that means, practically speaking, is that when your mother was just a fetus inside her mother, she already had developed one of the eggs that eventually became you.

ova
ovaries
fallopian tube
uterus
endometrium
cervix
cervical os
bladder
vagina

# CROSS-SECTION OF THE UTERUS

**Uterus:** The womb. A hollow, muscular, pear-shaped organ (about the size of a small lemon) that builds up and releases a blood-rich lining every cycle, and acts as an "incubator" for the developing fetus if conception occurs. In most women, the uterus curves forward.

**Fallopian tubes:** The 4–5-inch-long narrow tubes that transport the egg from the ovary to the uterus.

**Ova (ovum):** Granule-sized eggs stored in the ovaries, only one of which is usually released each cycle. The ovulated ova may unite with sperm during fertilization to form the eventual fetus.

**Ovaries:** Two almond-sized primary sex glands that contain up to a million immature eggs at birth. Each egg (or ovum) is surrounded by a group of cells called a follicle. The ovaries produce estrogen and progesterone during the reproductive years.

**Endometrium:** Lining of the uterus that builds up in preparation for a potential pregnancy and is shed every cycle in the form of menstruation.

**Cervix:** The lower opening of the uterus. The only part of the uterus that can be felt protruding into the upper vagina. Lined with channels which cyclically develop cervical fluid in which sperm thrive.

**Vagina:** The elastic 4–6-inch-long muscular passage between the vulva and cervix. During sexual arousal, the vagina expands to receive the penis during intercourse and stretches to become the birth canal during childbirth.

**Cervical os:** The small opening of the cervix that becomes larger around ovulation (referred to as "cervical tip" in this book).

One of the major differences between male and female anatomy has to do with when the sex cells (or gametes) are developed. As mentioned above, girls are born with all the eggs they will ever have. The eggs start to mature and be released at puberty, continuing to usually expel one egg per cycle until menopause. Boys, on the other hand, don't develop sperm until adolescence, but then continually produce sperm every day until they die. The box below reflects the three major differences between male and female fertility.

| DIFFERENCES BETWEEN MALE AND FEMALE FERTILITY | |
|---|---|
| **Males** | **Females** |
| Fertile all the time, since sperm are produced on a daily basis. | Fertile only a few days per cycle, since ovulation occurs only once a cycle. |
| Fertile from puberty until death. | Fertile from puberty until menopause (about 50 years old). |
| Do not develop any sperm until puberty. | Born with all the eggs they will ever have. |

## &#8766; EXTERNAL FEMALE REPRODUCTIVE ANATOMY

It is amazing how few women really know what their external anatomy looks like. Sadly, most girls are led to believe that they are "dirty down there," and are therefore reluctant to even examine themselves. Boys, however, are usually socialized to believe they possess a treasure in which to take pride.

Although the illustration on page 37 should be self-explanatory, there are several points I would like to make regarding external anatomy. One thing women should understand is that there are probably as many variations of sizes and shapes of vaginal lips as there are women. The enormous variation between women's vaginas and vaginal lips merely adds spice and uniqueness.

Aside from the obvious external difference between men and women, they also differ both sexually and in terms of certain potential physical problems.

# EXTERNAL FEMALE REPRODUCTIVE ANATOMY

**Vulva:** The external female genitalia.

**Mons Pubis:** The soft fleshy tissue beneath the pubic hair that protects the internal reproductive organs.

**Hood of Clitoris:** The protective covering of the clitoris, formed by the joining of the two inner vaginal lips.

**Clitoris:** The pea-sized organ that becomes filled with blood during sexual arousal, causing it to become firm and erect. The primary site of orgasm for the majority of women, since it is filled with more sexual nerve endings than any other part of the body. The female analog to the tip of the male penis.

**Vaginal lips (outer):** Soft padding, which contains oil-producing glands and a small amount of pubic hair.

**Vaginal lips (inner):** Folds of very soft, sleek skin. Typically covers the vagina unless the woman becomes sexually aroused, at which point the inner lips tend to fill with blood and blossom out to allow for insertion of the penis. They may also become full and separate around ovulation.

**Urethra:** The narrow tube that carries urine from the bladder out of the body.

**Vaginal opening:** The outer entrance to the vagina. The opening for the release of menstrual blood, as well as the site through which a baby's head comes out during childbirth.

**Vagina:** The elastic 4–6-inch-long muscular passage between the vulva and cervix, acting as the receptor of the penis during intercourse and the birth canal during childbirth.

**Perineum:** The membrane between the vaginal opening and the anus that is often cut during childbirth to facilitate passage of the baby out the vaginal opening.

Women, for example, tend to be more prone to urinary tract infections (UTIs). This is because a woman's urethra is shorter, so bacteria have less distance to travel from its opening to the bladder. In addition, its location so close to the vaginal opening makes it more vulnerable to external bacteria, as well as occasional irritation during intercourse. Finally, the contraceptive diaphragm can obstruct the flow of urine, creating a perfect medium for bacterial growth.

In addition to UTIs, women may develop occasional vaginal infections due to the delicate pH balance in the vagina. As you know, discharge from infections should not be confused with healthy cervical fluid which women usually produce every cycle around ovulation. (True vaginal infections are discussed in Chapter 15.)

Differences in anatomy affect the way men and women experience sexuality. This seems obvious on the surface, but there are so many subtle distinctions in this area that I have devoted much of Chapter 16 to discussing it. Still, one difference is certainly worth mentioning in this context: orgasms.

Women do not achieve orgasms the way men do. They're simply not built the same. A man's most sensitive nerves are just below the tip of the penis, which is the part most stimulated during sexual intercourse. It should come as no surprise that men achieve orgasm fairly easily due to the physical nature of intercourse.

Why do women not achieve orgasms during intercourse the same way men do? The answer is straightforward. The most sensitive sexual nerves in women are in the clitoris, which is outside and above the vagina. So during traditional intercourse (with the couple face-to-face in the missionary position), while the man is having a grand ol' time, the woman may be compiling a grocery list for dinner that night. It's not that the sensation of intercourse isn't wonderful for most women. And for the lucky 30% or so who achieve orgasms from intercourse, the experience can be fantastic. But the point is that women are built differently than men, plain and simple.

The most graphic way to explain this is by illustrating how a human being develops while in the uterus. Before a fetus evolves into a boy or girl, the exact same cells that would become the tip of the penis in the boy become the clitoris in the girl. And the same cells that would become the scrotum in the boy become the vulva in the girl. Perhaps the best way to help men understand women's sexuality would be to ask them whether they would be able to achieve an orgasm from merely being stroked on the scrotum. Who knows? Maybe, maybe not. Or maybe after, say, 2 hours! Yet high expectations cause men and women alike to get frustrated when women don't have orgasms as readily as men do.

## EMBRYONIC DEVELOPMENT OF FEMALE AND MALE GENITALIA

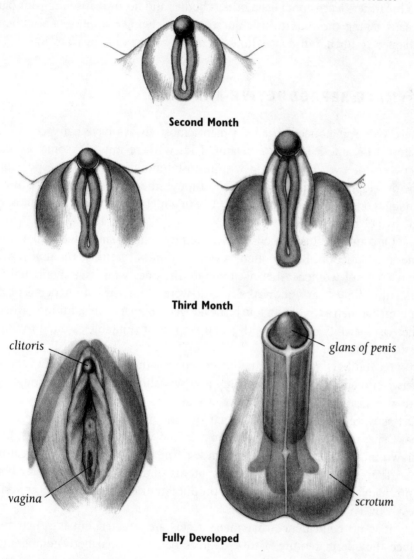

**Second Month**

**Third Month**

clitoris

glans of penis

vagina

scrotum

**Fully Developed**

If you could be a fly on the wall of bedrooms throughout the world, I think you'd be amused to discover how often women blame their partners for "lousy technique," which prevents them from having orgasms during intercourse. Meanwhile, men blame their partners for not being "womanly enough" to automatically have orgasms. Unfortunately, this often leads to conflict between the sexes.

Sex between men and women can be extremely sensual and gratifying if both partners learn about each other's bodies and needs. Satisfying your partner means taking the time to ask questions and being willing to be vulnerable. Chapter 16 further discusses how to enrich your sex life by charting.

## ꝏ MALE REPRODUCTIVE ANATOMY

Have you ever noticed that bald men almost always have hairy chests? Long before I became a fertility educator, I knew there must be some association between the two. It has to do with testosterone, the hormone responsible for the development of male sex traits. Although the exact mechanism is not fully understood, there is a correlation between a higher amount of testosterone and the two characteristics.

Of course, testosterone is also related to fertility, since it is responsible for sperm production. But so often, when we think of fertility, the tendency is to think only of women. After all, they are the ones who have menstrual cycles and ultimately bear children. Yet, if it weren't for the minor detail of men's sperm, women would obviously never get pregnant. In addition, whenever there is a fertility problem with a couple, it is attributable as often to the man as to the woman.

As you have seen from the last few pages, there are significant differences between men and women's fertility and sexuality. Interestingly enough, there are also distinct similarities between male and female reproductive anatomy. Just as women develop eggs in their ovaries, men produce the male counterpart, sperm, in their testes. And just as the woman's egg is picked up and drawn into the fallopian tube, a man's sperm travels through a tube called the vas deferens. Finally, the woman's uterus and the man's prostate, both in approximately the same location, produce nutrients for the egg and sperm, respectively.

It is no coincidence that men's testes are situated outside their bodies, since the sperm require 3 to 4 degrees below normal body temperature to develop. Apparently, that design works quite well, because most men produce 100 to 300 million sperm *a day!* To assure that the testicles remain cool, the scrotum that surrounds the testes thickens and thins in response to external temperature. For example, if a man jumps into a cold lake, the scrotum contracts, becoming very thick and pulling the testes against his body. But if he takes a hot shower, the scrotum thins out, allowing the testes to drop down. In this way, the body maintains a steady testicular temperature in various thermal conditions.

# MALE REPRODUCTIVE ANATOMY

**Bladder:** The muscular reservoir that stores urine before being released during urination.

**Prostate gland:** A walnut-sized gland which produces a thin, milky fluid that acts to nourish sperm and provide part of the substance which forms semen. Surrounds the junction of the vas deferens and the urethra.

**Cowper's gland:** Two pea-sized glands that produce a clear, lubricating fluid designed to provide nutrients for sperm survival. It also helps neutralize the acidity of any urine remaining in the urethra.

**Vas deferens:** A pair of approximately 15-inch-long tubes which carry sperm to the seminal vesicles. The inner channel is as thin as a hair.

**Penis:** The male organ through which urine and semen are emitted. Becomes erect for intercourse.

**Urethra:** The narrow 8-inch tube that can carry either urine or semen through the penis and out of the body.

**Testes (testicles):** The pair of oval-shaped sex glands that produce testosterone and an average of 200 million sperm daily. The left testes usually hangs lower than the right.

**Seminiferous tubules:** Microscopic tubes in the testes in which sperm are produced.

**Scrotum:** The loose, thin skin pouch surrounding the testicles, which thins out and contracts in response to external temperatures.

**Seminal vesicles:** Saclike structures which produce a nourishing substance for sperm and form about 65% of the seminal fluid in which sperm travel.

**Epididymis:** A 20-foot-long series of ultrathin, tightly coiled tubes that mature and store young sperm cells. Takes about 2 to 12 days for sperm to pass through, during which time they develop swimming ability and attain fertilization capability. Together the epididymis and vas deferens store about 700 million sperm at a time.

Even though sperm are produced on a daily basis, the production of individual sperm can take about 72 days to complete. They begin their reproductive journey inside the long, thin seminiferous tubules in the testes before going into "cold storage" in the epididymis, a series of 20-foot-long tightly coiled tubes that act as a school for sperm to perfect their swimming technique. It takes them anywhere from about 2 to 12 days to pass through the epididymus.

Before ejaculation, the cowper's gland releases a slippery, clear fluid designed to facilitate sperm survival and neutralize the acidity of the urethra. People often confuse these few drops of "leaking" with a man's inability to control his ejaculation. In reality, it is an absolutely healthy and necessary sexual function. But the pre-ejaculate may contain live sperm, which is why "withdrawal" is not recommended for birth control (though, in fact, it is more effective than having completely unprotected intercourse). At ejaculation itself, the prostate and seminal vesicles supply the nutrient-rich fluid in which sperm travel. One of the reasons it takes a while for men to be able to ejaculate again is that the seminal vesicle and prostate need time to manufacture more seminal fluid.

While we are on the subject of what men emit during ejaculation, you can rest assured that one of the things they do not emit is urine! One of the reasons it's difficult for a man to urinate when he is sexually aroused is that a muscular sphincter closes the opening of the bladder, preventing him from urinating and ejaculating simultaneously. Women can breathe a collective sigh of relief.

What does happen at ejaculation is that the sperm travel from the epididymis through the vas deferens and out the urethra. On the way, the fluid from the seminal vesicles also enters the vas deferens and mixes with the sperm. The seminal vesicles are two saclike structures that produce part of the seminal fluid in which the sperm travels. The other source of fluid for semen comes from the prostate gland.*

If a man ejaculates inside a woman, the length of time the sperm can survive is directly related to where the woman is in her cycle. If a woman is nowhere near ovulation, and is therefore infertile, the sperm won't survive more than a couple of hours or so. However, if she is approaching ovulation, and has wet-quality cervical fluid, sperm can live up to five days. This is discussed in greater detail later.

---

* Question: What did the epididymis say to the seminal vesicle? Answer: There's a vas deferens between us. (Thanks to Robert Mecklosky, New York City's most beloved science teacher.)

The initial gelatinlike consistency of the semen acts to prevent early leakage out of the vagina, while sugar within the gel provides instant energy for sperm motility. But once it has served this purpose, the gel tends to melt and leak out in the ensuing hours, much to the chagrin of many women.

Sperm comprise a surprisingly small fraction of the semen itself. The composition of semen is approximately as follows:

| | |
|---|---|
| Fluid from the seminal vesicles: | 65% |
| Fluid from the prostate gland: | 30% |
| Sperm and testicular fluid: | 5% |

Portions of the following list should shed light on why it is that many women who are trying to avoid pregnancy have good reason to be cautious:

| | |
|---|---|
| Number of sperm produced per day | 100–300 million |
| Typical number of sperm per ejaculate (2–6 ml) | 150–400 million |
| Typical number of sperm per milliliter | 20–200 million |
| Number of days sperm can live in fertile cervical fluid | 5 days |

The good news is that with a birth control method like FAM, women need not concern themselves with whether men produce one or a million sperm per minute. The point is that once women determine when they are not fertile themselves, it doesn't matter how many sperm the man produces. If there is no egg to be released, there is no physiological way a pregnancy can occur.

# CHAPTER 4

# Finally Making Sense of Your Menstrual Cycle

*K*eri and Brent are the classic example of educated people *being misinformed about normal cycle lengths. They weren't clients of mine, but Brent told me his theory about the effect of stress on women's cycles when he heard that I was writing a book on Fertility Awareness. He said his wife was so paranoid about getting pregnant that she would consistently worry herself into having delayed periods. Keri's anxiety would lead her to continually buy pregnancy tests that would always be negative, followed by menstruation within a day or two of the test. Based on this pattern, Brent deduced that anxiety itself was causing the delay, and that the reassuring news allowed her to finally relax enough for her period to start. Seems logical, right?*

Wrong. As you will learn, starting to worry about a pregnancy just a few days before your period is due will not delay it, since the time from ovulation to menstruation (the luteal phase) is a finite length that is not affected by external factors such as stress. In reality, what was undoubtedly happening was that Keri had longer than average cycles, perhaps 32 days or so. But since she was under the commonly held illusion that cycles were 28 days, she would start to panic when Day 30 or 31 arrived. Finally, by Day 32, she would take a pregnancy test, it would come out negative, and lo and behold, she would get her period the next day. But it wasn't the negative test results that were allowing her menstruation to begin. It was that her cycles were almost certainly about 32 days anyway.

"Then, when you're thirteen . . . a mysterious thing happens once a month, Shirley. . . . You begin to receive a MasterCard bill."

## 🖎 THE GREAT RACE

*There's a time when you have to explain to your children why they were born, and it's a marvelous thing if you know the reason by then.*
—HAZEL SCOTT (1920–1981)

Oh, yawn, here we go again . . . the menstrual cycle. Now, before you start whining about how boring this section is going to be, trust me. I promise, it's really one of the most remarkable things that happens within your body. The menstrual cycle is like a fine-tuned symphony, a fascinating interplay of hormones and physiologic responses. By the end of this chapter, I think you, too, will agree.

The bottom line is that your body prepares for a potential pregnancy every cycle, whether or not you want to actually conceive. In essence, your hormones do not always confer with your heart. They just do their thing regardless of your intentions.*

Every cycle, under the influence of Follicle Stimulating Hormone (FSH), about 15 to 20 eggs start to mature in each ovary. Each egg is encased in its own follicle. The follicles produce estrogen, the hormone necessary for ovulation to eventually occur. A race progresses for one follicle to become the largest. Eventually ovulation occurs when one ovary releases an egg from the most dominant follicle. (The other eggs that began to ripen disintegrate in a process called atresia.) It is fairly arbitrary which ovary ultimately releases the egg. Ovulation doesn't necessarily alternate between ovaries, as is often thought.

Although it averages about 2 weeks, this race to release an egg can take anywhere from about 8 days to a month or longer to complete. The primary factor that determines how long it will take before you ovulate is how soon your body reaches an estrogen threshold. The high levels of estrogen will trigger an abrupt surge of Luteinizing Hormone (LH). It's this LH surge which causes the egg to literally burst through the ovarian wall, usually within a day or so of its occurrence. After ovulation, the egg tumbles out into the pelvic cavity, where it is quickly swept up by the fingerlike projections of the fallopian tubes, called fimbria.

At this point, you may be thinking, what is she talking about? How many hormones are we dealing with here? Actually, a tidy little way for you to remember the general order of the hormones is through the expression FELOP, which stands for:

> **F**ollicle Stimulating Hormone
> **E**strogen
> **L**uteinizing Hormone (LH surge)
> **O**vulation
> **P**rogesterone

So the next time you are at a party and someone asks, you'll have a quick reply ready. Of course, things could get ugly if someone asks you for an even more detailed explanation of the menstrual cycle. For that, you should read the more comprehensive version of the cycle elaborated in Appendix E.

---

* Evolutionary biologist Margie Profet offers an altogether different theory as to why menstrual cycles occur. She believes the key function of menstruation is to actually rid the body of pathogens that are carried by the sperm and introduced into the woman's reproductive organs during sex. Her theory has caused considerable debate in the academic world, but she has maintained her sense of humor about it. "What they told you in kindergarten is true," she once told *Newsweek* (October 4, 1993), "boys really do have cooties."

## THE FOUR PRIMARY REPRODUCTIVE HORMONES

Once the egg tumbles into the pelvic cavity, the fimbria reach over and pick up the egg and draw it into one of the tubes. Occasionally the egg is not retrieved, and therefore pregnancy would not be possible that cycle. This would be true even if intercourse occurred when the woman was at the height of her fertile phase.

Following the release of the egg from the ovary, the follicle that held the egg collapses on itself, becoming a yellow body, or "corpus luteum." The corpus luteum remains behind on the interior ovarian wall, and starts releasing progesterone. The corpus luteum has a finite life span of about 12 to 16 days, rarely varying more than a couple of days within each individual woman. This is because its presence on the ovarian wall leaves it unaffected by the stresses of everyday life.

Thus, for example, if Myriam's luteal phase (the phase following ovulation) is normally 13 days, it may occasionally be 12 days, occasionally 14. Sometimes, luteal phases may be 11 or even 10 days. These are considered within a normal range, but phases less than 12 days can be *potentially* problematic if a couple is trying to get pregnant. (I discuss short luteal phases in greater detail in Chapters 11 and 12.)

Progesterone, the hormone released by the corpus luteum, is incredibly important for a woman's fertility because it does three things:

1. Prevents the release of all other eggs for that cycle.
2. Causes the uterine lining (endometrium) to thicken and sustain itself until the corpus luteum disintegrates 12 to 16 days later.
3. Causes the three primary fertility signs to change. These signs are waking temperature, cervical fluid, and cervical position.

In a small percentage of cycles, two or more eggs are released during ovulation, but always within a 24-hour period. This phenomenon, called multiple ovulation, is responsible for fraternal twins. The reason that more eggs cannot be released later that cycle is due to the powerful effects of progesterone mentioned above. *Progesterone quickly stops the release of all other eggs until the next cycle.* So a woman could not release an egg one day, get pregnant, then release an egg again weeks or months later. Her body protects that potential pregnancy by preventing her from being able to release more eggs following ovulation.*

## ᔥ OVULATION: THE DIVIDING LINE

The first part of the cycle, from Day 1 of menses to ovulation, is the follicular (or estrogenic) phase. Its length can vary considerably. The second phase of the cycle, from ovulation to the last day before the new period begins, is the luteal (or progestational) phase. It usually has a finite life span of 12 to 16 days. What this means is that, ultimately, it is the day of ovulation which will determine the length of your cycle.

For example, a woman could have an extremely delayed ovulation due to stress or other factors, not ovulating until Day 30 or so. This would result in about a 44-day cycle (30 plus 14). Thus, just because a woman is on Day 44 and hasn't gotten her period yet doesn't necessarily mean she's pregnant.

> *My brother Raymond was editing the manuscript for this book when he got*
> *a call from his good friend Marcela, who lives in Los Angeles. She appeared*
> *mildly panicked about possibly being pregnant, and was calling him for*

---

* In the United States, twin births occur in about one out of 83 deliveries. One-third of the time, they are identical twins, meaning that *one* fertilized egg splits in two. Two-thirds of the time, they are fraternal twins, meaning that *two* separate eggs are released and conceived within 24 hours of each other. Identical twins tend to be rare in nature in that there is no particular hereditary component involved. The birth of fraternal twins, on the other hand, may be influenced by heredity. What appears to be passed down is the propensity to release higher levels than average of FSH, which in turn may cause more than one egg to be released. In addition, older women may be more likely to release more than one egg, since FSH tends to increase as women get older.

Recent studies show that multiple ovulation may occur as often as 10% of all cycles, a much higher percentage than previously thought. While it is true that less than 1% of deliveries are fraternal twins, it must be remembered that most ovulations don't result in conception. In addition, new research has shown many more fraternal twins are actually conceived than delivered, but that in the majority of cases, one of the conceptions is spontaneously miscarried or reabsorbed, resulting in a single baby. Scientists refer to this as the phenomenon of the "vanishing twin." In any case, the fact that up to 10% of all cycles may have multiple ovulations highlights the importance of the various FAM rules for avoiding pregnancy that you'll learn later.

advice (Ray was accustomed to his friends' inquiries, since he possessed a certain expertise on fertility that few men do).

She explained that she was worried because she was on Day 42 and had never had a cycle longer than 32 days. Clearly enjoying his role as supportive friend and menstrual detective, Ray proceeded to record all the relevant information. Sex with her boyfriend on Day 5. "Sloppy withdrawal." No cycles ever less than 25 days. And so on.

The data convinced Ray that pregnancy was extremely unlikely. He then went on to explain to Marcela that if she had been sick, or traveled, or had experienced a lot of stress before she ovulated, it was possible ovulation could have been delayed days or even weeks, thus causing the extended cycle. She was not terribly reassured. "You must have been stressed out about something," he said. Marcela insisted that all was basically uneventful in her life, and that the only unusual anxiety she was experiencing had crept in just a few days earlier, about a week after her last period was "due."

Beyond being a menstrual detective, Ray was also an amateur historian. He loved dates. He took out his calendar and stared at it. "Marcela," he said coyly, "let me just verify. Your last period started on January 6, so you normally would've ovulated around January 20, give or take a few days."

"Yeah, I guess," she mumbled nervously.

"So, I'm just curious, on January 17, did you just sleep through the earthquake, or what?"

There was a pause.

"Oh God, I forgot about that! That was one of the scariest things I've ever been through. 6.7 on the Richter scale! It was awful." Ray laughed and told her to relax, that she almost certainly wasn't pregnant. Three days later Marcela called back, delighted to inform him that she had just gotten her period.

Ray suggested that the next time a massive quake strikes, the mayor should go on citywide TV. That way he could assure the women of L.A. that if their periods are late, it's quite possible there's nothing to worry about. It could just be your garden-variety, seismically delayed ovulation.

It should also be noted that a woman may occasionally not release an egg at all. This is referred to as an "anovulatory cycle." These types of cycles may range from very short to exceedingly long, and are discussed further in Chapter 7.

## ℘ᴀ **THE DRAMA OF CONCEPTION**

When the egg bursts through the ovarian wall, it's usually picked up by the fallopian tube. Once it's released, it can take as little as 20 seconds for the fimbria (the end of the fallopian tubes) to reach over and draw the egg into the tube itself. Assuming fertilization does not occur, the egg remains alive for a maximum of 24 hours, after which it simply disintegrates and either gets reabsorbed by the body or comes out in the menstrual flow. The egg is about the size of the period at the end of this sentence, hardly large enough to be seen reclining on the sanitary napkin.*

If fertilization does occur, it will take place in the outer third of the fallopian tube within a few hours of ovulation. (It does not take place in the uterus, as is popularly believed.) The lucky sperm may have journeyed up to several hours to reach its cherished date. The fertilized egg will then continue to be pulled toward the uterus by vibrating cilia, hairlike projections that line the fallopian tubes. After a week or so, it reaches its ultimate destination of the uterine lining, and begins the burrowing-in process. (See page 4 of color insert.)

In order for conception to occur, though, there must be three factors present: the egg, the sperm, and a *medium* in which the sperm can travel to reach the fallopian tubes. The medium is the fertile-quality cervical fluid, which acts as a living conduit to direct the sperm through the cervix. Women produce cervical fluid under the influence of increasing levels of estrogen in the first part of the cycle. Because the sperm can live up to 5 days in fertile-quality cervical fluid, it is actually possible to have intercourse on Monday, and get pregnant from that act on Friday. So, without wanting to burst anyone's bubble, you could enjoy a deliciously romantic, snowy evening making love in front of the fire, but not actually *conceive* until 5 days later, while you're jogging, and your sweetheart is flying off to a meeting in Kalamazoo.

The body's response to conception is truly amazing. If you became pregnant, it would be disastrous for the endometrium to begin to disintegrate and shed in the form of menstruation, as it does cycle after cycle. So the pregnant body has a means of preventing that from happening. As soon as the fertilized egg burrows into the lining, it starts releasing a pregnancy hormone, HCG,†

---

* A FAM instructor once told me that when she first began to menstruate, she would search every period for a blue egg that resembled a robin's egg, and would continually be disappointed when she couldn't find it.

† Human Chorionic Gonadotropin.

which sends a message back to the corpus luteum left behind on the ovarian wall. HCG signals the corpus luteum to remain alive beyond its usual maximum of 16 days, continuing to release progesterone long enough to sustain the nourishing lining. After several months, the placenta takes over, not only maintaining the endometrium, but providing all the oxygen and nutrients the fetus needs to thrive.

One of the reasons for "false negative" pregnancy tests is that the test is often done too soon, before the egg has had a chance to implant and start releasing HCG, or before the HCG has had time to reach a high enough level to be detected in the urine or bloodstream. Of course, the occurrence of such misleading results could be decreased if women charted their cycles and could identify for themselves when ovulation, and therefore implantation, most likely took place.

I hope the last few pages have convinced you that your menstrual cycle is an amazing orchestration of biological events. Far from being only about menstruation, it is a continual hormonal chorus working together toward the ultimate goal of releasing and nurturing a healthy egg. And as you will see in the next chapter, your body gives you conspicuous signs to help you understand on a daily basis what is transpiring within.

# CHAPTER 5

# The Three Primary Fertility Signs

*A*sk the typical woman whether she is aware that her own body is a walking biological computer revealing the most enlightening information about her fertility, and you're likely to meet a blank stare. But the truth is, all women of reproductive age can easily learn how to observe and chart three primary fertility signs that their bodies produce. This information can then be used to tell them numerous things about their cycle, the most obvious being whether they can or can't get pregnant on any given day.

As you know, the three primary fertility signs virtually all ovulating women produce are:

1. waking temperature
2. cervical fluid
3. cervical position

Let's take each sign individually.

## ❧ WAKING (BASAL BODY) TEMPERATURE

The easiest sign to observe is the waking temperature, for the simple reason that it is usually very graphic and objective. Many women who have charted their fertility for a few months find that it becomes a fun challenge to predict the day their temperatures will shift.

A woman's preovulatory waking temperatures typically range from about 97.0 to 97.5 degrees Fahrenheit, with postovulatory temperatures rising to about 97.6 to 98.6 degrees. After ovulation, they will stay elevated until her next period, about 12 to 16 days later. If she were to become pregnant, they would remain high throughout her pregnancy.

Temperatures typically rise within a day or so after ovulation, and are the result of the heat-inducing hormone, progesterone. Progesterone is released by the corpus luteum (the follicle that previously housed the egg before it burst out of the ovary, as discussed in the last chapter). So usually, by definition, the rise in temperature signifies that ovulation has *already* occurred. Waking temperatures within a cycle typically look like Chart 5.1 below.*

When interpreting temperatures, it is important that you train your eyes to "see the forest through the trees." The key to doing so is to look for a *pattern* of lows and highs. In other words, you'll find that your temperatures before ovulation will go up and down in a low range, and the temperatures after ovulation will go up and down in a high range. The trick is to see the whole, and not focus so much on the day-to-day changes.

I learned how helpful this concept is when I first taught at a women's clinic. Within a few weeks of the first class, I would inevitably start getting calls from clients who were convinced they must not be ovulating. But when they

**Chart 5.1. A typical waking temperature pattern.** Note the rise in temperature starting on Day 17, which means that for this particular cycle, ovulation most likely occurred on Day 16.

---

* A very small percentage of women won't have biphasic temperature patterns even if they are ovulating. In such a case, contraceptors wouldn't be able to use waking temperatures as a fertility sign, but they would still be able to use the Billings Method, which relies on cervical fluid alone. This method, though, is not quite as accurate, and often requires more days of abstinence to be effective. Pregnancy achievers whose temperatures don't reflect a shift will need to initially use other means of determining whether they are ovulating, such as cervical fluid patterns (which are not as conclusive), ovulation predictor kits, blood tests, ultrasound, or endometrial biopsies.

read me their temperatures over the phone, the pattern seemed perfectly evident. I couldn't understand why they didn't see what I saw. Then it dawned on me. They were not seeing the pattern, but were instead focusing on the fact that on Monday it was up, on Tuesday it was down, on Wednesday it was back up, and so on. Remember, stand back and see the whole picture. If you find that your temperatures are not obvious during the first cycle, I would encourage you to chart for several cycles before you depend on FAM as a method of birth control.

The preovulatory temperatures are suppressed by estrogen, whereas the postovulatory temperatures are increased by heat-inducing progesterone. In fact, one of the ways to remember that the second phase of the cycle is the "progesterone" phase is to think of it as the "pro-gestation" phase. In other words, this is the phase of the cycle that is warmer, as if designed to act as a human incubator to nurture an egg which may have just been fertilized.

I want to stress here that the rise in waking temperature almost always indicates that ovulation has already occurred. It does not reveal impending ovulation, as do the other two fertility signs, the cervical fluid and cervical position. You should also be aware that in only a minority of cycles will women ovulate at the lowest point of their temperature graph. Because a temperature dip is so rare, women should not rely on its occurrence for fertility purposes. Rather, they should use the cervical fluid and cervical position to indicate approaching ovulation.

You need to be aware of certain factors that can increase your waking temperature, such as:

- having a fever
- drinking alcohol the night before
- getting less than three consecutive hours of sleep before taking it
- taking it at a substantially different time than usual
- using an electric blanket or heating pad that you normally don't use

However, as you will see in the following chapter, you needn't worry about the occasional erratic temperatures that may result. This is because you can discount them without compromising the accuracy of the method. In any case, FAM gives you two other signs to daily cross-check your fertility.

## Temperatures, Stress Reduction, and the Dreaded Late Period

Waking temperatures can be extremely helpful in projecting how long a cycle will be, because they can identify if you've had a delayed ovulation that would cause your cycle to be longer than normal. Remember, once the temperature rises, it is typically a set 12 to 16 days until your period. And after you've charted for several months, you will be able to determine even more specifically what your particular postovulatory range usually is. (As previously discussed, for most women the phase after ovulation doesn't vary more than a couple of days.)

I, myself, experienced a classic delayed ovulation during a cycle when I was moving from one home to another. Three things were happening in my life that cycle, any one of which would have been enough to delay ovulation.

*It was November of '86, and I had all the signs that I was approaching ovulation. My cervical fluid was getting very wet, and my cervix was rising and becoming more open and soft. On Day 16 of my cycle, though, I had to completely move out of my old home and into the new one, meaning every speck of dirt had to be washed off the walls of the apartment, and all of my boxes moved into my new home. In addition, I had to lecture at a midwifery school across town before catching a plane during rush hour to lecture at a conference in another state the next morning. So what was going on? I was moving, traveling, and totally stressed out.*

*My body basically said: "Tell 'ya what. I think I'll just put your ovulation on hold until you're good and ready." In the end, as you can see from the chart below, I didn't even ovulate until about Day 24, and ended up with a 38-day cycle! Had I not been charting, I probably would have been completely panicked, thinking I was pregnant, since I had never in my life experienced such a long cycle.*

**Chart 5.2. A temperature pattern showing a delayed ovulation.** Note how the temperature shift didn't occur until Day 25.

This illustrates an important point. Women who don't chart are continually fearful when their periods seem "late," not realizing that long cycles are usually simply due to ovulating later, an occurrence that is very easy to identify through waking temperatures.

I have used my own experience above to exemplify the point that there are numerous things that can delay (or even prevent) ovulation, including stress, travel, moving, illness, medication, strenuous exercise, and sudden weight change. But by charting your temperature, you can accurately determine when you might be having a delayed ovulation. Whether you are trying to avoid or get pregnant, knowing this information is invaluable, sparing you needless stress and confusion.

## ❧ CERVICAL FLUID

One of the first things you'll probably be struck with when you start charting is the distinct pattern of cervical fluid throughout your cycle. And, if you are like most women who learn how to observe their fertility signs, the second thing you may experience is the sense of frustration and even anger when you realize how little you understood your body before. No, you were probably not experiencing recurring vaginal infections all the time. No, you were not dirty and in need of douching away the "discharge." In fact, the beauty of charting your cervical fluid is that you will be able to discern once and for all what is absolutely normal from the true symptomatic secretions which result from a vaginal infection. For this reason, I would suggest that you never use the "*d*-word" to describe your healthy cervical fluid. After all, we don't refer to men's healthy semen as "discharge."

*Cervical fluid is to the woman what seminal fluid is to the man.* Since men are always fertile, they produce seminal fluid continually. Women, on the other hand, are only fertile the few days around ovulation, and therefore only produce the substance necessary for sperm nourishment and mobility during that time. It is fairly intuitive. Sperm require a medium in which to live, move, and thrive—otherwise they will die. Once the sperm travel from the penis to the vagina, they need an analogous substance to sustain them. But the only time it is critical for the sperm to survive is around the time the egg is released. It is for this reason that women produce the substance that resembles semen for only a few days per cycle.

## THE CERVIX WITH MAGNIFICATION OF SPERM IN INFERTILE AND FERTILE CERVICAL FLUID

In essence, the fertile cervical fluid functions exactly like the seminal fluid. It provides an alkaline medium to protect the sperm in an otherwise acidic vagina. In addition, it provides nourishment for the sperm, acts as a filtering mechanism, and functions as a medium in which to move.

In a nutshell, a woman's cervical fluid starts to develop and resemble a man's seminal fluid in a very predictable way. After the woman's period and directly under the influence of rising estrogen, the cervical fluid typically starts to develop in the following pattern:

| Cervical Fluid | Symbol |
|---|---|
| (Menstruation) | ✳ |
| Nothing/dry | — |
| Sticky | S |
| Creamy | Ⓒ |
| Eggwhite | Ⓔ |
| Nothing/dry (or sticky) | — (or S) |
| (Menstruation) | ✳ |

In other words, right after your period, you may have a very dry vaginal sensation and observe *nothing* near the vaginal opening. Or you may notice a slight moisture similar to the way it would feel if you touched the inside of your cheek for a second. Your finger would have a dampness on it that would evaporate within a few seconds. This is the way the vaginal opening typically feels when there is no cervical fluid.

After perhaps a few days of this dryness, you may begin to develop a type of cervical fluid that is best described as *sticky,* like the paste you used in elementary school. Occasionally, it may even resemble drying rubber cement in that it is somewhat rubbery and slightly "springy," but the critical point is that it is *not wet.* The sticky and "rubber-cement" type of cervical fluid in themselves are not conducive to sperm survival, but are considered possibly fertile if found *before* ovulation.

The next type of cervical fluid you may notice for several days is *creamy* or lotionlike. It tends to feel rather cold at the vaginal opening, just as hand lotion itself feels cool to the touch. Sometimes the cervical fluid is so wet or watery that it is hard to physically handle (with a consistency similar to skim milk), but the obvious clue to your fertility at that point is the very wet vaginal *sensation* you will feel.

The final and most fertile cervical fluid resembles raw *eggwhite.* It's extremely slippery and usually stretches 1 to 10 inches. (This ability to stretch is called spinnbarkeit, or "spin," for short.) It's usually clear or partially streaked. It could also be very watery. The critical determinant of this quality cervical fluid is the extremely wet and lubricative vaginal sensation you usually feel. It may even leave a fairly symmetrical, round pattern of fluid on your underwear due to its high water content.*

---

* Women in their early 20s may have as many as 4 or 5 days of eggwhite, but by their mid-30s, most will only have a day or two.

Very fertile-quality cervical fluid often forms a fairly symmetrical round circle, due to its high concentration of water.

Nonwet-quality cervical fluid tends to form more of a rectangle or line on your underwear.

The most important feature of this extremely fertile cervical fluid is the lubricative quality. I cannot stress enough the importance of paying attention to the slippery sensation you will feel as you approach ovulation. You may even notice that the lubricative vaginal sensation continues a day or two beyond the actual eggwhite. *Pay close attention, because that sensation indicates that you are still extremely fertile.* Of course, vaginal sensation should not be confused with sexual lubrication. Vaginal sensation is something you simply feel throughout the day, without actually observing the cervical fluid.

| Cycle Day | 1 | 2 | 3 | 4 | 5 | 6 | 7 | 8 | 9 | 10 | 11 | 12 | 13 | 14 | 15 | 16 | 17 | 18 | 19 | 20 | 21 | 22 | 23 | 24 | 25 | 26 | 27 | 28 | 29 | 30 | 31 | 32 | 33 | 34 | 35 | 36 | 37 | 38 | 39 | 40 |
|---|---|---|---|---|---|---|---|---|---|---|---|---|---|---|---|---|---|---|---|---|---|---|---|---|---|---|---|---|---|---|---|---|---|---|---|---|---|---|---|---|
| Cervical Fluid | ✳ | ✳ | ✳ | ✳ | – | – | – | – | – | S | S | S | ⓒ | ⓒ | Ⓔ | Ⓔ | – | – | – | – | – | – | – | – | – | – | – | – | – | – | ✳ | | | | | | | | | |
| Peak Day | | | | | | | | | | | | | | | | | | | | | | | | | | | | | | | | | | | | | | | | |
| Vaginal Sensation | | | | | | | | | | dry | dry | sticky | cold | wet | wet | lube | | | | | | | | | | | | | | | | | | | | | | | | |
| Cervix | | | | | | | | | | | | | | | | | | | | | | | | | | | | | | | | | | | | | | | | |
| Cervical Fluid Description | | | | | | | | | | Scant, sticky | Scant, sticky | little more, still sticky | a lot more, lotiony | really wet, white cream | 1" stretchy eggwhite | 4" clear! | | | | | | | | | | | | | | | | | | | | | | | | |

**Chart 5.3. A typical cervical fluid pattern.** Note that there is usually a gradual progression from dry to sticky to wetter types, seen here in 2 days each of creamy and eggwhite. Also notice that the vaginal sensation generally corresponds with the cervical fluid ("lube" is used to signify a lubricative sensation at the vaginal opening). Finally, observe how she records Day 1 of the new menses on the same chart before repeating it again on a new chart. Every cycle is clearly delineated with a vertical closing line.

After estrogen has peaked and dropped, the cervical fluid changes abruptly, often within a few hours. This is due to the sudden drop in estrogen, combined with the surge of progesterone following ovulation. In other words, it may take up to a week for the fertile-quality cervical fluid to build up, but then it will usually dry up in less than a day. This sudden drying of the cervical fluid is the best way to know that estrogen has plummeted and that progesterone has taken over. The lack of wet cervical fluid will usually last the duration of the cycle. Note in the graphic below that the phases of cervical fluid buildup and subsequent drying are usually not symmetrical.

Finally, in the day or so before menstruation, women may occasionally notice a very wet, watery sensation, which in some women even resembles watery eggwhite. This is due to the drop in progesterone that precedes the disintegration of the lining of the uterus. The first part of the endometrium to flow out is typically water, hence, the very wet sensation. Obviously, this wet fluid immediately preceding menstruation does not indicate a fertile time.

A trick to help you identify the actual quality of the cervical fluid is to notice what it feels like to run your tissue (or your finger) across your vaginal lips. Does it feel dry, impeding movement? Is it smooth? Or does it simply glide across? When you are dry, the tissue won't pass across your vaginal lips smoothly. But as you approach ovulation, your cervical fluid gets progressively more lubricative, and thus the tissue should just glide easily.

The concept of paying special attention to wet sensations is especially important in women who seem to have some type of cervical fluid almost every day. In other words, for some women, their Basic Infertile Pattern (BIP) on either side of their fertile phase is to have sticky-quality cervical fluid rather than being truly dry. It is even more important for these women to learn how to identify that change to a fertile-quality cervical fluid, which I discuss in further detail in Appendix B.

## Knowing What's What

One of the saddest examples of a woman being misled about the nature of normal cervical fluid was a client that I had a few years ago.

*Brandy was a young woman who attended my class after having been on the Pill 6 years. Prior to my seminar she endured a traumatic, humiliating, and painful diagnostic test—all because of the unfortunate ignorance of her medical practitioner at the time.*

*Brandy noticed that every now and then when she would have a bowel movement, she would feel a slippery substance when she used the toilet paper. She became quite concerned that perhaps something was wrong with her intestinal tract, because she only noticed it after using the bathroom, and only periodically.*

*The doctor suggested she have a colonoscopy to rule out inflammatory bowel disease or polyps. She was required to fast a couple of days, have an enema, and then be subjected to one of the most painful experiences of her life. And why?*

*Because what she was experiencing was the absolutely normal and common occurrence of fertile eggwhite cervical fluid flowing from the vagina. Since that type is so slippery and profuse, it can easily be spread to the rectum with tissue paper. Of course, it is no wonder she only experienced this slippery substance every now and then, since she only produced eggwhite around the time of ovulation.*

Such accounts of unnecessary and demoralizing tests are what have motivated me to educate women about the simple signs their own bodies tell them about their reproductive health. This is not to say that women don't occasionally have genuine infections or other problems and medical concerns. But the point is that women should be taught what is normal so that they can better detect problems themselves.

You should also be aware that as with the temperature, there are certain factors that can potentially mask cervical fluid, such as:

- vaginal infections
- seminal fluid
- arousal fluid
- spermicides and lubricants
- antihistamines (which can dry it)

As for the seminal and arousal fluid above, women often wonder how cervical fluid differs from the two. Both seminal fluid and arousal fluid are much thinner and typically dry quicker on the finger, whereas cervical fluid tends to remain on your finger until you wash it off. I will discuss this in greater detail in the following chapter. Of course, once again, because you have three fertility signs to rely on, you can have the peace of mind of knowing that you can still interpret your fertility by cross-checking the other two signs if there is any ambiguity.

## 🙠 CERVICAL POSITION (OPTIONAL SIGN) *

Have you ever noticed that intercourse can sometimes be fairly uncomfortable in certain positions? Maybe you have wonderful memories of a lazy Sunday morning with your partner. You woke up that day feeling pretty amorous, and slid on top of him. But a week later, when you wanted to relive that wonderful day, you noticed that instead of experiencing the same delicious feeling, you felt a deep pain inside. What was going on? Why the discomfort this time?

Or have you ever noticed that there are times when it is quite easy to insert your diaphragm or cervical cap, but other times it seems almost impossible to find your cervix to insert it properly? Or worse yet, it seems like there is not even enough room to insert it? Or has your health practitioner ever commented that you appear fertile during a pelvic exam, even though she had done nothing more than insert a speculum?

All of this has to do with the fact that your cervix, the lower part of the uterus that extends into your vagina, goes through some amazing cyclical changes throughout your cycle, all of which can be easily felt. Your cervix is actually a wealth of information about your fertility, literally at your fingertips.

As with the cervical fluid, the cervix itself prepares for a pregnancy every cycle by transforming into a perfect "biological gate" through which the sperm can pass on their way to finding the egg. It does so by becoming soft and open around ovulation in order to allow the sperm passage through the uterus and on to the fallopian tubes. In addition, the cervix rises due to the estrogenic effect on the ligaments that hold the uterus in place.

After your period and directly under the influence of estrogen, your cervix typically starts to change.

One of the easiest ways to remember how your cervix feels as you approach ovulation is the acronym SHOW, as seen in the illustration on the opposite page.

---

* As you will read, "cervical position" as used in this book actually refers to more than just the height of the cervix in the vagina. However, it is easier to use this one term to describe the various cervical changes that occur in the cycle, particularly given that they're checked simultaneously, usually in a matter of seconds.

**CERVICAL POSITION CHANGES DURING THE CYCLE**

Around
Ovulation
↓

Menstruation      Firm            **S**oft          Firm            Menstruation
                  Low             **H**igh          Low
                  Closed          **O**pen          Closed
                  Nonwet          **W**et           Nonwet

Let's take each facet in the order listed above. The cervix is normally firm like the tip of your nose, and only becomes soft and rather mushy, like your lips, as you approach ovulation. In addition, it is normally fairly low and closed, feeling somewhat like a dimple, and only rises and opens in response to the high levels of estrogen around ovulation. And finally, it is the cervix itself that emits fertile-quality wet cervical fluid when the egg is about to be released. The chart below shows how to record your cervical changes.

| Cycle Day | 1 | 2 | 3 | 4 | 5 | 6 | 7 | 8 | 9 | 10 | 11 | 12 | 13 | 14 | 15 | 16 | 17 | 18 | 19 | 20 | 21 | 22 | 23 | 24 | 25 | 26 | 27 | 28 | 29 | 30 | 31 | 32 | 33 | 34 | 35 | 36 | 37 | 38 | 39 | 40 |
|---|---|---|---|---|---|---|---|---|---|---|---|---|---|---|---|---|---|---|---|---|---|---|---|---|---|---|---|---|---|---|---|---|---|---|---|---|---|---|---|---|
| Cervical Fluid | ✳ | ✳ | ✳ | ✳ | | | | | | | | | | | | | | | | | | | | | | | | ✳ | | | | | | | | | | | | |
| Peak Day | | | | | | | | | | | | | | | | | | | | | | | | | | | | | | | | | | | | | | | | |
| Vaginal Sensation | | | | | | | | | | | | | | | | | | | | | | | | | | | | | | | | | | | | | | | | |
| Cervix | | | | | ● | ● | ● | ● | o | o | O | O | o | ● | ● | ● | ● | ● | ● | ● | ● | ● | ● | ● | ● | ● | ● | | | | | | | | | | | | |
| | | | | | F | F | F | F | M | M | S | S | S | F | F | F | F | F | F | F | F | F | F | F | F | F | F | | | | | | | | | | | | |

**Chart 5.4. A typical cervical position pattern.** Note how the circles represent how open the cervix is and their position in the box represents how high it is. The letters below the circles stand for the firmness of the cervix—firm, medium, and soft.

## ❧ SECONDARY FERTILITY SIGNS

Many women are lucky enough to notice other signs on a regular basis, all of which are very helpful in being able to further understand their cycles. These signs are referred to as secondary fertility signs, because they do not necessarily occur in all women, or in every cycle in individual women. But they are still very practical for giving additional information to women to identify their fertile and infertile phases.

Secondary signs as ovulation approaches may include:

- Midcycle spotting
- Pain or achiness near the ovaries
- Increased sexual feelings
- Fuller vaginal lips
- Abdominal bloating
- Water retention
- Increased energy level
- Heightened sense of vision, smell, and taste
- Increased sensitivity in breasts and skin
- Breast tenderness

The first sign listed above, midcycle or ovulatory spotting, is thought to be the result of the sudden drop in estrogen just before ovulation. Because progesterone has not yet been released to sustain it, the lining often leaks a small amount of blood until the progesterone takes over. It's typically more common in long cycles.

*Courtney represented the classic example of a woman not understanding the distinction between different causes of bleeding. She called saying she wanted to use FAM for birth control, but thought she might not be an appropriate candidate for the method because she had "such short cycles." When I questioned her about them, she said they were "literally every 2 weeks, but alternated: heavy, light, heavy, light." Of course, what she was experiencing was a typical-length cycle with classic ovulatory spotting. I encouraged her to take my Fertility Awareness class. I don't know if she still uses FAM for contraception, but she certainly understands her body a lot better than before.*

As for the various pains that women often notice midcycle, there are several theories as to their causes. The important point is that you cannot say with certainty whether they are occurring before, during, or after you've actually ovulated.

| | |
|---|---|
| **Dull achiness:** | This is thought to be caused by the swelling of numerous follicles in the ovaries as the eggs race for dominance and ultimate ovulation. It is typically felt as a general abdominal achiness, since both ovaries swell with growing follicles as the woman approaches ovulation. |
| **A sharp pain:** | This could be the actual moment that the egg bursts through the ovarian wall and is usually felt on only one side. |
| **Crampiness:** | This is probably the result of irritation of the abdominal lining caused by leakage of blood or follicular fluid released from the ruptured egg follicle. It could also be due to contractions of the fallopian tubes around ovulation. |

Because there are several pains that may occur, none of them are considered primary fertility signs that can be depended on independently. But ovulatory pain in general is an excellent secondary fertility sign to corroborate the three primary signs. The pain is usually referred to as *mittelschmerz* (midpain) and is felt by about one-fifth of women around their ovulation. It typically lasts anywhere from a few minutes to a few hours, and on rare occasions, even a day or so.

In addition to those signs previously listed, you may find through charting that you yourself have some unique secondary fertility signs. I've certainly heard of many in my years of counseling women:

*Sandy gets hiccups as ovulation approaches. The skin on Cindy's thumb actually cracks in a somewhat painful lesion every cycle around ovulation. But through learning to chart, she was able to at least identify what caused it. And Kendel develops such a heightened sense of smell around ovulation that, as she describes it, if her chef-husband cooks something in their house during her fertile phase, she can smell it for days after and no amount of open windows will relieve her of the nausea. Likewise, if she eats potato chips, or anything with mustard on it, she practically sterilizes her hands afterwards, but unfortunately can still smell the residual effects. But if she is outside her fertile phase, he can whip up an onion-garlic casserole, and she's not the least bit affected by it.*

When women learn that all this is happening inside their bodies on a regular basis, they are often amazed. To think that all they were taught about their menstrual cycles in the sixth grade was whether to opt for tampons or sanitary napkins during their periods!

# CHAPTER 6

# How to Observe and Chart Your Fertility Signs

*"Monica's been on this marvellous self-examination course"*...

When some women first hear about observing fertility signs, their reaction is typically:

"You've got to be kidding me. Too much bother."
"There's no way. Take my temperature every day?"
"What a hassle. Who'd do it?"

I, too, had a similar response when I first heard about charting the cycle 13 years ago. But once I learned how simple it really was, I was chagrined. Today, I have a different attitude. Quite simply: *Charting is a privilege rather than a burden.*

How could I have been so ignorant about such a fundamental aspect of my body before I learned to be so aware? A cynic might question the time involved in checking every day. But I think many would agree that it is infinitely more appealing to take one's temperature in the morning before getting up than to stop lovemaking to insert a diaphragm or cervical cap, or to contend with numerous side effects and inconveniences of other methods. And for those frustrated in their desire to get pregnant, the time involved is minuscule compared to the inevitable office visits and procedures for those not educated in FAM.

To show how simple charting really is, let me make an analogy. If someone were to ask you to describe how to tie your shoelaces, you might begin:

> Let's see. Well, you take your right shoelace, and place it over the left one. Then take the left shoelace and twist it under the right, pulling both shoelaces away from each other to form a twisted knot. Then make a loop with the right shoelace, which was originally the left. Take the left shoelace and . . .

I'm exhausted just trying to write the rest of the directions. If you had to learn how to do something as simple as tie your shoes through following directions, you'd probably never get it right. Observing and charting your fertility signs is really no different. Once you learn the basic principles, it becomes second nature.

When reading this chapter on how to observe and chart fertility signs, refer to the sample chart on the opposite page. (Trust me. It's not as involved as it may first appear.) A blank master chart is on the last page of the book. It should be enlarged by about 125%.

## 🎝 WAKING TEMPERATURE

The first time I heard that FAM involved taking a temperature every day, I thought it wouldn't be worth it. But 4,745 temperatures later, I've lost sight of what the big deal was. In fact, it's nice to have an excuse to snuggle a minute, warm and cuddly—rather than feeling the need to bolt out of bed the second the alarm goes off.

Now granted, in order to get an accurate reading, you can't do 50 jumping jacks before taking it. Nor, for that matter, can you gab on the phone with your

# Fertility Cycle # 11

Last 12 Cycles:    Shortest **26**    Longest **31**    Month **February- March**    Year **'95**    This cycle length: **29**

| Cycle Day | 1 | 2 | 3 | 4 | 5 | 6 | 7 | 8 | 9 | 10 | 11 | 12 | 13 | 14 | 15 | 16 | 17 | 18 | 19 | 20 | 21 | 22 | 23 | 24 | 25 | 26 | 27 | 28 | 29 | 30 | 31 | 32 | 33 | 34 | 35 | 36 | 37 | 38 | 39 | 40 |
|---|---|---|---|---|---|---|---|---|---|---|---|---|---|---|---|---|---|---|---|---|---|---|---|---|---|---|---|---|---|---|---|---|---|---|---|---|---|---|---|---|
| Date | 2/19 | 20 | 21 | 22 | 23 | 24 | 25 | 26 | 27 | 28 | 3/1 | 2 | 3 | 4 | 5 | 6 | 7 | 8 | 9 | 10 | 11 | 12 | 13 | 14 | 15 | 16 | 17 | 18 | 19 | 20 | | | | | | | | | | |
| Day of Week | • | M | T | W | R | F | • | • | M | T | W | R | F | • | • | M | T | W | R | F | • | • | M | T | W | R | F | • | • | M | | | | | | | | | | |
| Intercourse | | ✓ | | ✓ | ✓ | | ✓ | | ✓ | ✓ | | | | | | | | ✓ | ✓ | | ✓ | | ✓ | | | | ✓ | ✓ | | | | | | | | | | | | |
| Birth Control Method Used | | | – | | – | | – | | – | – | | | | | | | | – | – | | – | | – | | | | – | – | | | | | | | | | | | | |

Time Temp Taken — 7:00 am (5:30), (9:00)

**Waking Temperature** — Temp Count 1 2 3

**Cervical Fluid:** ✱ ✱ ✱ (✱) — — — — S C C E E — — S — — — — S — ✱

**Peak Day:** PK 1 2 3 4

**Vaginal Sensation:** dry = = = = sticky moist cold wet lube lube dry = = = = = = sticky dry

**Cervix:** F F F F F F M M M S S F F F F

**Cervical Fluid Description:**
- red, small clots
- red, watery
- still watery
- light brownish
- sticky, white
- scant creamy
- thick cream
- a lot of wet cream
- slippery, no stretch > 1"
- 3" morn → 4" eve
- scant sticky
- slight crumbly

**Miscellaneous / Ovulatory Pain / PMS / Illness / Stress / Travel / Exercise / Breast Exam:**
- Up early to call Sara in N.Y.
- BSE
- Mardi Gras
- slept in - celebrated last night
- annual exam - 112 lbs
- right ovulatory twinge
- up all night - Kisha had kittens
- breast tenderness
- = =

| Cervical Fluid Symbols | ✱ Menses | (✱) Spotting | — No Cervical Fluid | S Sticky | C Creamy | E Eggwhite |
|---|---|---|---|---|---|---|
| | Bright Red | Pink or Brown | Nothing | Sticky, Crumbly, Gummy, or Rubbery Yellow or White | Creamy, Lotiony, Milky, or Smooth Yellow or White | Slippery and Usually Stretchy Clear, Streaked or Opaque |
| Vaginal Sensation | | Moist or Dry | Dry | Dry or Sticky | Wet and/or Cold | Lubricative and Very Wet, May Feel Humid |
| Cervix Symbols | • o O | | | | | |

F = Firm   M = Medium   S = Soft     • = Closed   o = Partly Open   O = Open

**Chart 6.1. Jane Responsible.**

Aunt Maria, or even get up to urinate first thing on awakening, even if you've downed two pints of lemonade the night before.

But on the positive side, taking your temperature will provide you with a wealth of information about your body that, when all is said and done, will have probably taken about a minute of your day. To fully appreciate what I am saying, let me list the benefits of taking your temperature every morning. You will be able to identify:

- If you are ovulating.
- When it would be safe to have deliciously natural intercourse without risk of an unplanned pregnancy.
- When you are *no longer* fertile, if you desire to avoid a pregnancy, or when you are *still* fertile if you desire to achieve one.
- When you will get your period.
- If there are potential problems in your cycle.

## Taking Your Temperature

**1.** Take your daily temperature first thing upon awakening, *before any other activity* such as getting up to use the bathroom, brushing your teeth, or talking on the phone. It should be taken throughout the cycle, ideally during menstruation, as well. (If you prefer, you may restrict temperature-taking to about one-third of the cycle, as discussed in Chapter 10 on Shortcuts. However, I would strongly discourage you from using shortcuts until you have charted several cycles.)

**2.** If using a digital thermometer, wait until it beeps, usually in about one minute. If using a glass basal body thermometer, leave it in for 5 minutes. Digital thermometers should reflect a clear pattern of lows and highs. But if the temperatures seem confusing, see page 266, or use a glass thermometer.

**3.** Take your temperature orally. (If you find that you don't get a clear temperature pattern, you may want to try taking it vaginally. Just be aware that it's important to be consistent and always take it from the same opening throughout the cycle.)

**4.** Take it about the same time every day, within an hour or so. However, you don't need to be a slave to your thermometer. If you sleep in on the weekends, or for whatever reason take it later or earlier, just be sure to note the time on your chart. For every half hour you sleep in, the temperature tends to creep up about one-tenth of a degree. (For how to handle the outlying temperatures that may result, see the Rule of Thumb, page 75.)

**5.** Take your temperature after *at least three consecutive hours* of sleep which, for most women, is first thing upon awakening in the morning. Note that if you normally take it at 8 A.M., but one morning you wake up at 6 A.M. and have to go to the bathroom, it is better to take your temperature at 6 and then get up. Otherwise, you will have only had 2 hours of sleep after getting up (from 6 to 8), which would make the reading inaccurate.

**6.** If you use a glass basal body thermometer, shake it down the day before. (This is because shaking the thermometer down upon awakening could raise your temperature.)

**7.** If you suspect you are getting sick, be sure to use a traditional fever or digital thermometer rather than the glass basal body type, since basal thermometers don't go above 100 degrees F. (Note that the high temperatures will be eliminated by the Rule of Thumb.)

## Charting Your Temperature

**1.** It's a good idea to record your temperature sometime in the morning. If this isn't practical, it doesn't need to be done until the evening, since most digital and glass thermometers will remain accurate until read or shaken down. (Just be sure to not leave your thermometer roasting on a hot window sill all day.)

**2.** If the temperature falls between two numbers on a glass thermometer, always record the lowest temperature.

**3.** Record and connect the temperatures with a pen.

**4.** Unusual events such as stress, illness, travel, or moving should be noted in the Miscellaneous column of the chart and taken into consideration when interpreting the temperature pattern. And temperatures taken earlier or later than usual should be noted in the Time Temp Taken column.

**5.** If you think a temperature is outside the normal range, wait until the next day to draw the connecting line. Omit any aberrant temperatures by drawing a dotted line between the normal temperatures. Record possible reasons for their aberrations. (See Chart 6.4 on page 75.)

## A GUIDE TO THERMOMETERS

### Digital Thermometers

The simplest, quickest type of thermometer is a digital. It usually requires only about a minute to register, and typically beeps when it is ready. For charting purposes, it should have memory capable of storing the last temperature until you retrieve it at the time you record. Also, it is imperative that it is accurate to as little as .1 degree F. (some are only to within .2 degrees). Be attentive to the possibility of needing to change its batteries.

While digitals may not be as accurate as the glass thermometers discussed below, you can rely on them as long as they clearly show the midcycle thermal shift that signals the passing of ovulation. If you are following all the method rules for birth control, using digitals shouldn't increase your risk of pregnancy, though it could force you to assume that you're fertile for more days than you really are. Thus, if your temperatures seem confusing, do not show a clear pattern of pre- and postovulatory lows and highs, or do not correlate closely with the other fertility signs, switch to a glass thermometer.

### Glass Basal Body Thermometers

Glass thermometers are considered the most reliable thermometer for detecting your waking basal body temperature (BBT). However, they do require a full 5 minutes to register an accurate reading. It must specifically say "basal body" as opposed to "fever thermometer." A basal body thermometer is easier to read because the temperatures are shown in increments of .1 rather than .2 degrees F. But BBT thermometers only go up to 100 degrees F., so if you have reason to think you are developing a fever, be sure to use a fever thermometer during those days.

### Ear Thermometers

The general consensus in the Fertility Awareness community is that ear thermometers are not reliable enough to be used for charting purposes (which is to say that they don't clearly show a thermal shift). This is unfortunate because they register temperatures in about a second. Perhaps in the future.

## Drawing the Coverline

Ultimately, the reason you are charting your temperature is to determine when you ovulated in any given cycle. Remember that after ovulation, temperatures quickly rise above the range of lows that preceded it. This thermal shift is often so obvious that you'll be able to spot it simply by glancing at the chart. However, in order to interpret accurately, you'll want to draw a *coverline* to help you differentiate between temperatures that are low (preovulatory) and high (postovulatory). The coverline is easily drawn using the following instructions:

1. Identify the first day your temperature rises at least two-tenths of a degree higher than it had been the previous six days.
2. Highlight the last six temperatures before the rise.
3. Locate the *highest* of those six highlighted temperatures.
4. Draw the coverline one-tenth of a degree above the highest of that cluster of six days preceding the rise. (Note that high temperatures during your period are irrelevant. It's not unusual to have high temperatures during menstruation due to the residual effects of progesterone lingering from the last cycle. Other aberrant high temperatures can also be discounted as seen by the Rule of Thumb on page 75.)

**Chart 6.2. A standard temperature pattern with coverline.** Note that the cluster of 6 temperatures before the thermal shift is highlighted. (An alternative way of drawing the coverline is discussed in Appendix H.)

**Chart 6.3a—The stair-step rise.** Note how the temperature rises in an initial spurt of about 3 days on Day 17 before rising further on Day 20.

**Chart 6.3b—The slow-rise.** Note how the temperature rises one tenth of a degree at a time, starting with Day 17 as the first temperature higher than the cluster of the six before it. Also notice that with this particular pattern, the coverline cannot be drawn using the standard instruction. (See page 272 for how you would do so.)

**Chart 6.3c—The fall-back rise.** Note how the temperature initially rises above the coverline on Day 17, but then falls back the next day before rising above again on Day 19.

## Types of Thermal Shift Patterns

Chart 6.2 on page 73 shows a coverline drawn with a *standard* thermal shift pattern. The standard pattern clearly shows the range of low temperatures, followed by a distinct thermal shift of at least two-tenths of a degree, followed by a consistent range of high temperatures that remain until the end of that cycle. Standard patterns are the easiest to interpret, and thus drawing their coverline is a breeze.

Most women tend to experience the same type of thermal shift patterns within their own cycles, although they may see variation now and then. While the standard shift is the most common, there are three other types that some women experience. They are shown in Charts 6.3 on the opposite page. While they can be a bit confusing initially, they are also easy to interpret once you are familiar with them. Pages 271–273 in Appendix A give further explanation should you find that you have these patterns.

## Outlying Temperatures and the Rule of Thumb

If you have an occasional temperature that is artificially high due to reasons such as fever, a restless night's sleep, or alcohol consumption the night before, you may cover the outlying temperature with your thumb when you are determining your coverline. Circle the outlying temperature as you would any other, but then draw dotted lines between the temperatures on either side, so that it doesn't interfere with your ability to interpret your chart. You essentially ignore the abnormal temperature, and thus still must count back the required six days, *not including the day eliminated,* in order to determine your coverline.

**Chart 6.4. Using the Rule of Thumb for aberrant temperatures.** Note the thumb covering the outlying temperature on Day 11. A dotted line should be drawn between the days on both sides of it. Also notice that Day 11 is not counted among the necessary six days to draw the coverline.

Also remember that if you occasionally sleep in, temperatures may tend to creep up, but again you can simply follow the guidelines above. However, pay special attention to temperature shifts after Daylight Savings, and after traveling to new time zones. This is because your temperatures could rise as much as ⅔₀ths of a degree for every hour that your body perceives itself as having slept beyond its usual waking time. In both situations, it may be simplest to record your temperatures, but to not count on their accuracy for the first few days.

Finally, you may on occasion experience a fever which lasts several days. How you will handle it will depend on when it occurs in your cycle, as discussed in Appendix A, page 276.

## How Temperature Patterns Predict Length of Cycles

The beauty of charting temperatures is that it can give you a sneak preview of how long your cycle will be simply by observing when the temperature rises. Remember that once your temperature shifts, it will remain basically the same length from the rise to your period. So, for example, if you experience a fever or a lot of stress during the first part of your cycle, you may experience a delayed ovulation that will be reflected in a late thermal shift. In such a case, you will still be able to count ahead to determine when you will menstruate.

*Cassandra and Everett were clients of mine. They were a young couple who were very much in love with each other. They both attended college but still lived at home to save money for their future marriage. One weekend, Cassandra's family went out of town, and they took the opportunity to finally be together without her younger siblings barging in on them.*

*A couple of months later, I met with them for their private follow-up consultation. One of the first things that struck me about her charts was that she was having a long cycle with a delayed ovulation. When I asked her whether she was experiencing stress, the two of them glanced at each other and burst into nervous laughter. With a little prodding, I soon discovered that several days after her parents had returned, her mother called Cassandra into her bedroom to inquire what a whipped cream cap was doing wedged between the mattress and the headboard. At least her charts would prevent her from worrying about a period that was sure to be late this cycle.*

**Chart 6.5.** Temperature charts showing one woman's cycles of 26, 30, and 38 days. Note that the preovulatory phase varies in length, whereas the postovulatory (luteal) phase remains consistent from cycle to cycle.

Chart 6.5 helps illustrate the point that the preovulatory phase can vary considerably both between women and within any one woman's pattern from cycle to cycle. The postovulatory phase, while varying somewhat from woman to woman, usually remains fairly constant for each individual woman (plus or minus a day or so).

## ༃ CERVICAL FLUID

Virtually all ovulating women experience an observable pattern of changes in their cervical fluid throughout their cycles. Once they learn to recognize these subtle differences, they realize that interpreting the pattern is really very simple. When a woman is extremely fertile, her cervical fluid becomes wet and humid. You could say it gives a whole new meaning to "feeling hot and steamy." Indeed, as you approach ovulation, the eggwhite-quality cervical fluid most women experience can feel so slippery that you may have a sensation of slip-sliding on your underwear as you sit down. Just as some women may initially balk at the idea of taking their temperature every morning, there are others who react similarly to the idea of checking their cervical fluid before urinating. But when you think about it, it only takes a second to touch the outside of your vagina, then feel its quality between your fingers.

For those of you who think of yourselves as too squeamish to do any of this, all I can say is that once you've checked a couple of times, you realize it's really no big deal. (And if you are even *considering* having a baby, I can assure you the world of diapers and infant regurgitation is a thousand times more traumatizing than cervical fluid!)

### Observing Your Cervical Fluid

**1.** Begin checking cervical fluid the first day after menstruation has ended.

**2.** Focus on vaginal *sensations* throughout the day (i.e., Does the outside of the vagina feel dry, sticky, wet? Does it feel like you are sitting in a puddle of eggwhite?). Vaginal sensations alone are extremely helpful in identifying fertility.

**3.** Try to check cervical fluid every time you use the bathroom, doing vaginal contractions called Kegels on the way. This will help to get the cervical fluid to flow down to the opening. Find creative times to do Kegels throughout the day, such as while washing dishes, or waiting for an annoying red light to change. (See page 85 for more on Kegels.)

**4.** Check cervical fluid at least three times a day, including the morning and night.

**5.** Be sure to check when you are not sexually aroused, since sexual lubrication can mask cervical fluid. (In other words, it would be highly ineffectual to whisper in your partner's ear after an hour of foreplay: "Let me just check my cervical fluid to see if I am fertile, hon.")

**6.** Learn to tell the difference between semen and cervical fluid. Semen sometimes appears as a rubbery whitish strand or slippery foam. It tends to be thinner, breaks easily, and dries on your fingers quicker. By contrast, eggwhite-quality cervical fluid tends to be clear, shimmering, and stretchy. Since the two are similar, though, it is imperative that you mark any ambiguity with a question mark in the Cervical Fluid column. Doing Kegels to eliminate semen should minimize any potential confusion.

**7.** Separate your vaginal lips and check your cervical fluid at the lower opening either with tissue or your fingers. (If using tissue, wipe from front to back to avoid spreading bacteria.)

**8.** Glance away before looking at the cervical fluid. Focus on the *quality* as you rub your fingers together. Does it feel dry? Sticky? Creamy? Slippery or lubricative (like eggwhite)?

**9.** Feel your cervical fluid. Then slowly open your fingers to see if it stretches, and if so, how much before it breaks.

**10.** After urinating, focus on how easily the tissue slides across your vaginal lips. Does it feel dry, smooth, or lubricative?

**11.** Note your underwear throughout the day. Remember that very fertile-quality cervical fluid often forms a fairly symmetrical round circle, due to its high concentration of water. Nonwet-quality cervical fluid tends to form more of a rectangular square or line on your underwear.

**12.** Around your most fertile time, look in the water while you use the toilet. You would be surprised how often eggwhite-quality cervical fluid flows out so quickly that you could miss it if not paying attention. In addition, it's interesting to see how eggwhite-quality cervical fluid often forms a ball when it hits the water, appearing like a cloudy marble sinking to the bottom.

**13.** If you find it hard to differentiate between cervical fluid and basic vaginal secretions, remember that cervical fluid is insoluble. A little trick that can help you initially learn to tell the difference is the glass of water test. Take the sample between two fingers and dip it into a glass of water. If it is true cervical fluid, it will usually form a blob that sinks to the bottom. If it's basic vaginal secretions, it will simply dissolve.

**14.** Note the quality and quantity of the cervical fluid (i.e., color, consistency, and amount).

**15.** Pay special attention to cervical fluid after a bowel movement, since that is when it is most likely to flow out. Of course, to prevent infections while checking, you must always use two separate tissues, wiping the vaginal opening from front to back first.

**16.** If you find that it is difficult to detect any cervical fluid at your vaginal opening, you can check internally by using your index and middle fingers to draw out the cervical fluid from the cervix itself.

Keep in mind, though, that if you choose to check internally, you should be consistent in doing so. You shouldn't alternate external-internal checking. In addition, remember that you will always notice a moistness on your finger if you check internally. But this is different from actual cervical fluid, which does not dissipate within a few seconds the way natural vaginal moisture does.

## Charting Your Cervical Fluid

**1.** Day 1 of the cycle is the first day of red menstrual bleeding. If you have brown or light spotting on the day or two before the flow, it is usually considered part of the previous cycle. (See page 259.)

**2.** The following symbols are used for the cervical fluid seen throughout the day, and are recorded in the Cervical Fluid column (alternative symbols are listed in Appendix I). Note that menses is marked by ✳, while spotting is marked by (✳) to show the latter is not red blood. Also, note that the wet days are circled:

> **Menses:**    Red blood flow.
> ✳
>
> **Spotting:**   Brown, pink, or discolored.
> (✳)
>
> **Nothing:**    Dry. No cervical fluid present. May feel dampness
> —             on finger that quickly dissipates after you check
>               your vaginal opening.

**Sticky:**
S

Opaque white or yellow, occasionally clear. Can be fairly thick. Critical quality is its stickiness or lack of true wetness. May be crumbly or flaky like paste, or gummy and rubbery like rubber cement. May form small peaks when you separate your fingers.

**Creamy:**
ⓒ

Milky or cloudy, white or yellow.
Creamy or lotiony.
Wet, watery, or thin.
When separating fingers, doesn't form peaks, but remains smooth like hand lotion.

**Eggwhite:**
Ⓔ

Usually clear but can have opaque streaks in it.
Very slippery and wet, like raw eggwhite. Causes extremely lubricative feel at vaginal opening. May stretch from 1 to 10 inches.

**3.** Record the most *fertile-* or *wet*-quality cervical fluid of the day, even if you are dry all day except for one single observation. (Obviously, any spotting should also be recorded.) The cervical fluid column will appear similar to Chart 6.6 below.

**4.** Treat all signs of semen or residual spermicide as a question mark in the Cervical Fluid column, since they can mask cervical fluid. Remember, doing Kegels following intercourse will usually get rid of both.

**Chart 6.6. A typical cervical fluid pattern.** Note how cervical fluid becomes progressively wetter as ovulation approaches.

**5.** The vaginal *sensation* you notice throughout the day is an extremely important indicator of your fertility. Don't be surprised if the cervical fluid seems to disappear a day or so before the slippery, lubricative vaginal *feeling* dissipates.

## Identifying Your Peak Day

Once you have learned to chart your cervical fluid, you will want to use this information to determine your most fertile day. Generally speaking, this is considered the last day that you produce fertile cervical fluid *or* have a lubricative vaginal sensation for any given cycle. It is called the "Peak Day," because it denotes your peak day of fertility. It most likely occurs either a day before you ovulate or on the day of ovulation itself (the only way to know for certain would be to have an ultrasound). Practically speaking this means that your Peak Day will usually occur one or two days before your temperature shift.

You may have already noticed that you will only be able to determine the Peak Day in retrospect, on the following day. This is because you can only recognize it after your cervical fluid and vaginal sensation have already begun to dry up. This concept should become intuitive fairly quickly. Also be aware that the Peak Day is not necessarily the day of the greatest quantity of cervical fluid. In fact, the "longest eggwhite stretch" or greatest amount could occur a day or two before, as seen in Chart 6.6.

Knowing how to accurately determine your Peak Day is critical if you are to correctly follow the rules for both birth control and pregnancy achievement, so please read carefully and internalize the following guidelines:

**I.** Your Peak Day is the *last* day of either:

- **eggwhite-quality cervical fluid** (which is slippery and usually stretchy)
- **lubricative vaginal sensation** (which is wet and slippery, but may not be accompanied by any cervical fluid), or
- **any midcycle spotting**

This means that if your last day of eggwhite is on a Monday but you still have one more day of lubricative vaginal sensation (or spotting) on Tuesday, your Peak Day is Tuesday. Of course, the reverse applies as well.

**2.** If you don't have eggwhite cervical fluid, you would count the last day of the wettest-quality cervical fluid that you do have, which would probably be *creamy*. (Of course, once again, if your last day of creamy is on a Monday but your last day of wet vaginal sensation is on a Tuesday, your Peak Day would be Tuesday.)

**3.** Some women will occasionally have a day of creamy cervical fluid after their last eggwhite day. Most Fertility Awareness instructors still consider the last day of eggwhite as the true Peak Day.

**4.** Once you have identified the Peak Day, you should write "PK" in the Peak Day column of your chart. Charts 6.7 below show the most common cervical fluid patterns and how their corresponding Peak Days would be recorded.

**Chart 6.7a.** The classic cervical fluid pattern, with the last day of eggwhite as the Peak Day. In this case Day 17.

**Chart 6.7b.** The same pattern of cervical fluid as Chart 6.7a above, except she still has a lubricative vaginal sensation the day *after* her last day of eggwhite (recorded as "lube"). Thus, her Peak Day is Day 18.

**Chart 6.7c.** A common cervical fluid pattern in which eggwhite is never observed. Her Peak Day is therefore Day 13, the last day of creamy cervical fluid.

**Chart 6.7d.** A cervical fluid pattern in which a day of creamy follows the last day of eggwhite. In this case, the Peak Day is still considered Day 15, that last eggwhite day.

### KEGEL EXERCISES

Kegel exercises strengthen the vaginal muscles, which are usually referred to as pubococcygeus muscles, or thankfully, just PC muscles. Strengthening them serves many useful purposes, including aiding in:

a. Increasing sexual pleasure.
b. Pushing cervical fluid down to the vaginal opening.
c. Pushing semen out of the vagina (see SETs, below).
d. Restoring vaginal muscle tone following childbirth.
e. Maintaining urinary continence in older women.

**How to Identify the PC Muscle**

Sit on a toilet and stop and start the flow of urine without moving your legs. Your PC muscle is what is turning the flow on and off.

**Kegel Exercises**

When you are first learning to chart, you may want to do Kegel exercises at set times to get used to strengthening your vaginal muscles. But soon it will become such habit that you'll find yourself doing them throughout the day without even thinking about it.

Slow Kegels:  Tighten the PC muscle as you did to stop the urine. Hold it for a slow count of three. Relax. Repeat.

Fast Kegels:  Tighten and relax the PC muscles as rapidly as you can. Repeat.

**When to Do Kegels**

You can do Kegels any time during your daily activities. Be creative and find times throughout the day, such as while driving your car, watching television, or washing dishes.

**What You May Initially Experience When You Start Doing Kegels**

When you first start practicing Kegels, you will probably notice that the muscle doesn't want to stay contracted during the slow exercises and that you can't do the quick ones as fast or evenly as you'd like. In addition, sometimes the muscle will start to feel a little tired, which is not surprising. You probably haven't used it much before. Take a few seconds and start again. In a week or two you will probably notice that you can control them quite well.

A good way to check how you are doing is to insert one or two fingers into your vagina and feel if you are able to tighten your PC muscle around your finger.

**Semen Emitting Technique (SETs)**

The first time you urinate following intercourse, push out as much semen as possible, absorbing the rest with tissue. The next couple of times, stop and start the flow with Kegels, wiping away the semen after each contraction. You will usually be able to eliminate the semen by the time you are through urinating. (This technique should work for residual spermicide, as well.)

## ❧ CERVICAL POSITION (OPTIONAL)

The cervical position is the one fertility sign that often takes more than one cycle to grasp, since you probably haven't had experience feeling your cervix. It may take a few cycles to be able to tell the difference between high and low, soft and firm, or open and closed.

You should notice that as you approach ovulation, your cervix tends to rise, soften, and open. It progresses from feeling firm like the tip of your nose (when not fertile) to feeling soft like your lips as you approach ovulation. Your cervix will drop abruptly into the vagina when estrogen levels fall, and progesterone becomes dominant after ovulation. By simply inserting your clean middle finger, you can detect these subtle changes.

The cervical position is an optional sign, but it is especially helpful if either of the other primary signs are confusing in any particular cycle. It should never be relied on alone. The best time to observe dramatic changes are right around ovulation, when the cervix shifts the most abruptly.

Some women may be initially squeamish about checking the cervix. This is understandable, since it is not something they are accustomed to feeling. Simply breathe slowly and let your body relax. You'll probably find that it can be fascinating to observe how it varies throughout the cycle. And once you become familiar with the various changes, you can restrict your cervix checking to about a week per cycle (see Shortcuts, Chapter 10).

Remember, the cervix is an optional sign, so you may decide you'd rather not check it at all, though I do recommend it for the following people:

1. Those women whose temperature patterns do not reflect a completely obvious thermal shift. The cervix in such cases would provide corroborating evidence of fertility.
2. Those whose cervical fluid or temperatures are not easy to interpret.
3. Those who are willing to take slightly increased risks in order to extend the time they consider themselves infertile.
4. Those people who absolutely cannot risk an unplanned pregnancy and want a third sign to confirm infertile days.

## Observing Your Cervix

**1.** Begin checking your cervix once a day after menstruation has ended.

**2.** Always wash your hands with soap first.

**3.** Try to check about the same time each day. Checking just after a morning or evening shower is convenient, since your hands are clean, and you don't have to bother with clothing.

**4.** The most effective position in which to check is squatting, since this pushes the cervix closest to the vaginal opening. However, some women prefer to check while sitting on the toilet, or putting one leg on the bathtub. The most important thing is to be consistent about the position you choose, since different positions will change the cervical height.

**5.** Use your finger as a convenient gauge. Insert your middle finger (nails should be trimmed) and observe the following conditions of the cervix in this order: *

    a. **height** in the vagina (low, midway, or high)
    b. **softness** (firm, medium, or soft)
    c. **opening** (closed, partly open, or open)
    d. **wetness** (nothing, sticky, creamy, or eggwhite)
       (Technically, wetness is a quality of the cervical fluid and not the cervix, but it is included here since, when checking the cervix, you can't help notice whatever fluid there is.)

**6.** Note that women who have vaginally delivered children will always have a slightly open cervix. It will feel more oval and usually shaped like a horizontal slit, so it is important to focus on the subtle variation throughout the cycle.

Woman who has never
vaginally delivered children
      
Woman who has
vaginally delivered children

**7.** The best time to begin observing cervical changes is when the wet-quality cervical fluid starts to build up in the days before ovulation. You should continue observing at least until the cervical fluid and cervix abruptly revert back to their infertile quality. Cervical changes will become easier to observe with practice.

**8.** Don't be surprised if you notice small firm bumps that feel like granules of sand under the skin of your cervix. These are called nabothian cysts, and typically come and go without treatment (see illustration on page 203).

**9.** Obviously, you should not check your cervical position if you have genital sores or vaginal infections.

---

* While SHOW is a convenient mnemonic device to remind you of the cervical qualities, the order listed is the way in which you'll most likely notice your own cervix.

| Cycle Day | 1 | 2 | 3 | 4 | 5 | 6 | 7 | 8 | 9 | 10 | 11 | 12 | 13 | 14 | 15 | 16 | 17 | 18 | 19 | 20 | 21 | 22 | 23 | 24 | 25 | 26 | 27 | 28 | 29 | 30 | 31 | 32 | 33 | 34 | 35 | 36 | 37 | 38 | 39 | 40 |
|---|---|---|---|---|---|---|---|---|---|---|---|---|---|---|---|---|---|---|---|---|---|---|---|---|---|---|---|---|---|---|---|---|---|---|---|---|---|---|---|---|
| Cervical Fluid | ✕ | ✕ | ✕ | ✕ | ✕ | | | | | | | | | | | | | | | | | | | | | | | ✕ | | | | | | | | | | | | |
| Peak Day | | | | | | | | | | | | | | | | | | | | | | | | | | | | | | | | | | | | | | | | |
| Vaginal Sensation | | | | | | | | | | | | | | | | | | | | | | | | | | | | | | | | | | | | | | | | |
| Cervix | | | | | | F | F | F | F | M | M | M | S | S | F | F | F | F | F | F | F | F | F | F | F | F | F | | | | | | | | | | | | | |

**Chart 6.8. A typical cervical position pattern.** Note that the cervix quickly reverts back from its Peak Day of fertility, and thus in this case is closed and low by Day 16.

## Charting Your Cervix

1. Use a circle to represent the cervical opening (called the cervical os).

   = low, closed, and firm (F)

   = midway, partly open, and medium (M)

   = high, open, and soft (S)

2. The general cervical pattern will look like Chart 6.8, above.

## 🙰 PUTTING IT ALL TOGETHER: A SUMMARY

The time it takes to actually check all three signs is negligible compared to the advantages to be gained. The following, then, is a summary of how to observe and chart the three fertility signs:

## Taking Your Temperature

1. Take your daily temperature first thing upon awakening *before any other activity* and record throughout the cycle.
2. If using a digital thermometer, wait until it beeps, about a minute. If using a glass basal thermometer, leave it in for 5 minutes.
3. Take your temperature orally or vaginally, but always *from the same opening* throughout the cycle.
4. Take it about the same time every day, within an hour or so.
5. Take your temperature after *at least three consecutive hours* of sleep.
6. If you use a glass basal body thermometer, shake it down the day before.
7. If you suspect you are getting sick, be sure to use a traditional fever or digital thermometer.

## Charting Your Temperature

1. Try to record your temperature sometime in the morning, although it can be done later.
2. If the temperature falls between two numbers on a glass thermometer, always record the *lowest* temperature.
3. Record and connect the temperatures with a pen.
4. Note unusual events such as stress, illness, or fever in the Miscellaneous column. Temperatures taken earlier or later than usual should be noted in the Time Temp Taken column.
5. Omit any temperatures that are out of line by drawing a dotted line between the normal temperatures.

## Drawing the Coverline

1. Identify the first day your temperature rises at least two-tenths of a degree higher than it had been the previous 6 days.
2. Highlight the last six temperatures before the rise.
3. Locate the *highest* of those six highlighted temperatures.
4. Draw the coverline one-tenth of a degree above the highest of that cluster of 6 days preceding the rise. (Days eliminated by the Rule of Thumb are not counted as part of the previous 6.)

## Observing Your Cervical Fluid

1. Begin checking cervical fluid the first day after menstruation has ended.
2. Focus on vaginal *sensations* throughout the day.
3. Try to check cervical fluid every time you use the bathroom, doing Kegels on the way.
4. Check cervical fluid at least three times a day, including the morning and night.
5. Don't check cervical fluid while you are sexually aroused.
6. Learn to differentiate between semen and cervical fluid (and learn to do Kegels to get rid of the semen, as discussed on page 85).
7. Separate your vaginal lips and check your cervical fluid at the lower opening either with tissue or your fingers.

8. Glance away before looking at the cervical fluid. Focus on the *quality*. Does it feel dry? Sticky? Creamy? Slippery or lubricative (like eggwhite)?

9. Feel your cervical fluid. Then slowly open your fingers to see if it stretches.

10. After urinating, focus on how easily the tissue slides across your vaginal lips.

11. Note your underwear throughout the day.

12. Around your most fertile time, look in the water while you use the toilet.

13. If you find it difficult differentiating between cervical fluid and basic vaginal secretions, do the glass of water test by inserting the cervical fluid in the water.

14. Note the quality and quantity of the cervical fluid (i.e., color, consistency, and amount).

15. Pay special attention to whether you see cervical fluid after a bowel movement, since that is when it is most likely to flow out.

16. If you find that it is difficult to detect any cervical fluid at your vaginal opening, you can check internally by using your index and middle fingers to draw out the cervical fluid from the cervix itself.

## Charting Your Cervical Fluid

1. Day 1 of the cycle is the first day of true menstrual bleeding.

2. Use the following symbols recorded in the Cervical Fluid column (or use the alternative symbols in Appendix I). Note that the wet days are circled:

| | | | | | |
|---|---|---|---|---|---|
| * | (*) | — | S | Ⓒ | Ⓔ |
| Menses | Spotting | Nothing | Sticky | Creamy | Eggwhite |

3. Record the most *fertile- or wet-*quality cervical fluid of the day, as well as any spotting. Your cervical fluid will become progressively wetter as you approach ovulation.

4. Treat signs of semen or spermicide as a question mark in the Cervical Fluid column.

5. The vaginal sensation you notice throughout the day is an extremely important indicator of your fertility.

## Identifying Your Peak Day

1. Your Peak Day is the last day of eggwhite cervical fluid or lubricative vaginal sensation, or midcycle spotting.
2. If you don't have eggwhite, you would count the last day of your wettest-quality cervical fluid or wet vaginal sensation.
3. If you have a creamy day after your last day of eggwhite, that last day of eggwhite is still considered your Peak Day.
4. Once you have identified the Peak Day, you should write "PK" in the Peak Day column of your chart.

## Observing Your Cervix

1. Begin checking the cervix once a day after menstruation has ended.
2. Always wash your hands with soap first.
3. Try to check about the same time each day.
4. The most effective position in which to check is squatting.
5. Insert your middle finger and observe the conditions of the cervix (height, softness, opening, and wetness).
6. Women who have vaginally delivered children will always have a slightly open cervix that feels more oval.
7. The best time to begin observing cervical changes is when the wet-quality cervical fluid starts to build up in the days before ovulation.
8. Don't be surprised if you feel nabothian cysts on the cervix.
9. Do not check your cervical position if you have genital sores or a vaginal infection.

## Charting Your Cervix

1. Use a circle to represent the cervical opening.

   $\boxed{\substack{\cdot \\ F}}$ = low, closed, and firm (F)

   $\boxed{\substack{o \\ M}}$ = midway, partly open, and medium (M)

   $\boxed{\substack{O \\ S}}$ = high, open, and soft (S)

2. The general cervical pattern after menstruation will typically progress gradually from low, closed, and firm before ovulation to high, open, and soft around ovulation, before abruptly returning to its original position.

## ❧ NOW THAT YOU KNOW

Congratulations! If you have understood this chapter, you are now ready to apply your newfound knowledge toward either avoiding pregnancy naturally, achieving pregnancy, or simply taking control of and understanding your body.

# CHAPTER 7

# Why Women Don't Always Ovulate or Menstruate

*N*one of us are Barbie dolls. As much as Madison Avenue tries to convince us that all women should be 5 feet 9 inches and thin as a rail, the reality is that there is tremendous variety among women. Even the standard (not-so-wise) wisdom out there is that all women should have 28-day cycles and ovulate on Day 14. Of course, you know by now that's not true.

Not only can a woman have cycles that vary—but a woman's cycles may be different depending on whether she is an adolescent, just coming off the Pill, breastfeeding, or approaching menopause. Her cycles may also vary depending on other temporary factors such as illness, travel, stress, or exercise.

The beauty of charting your cycles, though, is that you can take control and understand what is transpiring in your body on a daily basis, regardless of your particular circumstances. You may find that you'll go through months or even years with only intermittent ovulation. If you are using FAM as birth control, it's important to realize that anytime you don't ovulate, you need to treat each day as if you were in a *pre*-ovulatory state. Thus, the presence of any cervical fluid must be very carefully observed to see if it is potentially fertile.

There are differences in the way your fertility signs are reflected over time, depending on whether you are ovulating:

**A typical cycle:** In a normal cycle, your body prepares for the release of an egg in a fairly timely, predictable manner. After your period, under the influence of rising estrogen, you'll usually have several days of no cervical fluid, followed by days building up to a progressively wetter fertile-quality cervical fluid. After the egg is released, your cervical fluid will rapidly dry up until you start the pattern over again the next cycle.

**An anovulatory phase** (breastfeeding, premenopause, etc.): This refers to those periods of time when women take longer to release an egg. In such special circumstances, your body may need months or even years to build up to a high enough level of estrogen to trigger an ovulation. It's almost a one-step-forward, two-steps-back situation. Your body may make several attempts to ovulate before it finally is able to do so, as seen in the graphic below:

During this time, you may notice what are referred to as "patches of cervical fluid." Instead of the classic buildup typical of normal cycles, you may see a series of patches of wetness interspersed with drier days.

This chapter is devoted to what transpires in your body during these special circumstances when you don't ovulate. Appendix B discusses how to use FAM for birth control during such times.

## ๛ DIFFERENT PHASES OF ANOVULATION IN WOMEN'S LIVES

### Adolescence

American girls typically start to menstruate between 12 and 14 years old. But the onset of periods doesn't necessarily mean the release of eggs every cycle. In fact, one of the factors that characterizes menstrual cycles in teenagers is irregularity due to fluctuating estrogen levels, and thus, cycles don't automatically start out predictably. It is a gradual process that can take several years while the hormonal feedback system matures. During this time, then, an adolescent's cycles may vary considerably, with many anovulatory cycles dispersed throughout.

## *Pregnancy and Breastfeeding*

If you were to take a survey of pregnant or breastfeeding women, one of the things they would probably tell you they enjoy about their condition is that their periods have stopped. Of course, it makes sense physiologically for the woman's body to be incapable of getting pregnant again following conception. Once a woman becomes pregnant, she won't ovulate until after the baby is born.

And if she is breastfeeding "on request," that is, virtually every time the baby cries to be fed, she may not resume ovulating again for many months after the baby's birth. This is because every time a baby suckles at the breast, it indirectly suppresses the hormones that trigger ovulation. But in order for breastfeeding to efficiently prevent the release of eggs, the baby must suckle consistently throughout the day and night.

A breastfeeding woman could go up to a year or so without a thermal shift, and experience the same cervical fluid, whether it be dry, sticky, or a combination, day after day. The reason she usually won't see wet-quality cervical fluid initially is that the low estrogen levels which are indirectly caused by the prolactin will also keep the fertile-quality cervical fluid from being produced. The trick is for breastfeeding women to be attentive to the *change* in the quality of cervical fluid that indicates that ovulation will be resuming soon. Because cycles while breastfeeding can be either nonexistent or quite confusing, you should read Appendices B and C, if you plan to use FAM during these times.

## *Premenopause*

Menopause is the time in a woman's life when she ceases ovulating and having menstrual periods altogether. It typically occurs around age 50. But the time leading up to menopause can take several years. During this phase, her cycles may start appearing very different than anything she is used to. The cycles tend to initially shorten due to a combination of more frequent ovulations combined with shortening luteal phases. Eventually, though, the cycles become longer and longer as the number of times an egg is released becomes less frequent. Finally, cycles cease altogether. A woman is generally said to have completed menopause if she is in her 40s or older, and has gone for a full year without a period.

It used to be that the concept of menopause was taboo, shrouded in mystery and misinformation. Luckily, today much more is known about menopause, and women are reaping the benefits of such newfound knowledge. As with breastfeeding, though, cycles while approaching menopause can be fairly tricky. You should read Chapter 19 and Appendix B carefully for how to use FAM as contraception during the premenopausal phase.

## 🐚 CAUSES OF TEMPORARY ANOVULATION

There is a huge difference between cycles in which the woman may ovulate but not get her period, and one in which she gets her period but doesn't ovulate. Stop and think. What is the difference? In the former case, the woman is almost certainly pregnant! In the latter case, she has had an anovulatory cycle. The two charts below show how very different the two scenarios look on paper.

**Chart 7.1. A typical temperature pattern for pregnancy.** Note that Rena almost certainly ovulated by Day 17 as seen by that morning's thermal shift. Her chart shows more than 18 high temperatures following the shift, thus confirming her pregnancy.

**Chart 7.2. A typical temperature pattern with anovulation.** Note that there is no thermal shift reflecting ovulation, and thus the "period" that follows on Day 40 is actually anovulatory bleeding, which is technically not menstruation.

In anovulatory cycles, noncharting women may assume that they are menstruating normally. So why would they continue to experience bleeding if ovulation has not occurred? Such bleeding results when estrogen production continues to develop the uterine lining without reaching the threshold necessary to trigger ovulation. In such a case, one of two things may happen that lead to what *appears to be* a menstrual period: (1) The estrogen will build up slowly to a point below the threshold and then drop, resulting in "estrogen withdrawal bleeding." Or (2), more commonly, the endometrium builds up slowly over an extended period of time, eventually to the point where the resulting uterine lining is so thickened it can no longer sustain itself. This is known as "estrogen breakthrough bleeding."

In either case, if you weren't charting, you might think you were simply menstruating, though you may notice a difference in the type of bleeding. Specifically the flow can be either unusually heavy or light, and of course, the timing can result in cycle lengths all over the map, or the chart, as it were.

The following are common reasons why women may temporarily not ovulate:

## Coming Off the Pill or Other Hormones Such as Norplant or Depo-Provera

Women who discontinue hormones are often surprised that their cycles don't necessarily resume in the same clockwork manner that they had become accustomed to while taking hormones. But you must remember that cycles on hormones are artificially induced to be perfect. Ovulation doesn't necessarily resume immediately, usually because of the oversuppression of the feedback mechanism of the hypothalamus and pituitary gland.

When a woman comes off the Pill or other hormones, her cycles will eventually revert back to the way they were before. However, the length of time it takes varies tremendously among women. For some, it is almost immediate. But for most women, there is at least a short delay. And for others, it could take many months. This variation is a function of the type and dosage of hormones used, as well as the basic physiology of the woman.

Those who tend to take longer to clear the drug from their systems, and therefore take several months to resume cycling after hormones, are often young or thin (especially those who lost weight while on hormones). Those who were irregular before hormones typically return to their irregular pattern after. In addition, you should be aware that once women do resume natural cycling, they may experience short luteal phases for the first few months. This will usually be reflected in high temperatures of fewer than 10 days after the thermal shift.

Once they discontinue hormones, but before their cycles start showing the classic buildup of fertile-quality cervical fluid, they may notice a somewhat milky-quality cervical fluid. Some experience a type that is a combination of both sticky and wet. Because the cervical fluid can be confusing initially, it is imperative that women not rely on FAM as the sole method of birth control until they feel confident in being able to interpret their fertility signs.

## Illness

Being sick does not necessarily affect your cycle, but if it does, its impact is usually influenced by which phase you are in when you get sick. If your illness occurs before ovulation, it may delay it or even prevent it altogether (see page 276). If it occurs after, it will almost never affect your cycle, because the luteal phase has a consistent life span of 12 to 16 days that is typically not affected by factors such as sickness, travel, or exercise. (For each individual woman, the luteal phase is even more consistent and will generally not vary more than a day or so.)

In any event, you needn't worry that a fever will affect your ability to interpret your chart. For one thing, you can usually depend on the other two fertility signs. In addition, the temperatures will indeed indicate if fever has affected your cycle by either delaying or preventing ovulation. Remember, if getting sick affects your cycle at all, it will depend on when it happens.

## Travel

Traveling is notorious for affecting cycles. There's nothing like wearing a pair of crisp white walking shorts while strolling down the Champs-Elysées in Paris when . . . uh-oh, surprise, surprise. Although many women are blessed with cycles that continue like clockwork while vacationing, many others are faced with the challenge of trying to figure out if or when they will get their periods.

As delightful as a vacation may be for you, your body still interprets it as a type of stress. Many women find that their cycles become extremely long due to delayed ovulations. Others actually stop ovulating and getting periods altogether. Once again, charting your cycle can be very helpful in determining what is happening with your body. Keep in mind though, that traveling is a time when it is especially helpful to chart all three signs in order to understand any ambiguities that result from the disruption in your life. In particular, always be on the lookout for factors which may affect your temperature.

*Years ago, my college roommate seemed to redefine the limits of travel-related anovulation. Cathy spent her junior year in England. She had a period just before she arrived in London, then didn't menstruate for the 10 months she lived there. But sure enough, the month she returned home, she got her period again.*

## Exercise

Strenuous exercise has the potential to delay or even prevent ovulation altogether. Although you may be tempted to use this as an excuse to not exercise, don't! It seems to affect mostly those who are competitive athletes with a very low ratio of body fat to total body weight. The women most affected are runners, swimmers, and ballet dancers. But what is somewhat inconclusive about studies of these athletes is that they have been unable to separate the effects of fat ratio from physical and emotional stress, diet, and even changes in thyroid metabolism. It appears that all of these can affect a woman's cycle.

## Weight Gain or Loss

In order for the average woman to maintain normal ovulatory cycles, she should have a minimum of about 18% body fat. The purpose of the fat is to store estrogen as well as convert androgens (another hormone) to a type of estrogen needed for ovulation to occur.

Extremely thin women, particularly those with the eating disorder anorexia nervosa, often stop having periods altogether. It is thought that this occurs because their bodies are unable to pass above the estrogen threshold necessary to cause an egg to be released. In addition, women who lose 10 to 15% of their total body weight (or about one-third of their body fat) may also cease having periods. And as mentioned above, female athletes often stop menstruating because of the combination of lean body fat and stress caused by competition.

*Among my clients was a French couple who had been trying to get pregnant for 5 years. They asked to meet with me privately rather than take a group seminar because he was a doctor and felt the class might be too elementary for them. When they arrived at my office, I sensed a potential fertility problem immediately.*

*The woman was tall and fit, but extremely thin. I asked her whether she would consider gaining a little weight to alter her cycles, but she said she was adamantly opposed to consuming any fat in her diet. They both claimed they were totally perplexed as to why she wasn't getting pregnant, since she took such good care of herself. But when I asked her to describe her cycles to me, she said there weren't any to describe—she hadn't had a period in 5 years!*

*I was stunned. Here were two educated people, one of them a doctor, yet they couldn't understand why she wasn't getting pregnant even though she wasn't menstruating. I questioned why they thought she was fertile if she hadn't had a period in all those years. Their answer amazed me. Years prior, when they were trying to avoid pregnancy, her physician asked her what form of contraception she used. She said they didn't use birth control because she wasn't menstruating. Her physician at the time insisted that she protect herself anyway, since, as he rightly pointed out, she could still ovulate at any time. Based on that one comment, that she could ovulate at any time, she interpreted that to mean she was indeed fertile.*

*I was able to explain to them that the odds of pregnancy must be seen differently, depending on the desires of the couple. From the contraceptive perspective, it's imperative that women protect themselves because ovulation always occurs before menstruation. But if a woman is trying to get pregnant, and is not menstruating, then clearly she is not ovulating. Their experience taught me how easy it is to confuse the risk of an unwanted pregnancy with the slight possibility of one that is wanted. Unfortunately, I never did learn what happened to them because they returned to France shortly after we met, but I assume that they at least sought treatment for her anovulatory condition.*

On the other end of the spectrum are women who tend to be overweight. They too may stop ovulating. At this point, you may be thinking, "Wait a second. She said that it could be problematic if the woman is too thin, and now she's saying it could be a problem if she's too heavy." Such is the nature of women's bodies! With obesity, excess fatty tissue can cause too much estrogen, disrupting the hormonal feedback system that tells the egg follicles to mature.

## Stress

One of the most common causes of occasional long cycles is stress, both physiological and psychological. If stress affects a cycle at all, it tends to delay ovulation, not accelerate it. As you know, the timing of ovulation will determine the length of the cycle—the later it occurs, the longer the cycle will be. Occasionally, if stress is severe, it can actually prevent ovulation from occurring altogether.

*Medical Conditions*

In addition to the various temporary factors listed above, there are a variety of medical conditions such as pituitary gland problems and polycystic ovarian disease that may cause women to stop ovulating indefinitely. Many of these conditions can be treated, but all will require consultation with a physician.

## ৪৯ PUTTING ANOVULATION IN PERSPECTIVE

As you can see, there are many reasons why women don't necessarily ovulate every cycle. Some involve particular phases in a woman's life, such as adolescence, pregnancy and breastfeeding, or menopause. Others are due to more transitory factors such as coming off the Pill and other hormones, stress, illness, exercise, body weight, and travel. And finally, some are caused by more serious physiological conditions. The important point is that anovulatory cycles should be understood in the right context. At times, they are completely normal and even predictable. But if you think you have a serious medical problem, your charting may help your doctor to diagnose it.

## ৪৯ FERTILITY AWARENESS AND ANOVULATION

If you plan to use Fertility Awareness for contraception during periods of anovulation, you need to be aware that the rules are somewhat more involved than the normal ones you will be learning in Chapter 9 of this book. Remember that while you are ironically less fertile, you need to treat every day as if you were in your preovulatory phase. Depending on your own particular anovulatory pattern, this may or may not be difficult. I suggest that you finish reading the normal rules discussed in Chapter 9, then if you have determined that you are in an anovulatory phase of your life, you should carefully read Appendix B.

# PART THREE

# Natural Birth Control

# CHAPTER 8

# Fertility Awareness in the Age of AIDS

*B*efore you use Fertility Awareness as a method of birth control, you must take the appropriate precautions needed to eliminate the risk of AIDS and other sexually transmitted diseases (STDs). In particular, I must state what I hope is obvious: As a form of contraception, FAM is only advisable for those people involved in a monogamous relationship in which neither partner has an STD.

I have talked to many people who have told me that as wonderful as Fertility Awareness is, they aren't sure its promotion is compatible with today's essential "safe sex" message. As a woman's health educator, my primary concern is that women are given the information they need to take control of their own health and well-being. Certainly, this includes developing the knowledge and self-esteem necessary to minimize the risk of contracting the various STDs that now exist. However, it does not mean that Fertility Awareness is irrelevant given the realities of today's world. Simply put, FAM *is* compatible with safe sex, as long as the sex in question is *with a safe partner*. I would like to spend the rest of this chapter discussing the real-world decisions that this last statement suggests.

Before entering into a new sexual relationship in which you would like to use Fertility Awareness as your method of contraception, it is best to act as if your new partner were HIV positive until proven otherwise.* This means using condoms every time, to protect both you and him. The condoms should be made of latex, and come with a spermicidal lubricant such as nonoxynol-9. Be sure you both know how to use them correctly.

---

* HIV stands for human immunodeficiency virus, the virus that causes AIDS. If a person is HIV positive they have the virus in their blood, though they may have no symptoms of illness, and in fact they may not get sick for years. If a person is HIV negative they do not have the virus in their blood and, therefore, there is no threat of passing it on to another person.

After an appropriate amount of time, you might be considering a long-term relationship. If you feel intimate enough to trust your partner, you may be ready to take the most important step. Note again that for the purposes of Fertility Awareness, trustworthiness is critical, because as has often been noted, "cheating" today means more than risking just the other person's feelings. Thus, at a minimum, monogamy is necessary if you're going to use FAM. And before every new relationship, both you and your partner should undergo an HIV-antibody test.

There are numerous reasons to verify HIV-negative status before giving up condoms. Perhaps most important, the HIV-antibody test is accurate, inexpensive, and can be taken anonymously. Until recently, people in many areas of the country were advised against taking the test if they did not fit into an identifiable high-risk group because the chances of receiving a false-positive result were greater than actually being HIV positive. While this may be statistically true, studies still show that the chance of a false-positive reading on the most common antibody test is below 1%. And while no doubt one could suffer great emotional turmoil if told such misleading information, false positives are quickly shown to be negative by the routine administering of follow-up tests.

Thus, even if both partners find themselves in a relatively low-risk group, I would still recommend the test for each. It's true that the highest-risk partners for women are those men who have engaged in homosexual acts, have used intravenous drugs, or have received a blood transfusion between the late 1970s and 1985. Yet it is also true that risk is always a *relative* concept. A male partner may never have had sex with other men, but if he's slept with numerous women and only used condoms sporadically, he still poses a greater risk than a virgin. You should also be very aware that the danger of HIV transmission from women to men appears to increase substantially when other cofactors exist, most important, the presence of other STDs. This is because the open genital sores caused by certain STDs may allow an easier pathway for HIV to get into a man's blood.

With all this in mind, the slight chance of receiving a false-positive scare is worth taking in order to minimize any possibility of spreading the HIV virus. This is hardly a controversial position given that the virus in question can cause a fatal disease for which there is presently no known cure. It signals a sense of responsibility and seriousness on the part of each partner to the other, and thus confirms qualities that one would hope are present in any monogamous relationship in which you would find yourself. In addition, testing allows you to solidify the closeness of a developing relationship by giving both of you the medical confirmation to move beyond condoms to the more natural and enjoyable lovemaking Fertility Awareness allows. This is not to say that if one partner were to test positive for HIV that a completely loving and full relationship could not blossom, but only that HIV-positive status requires taking very real precautions to protect the health of the other partner. And for those couples who test HIV negative, a relationship can begin anew in which the fear of AIDS is put behind them, freeing them to look forward to the benefits of effective and completely natural contraception.

Assuming you decide to take the test, the next big decision is when to do so. This is because it generally takes a few months for HIV antibodies to show up in the blood, and thus it would be pointless to undergo a test just a few days after risking infection. If people who are HIV positive take the test too early, they may get a false-negative result. Scientific studies have shown that a large majority of HIV-positive people develop antibodies within 3 months of exposure, but it is generally recommended that you wait 6 months before relying on an HIV-negative result. This is particularly true if the person's last exposure falls into what is considered one of the high-risk activities.

The major HIV-antibody test is called the ELISA, or Enzyme Linked Immuno-Sorbent Assay. It is a reliable blood test that is simple to administer. It is offered at health department clinics, HIV testing and counseling centers, and some private doctors' offices. Depending on where the test is performed, results are given back in anywhere from a day to a couple of weeks. Many clinics will offer free, anonymous testing. Private doctors may charge $50 or more, but usually get you the results more quickly. If an ELISA test were to turn up HIV positive, another ELISA would be performed to check for false positives. After two ELISA tests in which the results are HIV positive, a different and final test called a "Western Blot" will usually be performed in order to absolutely verify HIV-positive status.

There is one other type of HIV test that you may have heard of, called the Polymerase Chain Reaction (PCR). Unlike the others, it is designed to detect parts of the virus itself, and not just HIV antibodies. The great advantage of this test is that it reveals HIV in the blood almost as soon as the HIV enters the body, thus eliminating the need for a waiting period between the last exposure and the time of testing. It is also considered an extremely accurate test in which an HIV-negative result virtually guarantees that you are indeed HIV negative.

Unfortunately, as of this writing, PCR testing in the United States is still limited to very select circumstances. This is because until recently, its heightened sensitivity had made it a fairly expensive and impractical test to administer. In addition, it also produced a somewhat greater number of false positives than the ELISA. Hopefully, these drawbacks will be corrected by the development of more advanced technologies, and thus it's possible that PCR will eventually be used with greater frequency.

Of course, before taking any type of HIV test, it is necessary that you and your partner be physically and emotionally prepared. You should never feel pressured to take it, but if you don't, you obviously should continue using condoms. In addition, I suggest that you only undergo HIV testing where your anonymity is protected, and where counseling services are available should they be needed.

Finally, if the two of you have arrived at the point where your commitment to each other results in a decision to undergo HIV testing, you have probably reached a level of communication where open and honest discussion about all aspects of your sexual health is possible. That is both good and necessary, because the reality is that for the vast majority of you, the risk of contracting several other STDs is much greater than contracting AIDS.

Before giving up condoms, you should discuss with your partner all possible symptoms of any sexually transmitted diseases that either you or he may have acquired. Anything suspicious may merit a trip to a health clinic for some quick testing, or at minimum a review of the latest informational pamphlets available there. Of particular concern is chlamydia, which although not as well known as syphilis or gonorrhea, is the most common STD today. It is easily treated, but if left undetected can cause infertility in both men and women. This is important to keep in mind, since its usual symptoms, burning or an oozing when urinating, are occasionally so mild that people are not even aware that they have it.

There are two other prevalent STDs of which you should definitely be aware: genital warts, which are caused by the human papilloma virus (HPV), and genital herpes. There are two particular types of HPV that could lead to cervical cancer. This simply gives you another reason to get an annual Pap test, for if caught early, the disease is highly curable. (It's worth pointing out that the vast majority of HPV strains do not lead to cancer, and in fact the majority of infections will disappear on their own.) You should also know that in certain cases herpes can be dangerous to a developing embryo, so if you get pregnant and have it, you should inform your doctor.

Those risks aside, HPV and herpes are usually more of a nuisance than a real medical danger. Today, warts are easily removed through laser surgery or by freezing them off with liquid nitrogen. Herpes is more treatable than in the past, in that the occasional outbreaks of genital sores associated with the disease can often be reduced in severity and frequency with various drugs. For both genital warts and herpes, risk of sexual transmission to a partner is dramatically reduced if surface warts are removed or open sores are in remission. However, the risk is never completely eliminated, a fact worth keeping in mind given the prevalence of both in the general population. If you suspect that you or your partner have either of these viruses, you should discuss the situation with a doctor before giving up condoms.

I would like to conclude by stating that although I have been talking about the danger of AIDS and other STDs when *beginning* a new relationship, one certainly needs to be aware that the risk could exist for all couples, no matter how long they have been monogamous. The obvious question is whether either partner had contracted HIV or something else before the present relationship began (or by nonsexual transmission at any time in the past).

Clearly many of you reading this will be in a situation where you have been in a long-term relationship, and you may be desiring to use FAM instead of your old method, which might have been any number of other methods such as the Pill or diaphragm. The fact is that probably most of you are not in a high-risk group for HIV infection, and given your previous decision not to use condoms, I can't honestly say I believe you should immediately run out and get an HIV-antibody test. That's a decision that you can best make yourself, but it is important that every person intelligently analyze the risks, however small they may be. It's also worth remembering that for those who plan to use FAM as a method of pregnancy achievement, there is the danger of an HIV-positive mother passing on the virus to her baby.

All of this information is important to know so that each individual can make those decisions that are most advisable for their emotional and physical well-being, particularly as related to one's reproductive health. I have no doubt that using Fertility Awareness is consistent with a lifestyle that is both empowering and healthy, but for it to be truly either of these, it simply must be practiced *responsibly*.

# Natural Birth Control Without Chemicals or Devices

*Contraceptives should be used on every conceivable occasion.*

—SPIKE MILLIGAN

*here are certain clients I will never forget. One particular couple was given my seminar on natural birth control as a wedding gift by the woman's parents. Although they seemed thoroughly absorbed in the class, I was soon to discover that they failed to internalize the most fundamental concept of the method. A month after the seminar, I met with them for their follow-up consultation. Everything seemed to go just fine. Her charts looked great. She recorded her fertility signs perfectly.*

*But I noticed that even though they had had intercourse throughout her cycle, they didn't record what method of birth control they used in the "method" column of the chart. In other words, they didn't record whether they used condoms, for example, during her fertile phase. So as they were getting up to leave, I casually reminded them to be sure to record what contraceptive they use every time they have intercourse during her fertile phase. She gave me a completely puzzled look, quizzically glanced at her husband, then looked back toward me with a blank stare.*

*Silence.*

*I said, "In other words, every time you have intercourse, just be sure to record whether you specifically chose not to use birth control because you are infertile at the time, or record what method you used while you were fertile." Again, the glazed-over look.*

*And again, more silence.*

*"What do you mean, 'what method'? I thought this was a method of birth control." The hair stood up on my arms. It was only then that I realized that this couple actually thought that by merely recording her fertility signs, they were using a reliable method of birth control!*

Needless to say, the Fertility Awareness Method only works as a contraceptive if, during your fertile phase, you choose to either postpone intercourse or use a barrier method. Statistically speaking, though, you should be aware that the method is much more effective if you choose to abstain during your fertile phase. The reason for this is:

1. If a barrier method is going to fail, it's going to fail when you're in your *fertile* phase. And all contraceptives have a failure rate.
2. Using barriers with spermicide during the fertile phase can mask cervical fluid. (This is one of several reasons why I recommend condoms if you are not going to abstain.)

Ideally, then, the method would be most effective if you only have intercourse when you're infertile. Actually, while it may seem difficult to do, many users of natural birth control feel that this creates a "courtship and honeymoon" effect. This is to say that every cycle, there is a phase when the couple finds creative ways to sexually express themselves, knowing that within a few days, they can resume intercourse again. By choosing to postpone sex rather than use a barrier method during the fertile phase, people often feel they're living in harmony with their fertility, rather than fighting it.

Part of this harmony with your fertility is simply learning to understand how your body works. A way to conceptualize the length of a woman's fertility is to remember that it is totally dependent on the man's fertility. In a vacuum, a woman would only be fertile a maximum of 24 hours, or 48 hours if two or more eggs were released at ovulation. But think of fertility in terms of a range that combines the viability of both sperm and egg. The only reason a woman is fertile for longer than 24 to 48 hours is because sperm can live up to 5 days.

In essence, then, the first part of the woman's fertile phase is determined by the survival of the sperm, the second part by the viability of the egg. When FAM is used for birth control, this typically adds up to about 9 or 10 days, during which abstinence or a barrier method of contraception is called for. This fertile phase includes a significant safety margin on both sides of the woman's fertile phase.*

---

* The maximum ova viability of 2 days is calculated by assuming a 24-hour life span for each egg, the last one being released a full 24 hours after the first. In reality, this is highly unlikely in that ova probably live closer to 12 hours, and multiple ovulations probably occur closer together. And while you must count on sperm survival of 5 days, 2 to 3 is much more probable. Sperm viability of longer than 5 days has been documented, though this is extremely rare, and in any case would not affect the contraceptive principles of FAM given that sperm without cervical fluid present will live at most a few hours.

"I'm only gonna say this one more time: Our
only chance is self-control."

By thinking of female fertility as a range, you should see that even experienced FAM users can only identify when their fertility begins and ends, and not the exact day of ovulation. In order to use the method effectively, though, it isn't necessary to pinpoint the precise moment that the egg is released.

For most women, the cycle can basically be divided into three parts. Note that the four FAM rules identify the beginning and end of the fertile phase, the time that unprotected intercourse can result in pregnancy.

| THE THREE PHASES OF THE CYCLE | | |
|---|---|---|
| **Preovulatory Infertile Phase** | **Fertile Phase** | **Postovulatory Infertile Phase** |
| | **The Four FAM Rules** | |
| 1) First 5 Days Rule | | 3) Temperature Shift Rule |
| 2) Dry Day Rule | | 4) Peak Day Rule |

What follows are the contraceptive rules you must employ to use the Fertility Awareness Method with maximum safety. While they may be a bit tricky to internalize on a first reading, they should become intuitive if you've understood the basic biological principles presented earlier in the book. I suggest you read this section slowly and several times, as well as carefully review all of Chapter 6. It's basically easy but as with any new process, it requires a little patience.

To be safe, I strongly suggest that you chart at least two full cycles before relying on these rules for birth control. The peace of mind you'll gain will be more than worth it. If you still find you need further clarification, I would encourage you either to take a class on the Fertility Awareness Method or meet with a qualified instructor. Finally, a guiding principle is that if you encounter any ambiguity, be conservative. All four rules should indicate that you are infertile before you consider yourself safe. If in doubt, don't!

## ❧ THE FOUR FAM RULES
## PREOVULATORY INFERTILE-PHASE RULES

### I. FIRST 5 DAYS RULE

> You are safe *the first 5 days* of the menstrual cycle *if* you had an obvious temperature shift 12 to 16 days before.

The First 5 Days Rule applies to the first 5 days of the cycle, *regardless* how many days you actually bleed. Any bleeding after the 5th day of the cycle should be considered fertile, since it could mask your ability to check cervical fluid.

By noting an obvious thermal shift 12 to 16 days before you bleed, you have strong evidence that ovulation occurred that previous cycle. This confirms that the bleeding within the first 5 days of the new cycle is true menstruation and not ovulatory spotting or abnormal bleeding unrelated to menses.

| Cycle Day | 1 | 2 | 3 | 4 | 5 | 6 | 7 | 8 | 9 | 10 | 11 | 12 | 13 | 14 | 15 | 16 | 17 | 18 | 19 | 20 | 21 | 22 | 23 | 24 | 25 | 26 | 27 | 28 | 29 | 30 | 31 | 32 | 33 | 34 | 35 | 36 | 37 | 38 | 39 | 40 |
|---|---|---|---|---|---|---|---|---|---|---|---|---|---|---|---|---|---|---|---|---|---|---|---|---|---|---|---|---|---|---|---|---|---|---|---|---|---|---|---|---|
| Cervical Fluid | ✳ | ✳ | ✳ | ✳ | ✳ | (✳) | - | - | S | S | © | © | © | © | - | - | S | S | - | - | - | S | - | - | - | - | - | ✳ | | | | | | | | | | | | |

**Chart 9.1. The First 5 Days Rule.**

This rule is highly effective because the combined risk of ovulation occurring on Day 10 or earlier and sperm living long enough to fertilize the egg is, statistically speaking, extremely rare. Remember, sperm can generally survive a maximum of 5 days, and even that is only in fertile quality cervical fluid. Still, the rule should be modified for women with a recent history of very short cycles, and it should not be relied upon for women with premenopausal signs:

**1.** If any of your last 12 cycles have been 25 days or shorter, you should only assume that the first 3 days are safe. This extra precaution is taken because of the increased risk of a very early ovulation. If cervical fluid were to develop while you were menstruating, you would be unable to detect it through the blood, and thus sperm could theoretically survive the few days necessary to fertilize the egg. There is some disagreement in the FAM community over the necessity of this conservative guideline, but I would personally recommend it.*

**2.** Women approaching menopause with such signs as hot flashes and vaginal dryness should not rely upon this rule at all. This is because premenopausal women are subject to major hormonal changes which could result in dramatically early ovulations (see page 247).

## 2. DRY DAY RULE

> Before ovulation, you are safe the evening of every dry day.

| Cycle Day | 1 | 2 | 3 | 4 | 5 | 6 | 7 | 8 | 9 | 10 | 11 | 12 | 13 | 14 | 15 | 16 | 17 | 18 | 19 | 20 | 21 | 22 | 23 | 24 | 25 | 26 | 27 | 28 | 29 | 30 | 31 | 32 | 33 | 34 | 35 | 36 | 37 | 38 | 39 | 40 |
|---|---|---|---|---|---|---|---|---|---|---|---|---|---|---|---|---|---|---|---|---|---|---|---|---|---|---|---|---|---|---|---|---|---|---|---|---|---|---|---|---|
| Cervical Fluid | ✗ | ✗ | ✗ | ✗ | – | – | – | – | – | – | S | S | ⓒ | ⓔ | ⓔ | – | – | – | – | S | – | – | – | S | S | – | – | – | ✶ | | | | | | | | | | | |
| Peak Day | | | | | | | | | | | | | | | | | | | | | | | | | | | | | | | | | | | | | | | | |
| Vaginal Sensation | | | | | dry | · | = | = | · | = | sticky | = | wet | wet | wet | dry | · | = | = | = | ◦ | · | = | = | = | = | = | | | | | | | | | | | | | |

**Chart 9.2. Dry Day Rule.** Note that she is safe the evening of every preovulatory dry day, which in this chart occurs on Days 5 to 10.

* Unlike the other three rules in this chapter, a part of the First 5 Days Rule admittedly relies on past cycles to estimate a possibly increased risk of present fertility. However, there is a fundamental difference between this particular guideline and the Rhythm Method. The likelihood of conception occurring from intercourse on Day 5 or before is very remote, whereas the chances of ovulation varying widely from Day 10 onward is extremely high. The principle here is to simply add one more buffer for women who may have a somewhat higher risk than the statistical average.

For the record, it is likely that the vast majority of women who truly conceived from sex during their period had intercourse at the end of a long menstruation, on Day 6 or after. There is also a definite possibility that what was perceived as sex during menses actually took place during ovulatory spotting.

**I.** Before ovulation, you are safe for unprotected intercourse the evening of every dry day (after 6 P.M.).* Dryness is determined by checking throughout the day and observing that no cervical fluid or wetness is present at any point during the day. But as soon as you see even *sticky*-quality cervical fluid, you should consider yourself potentially fertile.

It may surprise you that you must consider sticky cervical fluid as potentially fertile before ovulation. It's true that it's very difficult for sperm to survive in it. However, the rules are extremely conservative, and take into consideration the fact that a woman may not be able to differentiate between sticky cervical fluid and the beginning phases of the wetter, creamier quality. In addition, this eliminates the risk of wetter fluid dripping down from the cervical tip in time to save the few hearty sperm that may have survived.

Therefore, before ovulation, the only days that are considered safe are those dry days in which there is no cervical fluid present. (Note that women will always notice a slight dampness or moistness at the vaginal opening, which quickly dissipates from the finger. These days are still considered dry if you have no cervical fluid.)

**2.** The day after intercourse is marked with a question mark if semen or spermicide is present, because they can mask the presence of cervical fluid. The evening of a "Semen Day" is considered fertile since there is no way to prove that day is indeed dry. (For recording semen, see Chart 9.3 below. Better yet, for an efficient way to eliminate semen, refer back to page 85 on SETs.)

If, by the end of the day after intercourse, you are dry all day, you are safe for unprotected intercourse again that evening. There are two reasons why you can have peace of mind using the Dry Day Rule before ovulation:

a. Sperm can't survive if there's no cervical fluid present to sustain them. At longest, they will live a few hours. And because the

**Chart 9.3. When semen masks cervical fluid.** Note that she is safe on the evenings of preovulatory dry days, but any day with residual semen must be recorded with a question mark, as she did on Days 6 and 8. These days are considered potentially fertile.

* If you are tempted to have sex before 6 P.M., see page 314.

sticky-quality cervical fluid that develops before wetter types is just about as inhospitable to sperm as a completely dry vaginal environment, the risk of conception is extremely low.

    b. If you don't have cervical fluid, it's an indication that your estrogen levels are so low that you're not near ovulation. Remember that ovulation is preceded by a buildup of wet-quality cervical fluid.

The above two reasons should reduce fears that you might have regarding the issue of sperm surviving long enough for an egg to pop out. To exaggerate the point, even if sperm could live *10* days in ideal conditions *and* ovulation occurred the day after intercourse, it's extremely unlikely you would get pregnant if your lovemaking was on a dry day. Of course, this scenario would probably never happen, but I want to stress the concept of sperm needing fertile cervical fluid in order to survive and move.

Finally, you should realize that because sperm can survive for 5 days if fertile-quality cervical fluid *is* present, you absolutely cannot rely on ovulation predictor kits, which only give about one day's warning of impending ovulation. And just for the record—no, arousal fluid and lubricants don't provide the necessary environment for sperm survival.

**3.** After a couple cycles of charting you may notice that immediately after your period ends you don't have any dry days. Rather, you have a sticky-quality

**Chart 9.4. Basic Infertile Pattern of sticky cervical fluid.** After charting a couple of cycles, Kelly notices that her Basic Infertile Pattern is sticky rather than dry immediately following her period. Because this is her preovulatory pattern, she may treat Days 6 to 11 above as if they were dry and follow the Dry Day Rule. In order to minimize the risk of pregnancy, she verifies that no *wet* cervical fluid is present at her cervical tip before having intercourse.

cervical fluid that starts just after menstruation and continues day after day until you see the *change* into a wetter quality. This just means that your Basic Infertile Pattern (BIP) during your infertile phase is *sticky* rather than dry. If this is the case, you may be able to apply the Dry Day Rule on those days of sticky cervical fluid, treating the sticky days as if they were dry. Of course, the first sign of wet cervical fluid is considered fertile.

This exception, though, only applies to those who never experience dry days preovulatory. And even then, you should be aware that you may be taking a somewhat increased risk in following this modified guideline. Because of this, I strongly suggest that if you are using FAM with a sticky BIP, you verify that there is no wet cervical fluid at your cervical tip before having intercourse. (See Chart 9.4 on opposite page.)

## 🐚 POSTOVULATORY INFERTILE-PHASE RULES

### 3. TEMPERATURE SHIFT RULE

> You are safe the evening of the third consecutive day your temperature is above the coverline.

**Chart 9.5. Temperature Shift Rule.** Note that she had a thermal shift on Day 18 and then drew the appropriate coverline. She then recorded 1,2,3 in the Temp Count column and started her infertile phase the evening of Day 20 after three consecutive high temperatures above the coverline.

### The Coverline and Your Thermal Shift

You may want to review page 73 on how to draw a coverline. The following rules assume that you have already internalized that information.

**1.** You are considered infertile starting at 6 P.M. the third *consecutive* night that your temperature remains *above* the coverline. Record the 1,2,3 in the Temp Count column of your chart. Draw a vertical line between Days 2 and 3 of high temperatures to indicate that you are safe from the third evening on. (See Chart 9.5 on previous page.)

**2.** If a temperature falls *on or below* the coverline during the 3-day count, you must start the count over again once it has risen back above the line (I know, I know, boo, hiss). However, you don't have to draw the coverline again.

**3.** If you are sick, you should not consider yourself safe until you have recorded three consecutive normal temperatures above the coverline without having a fever. (Page 276 explains how illness can affect fertility.)

You should review the Rule of Thumb on page 75 to see how to handle outlying preovulatory temperatures caused by such factors as alcohol consumption and lack of sleep (as well as a fever). Remember that the resulting temperatures can be discounted, but in order to determine your coverline, you must count back six low temperatures, not including the days eliminated. Also remember to compensate for any possible temperature rise caused by Daylight Savings or travel to another time zone.

If you notice that your temperature has risen either higher than normal or earlier than you would expect, pay close attention. This is an important time to observe your other fertility signs as well. Ovulation is virtually always preceded by a buildup of wet cervical fluid and changes in the cervix. If you didn't observe the fluid changes, you shouldn't assume that you've already ovulated.

| Cycle Day | 1 | 2 | 3 | 4 | 5 | 6 | 7 | 8 | 9 | 10 | 11 | 12 | 13 | 14 | 15 | 16 | 17 | 18 | 19 | 20 | 21 | 22 | 23 | 24 | 25 | 26 | 27 | 28 | 29 | 30 | 31 | 32 | 33 | 34 | 35 | 36 | 37 | 38 | 39 | 40 |
|---|---|---|---|---|---|---|---|---|---|---|---|---|---|---|---|---|---|---|---|---|---|---|---|---|---|---|---|---|---|---|---|---|---|---|---|---|---|---|---|---|
| Cervical Fluid | ✱ | ✱ | ✱ | ✱ | – | – | – | – | – | – | – | S | ⊙ | ⊙ | Ⓔ | Ⓔ | Ⓔ | – | S | – | S | – | – | – | S | – | S | – | – | – | S | – | ✱ | | | | | | | |
| Peak Day | | | | | | | | | | | | | | | | | PK | 1 | 2 | 3 | 4 | | | | | | | | | | | | | | | | | | | |
| Vaginal Sensation | | | | | dry | = | = | = | = | = | sticky | wet | wet | humid | humid | wet | dry | = | = | | ↑ = | = | = | = | sticky | dry | . | = | = | . | sticky | dry | | | | | | | | |

**Chart 9.6. Peak Day Rule.** Her last day of wet cervical fluid was Day 17. She marked "PK" (for "Peak") under it, then recorded 1,2,3,4 on the subsequent days in the Peak Day column. She considered herself safe the fourth evening after her Peak Day, on Day 21. Note that even though she had sticky cervical fluid on the fourth day, she is still considered safe as long as wet cervical fluid does not reappear during the 4-day count.

## 4. PEAK DAY RULE

> You are safe the evening of the 4th consecutive day after your Peak Day.

**I.** Identify your Peak Day (the last day of wetness, as described on page 83). Mark "PK" below it, in the Peak Day column. Subsequent days should be labeled "1,2,3,4" in that same column. But it is best to record them in the evening after having observed your cervical fluid each day. You will only know it is the peak the following day, when your cervical fluid and lubricative vaginal sensation have already started to dry up.

Remember that if your last day of eggwhite is on a Monday, but you still have one more day of lubricative vaginal sensation (or spotting) on Tuesday, your Peak Day is Tuesday. Of course, the reverse applies as well.

**2.** You are considered safe after 6 P.M. the evening of the 4th consecutive day following the Peak Day. Draw a vertical line between Days 3 and 4 to indicate that you are safe from the 4th evening on. (Note that you are still considered infertile even if you have sticky days after you've drawn the vertical line.)

**3.** If you have a cervical fluid pattern in which you have a day of creamy after your last day of eggwhite (most women have nothing or sticky), your Peak Day is still considered that last day of eggwhite. However, if you cannot identify an obvious thermal shift by the second morning after the last eggwhite day, or your creamy days continue, you should be conservative and consider the last creamy day that you have as your Peak Day.

**Chart 9.7. Split peaks.** Note that she had what is referred to as a split peak. Her body prepared to ovulate by producing fertile-quality cervical fluid starting on Day 11, but then stress or some other factor delayed her ovulation. In this case, it appeared that her Peak Day was Day 14, but after only a couple of days she started producing wet cervical fluid again, so she had to start the count over. Her true Peak Day was then Day 18, after which she counted 1,2,3,4 and considered herself safe starting on the evening of Day 22. While these split peaks can be confusing, a thermal shift will clarify the picture and allow you to determine whether ovulation has actually occurred.

**4.** Usually, any wetness will dry up until the next cycle, but if wet cervical fluid or vaginal sensations reappear during the 4-day count, as in the chart above, wait until the wetness ends to reestablish the Peak Day. Begin the count over again. This type of recurring pattern is sometimes referred to as a "split peak" and is often caused by stress or illness. A delayed thermal shift will ultimately confirm when you have finally ovulated.

### A Word About Vaginal Infections

Almost all women will experience real vaginal infections at various points in their lives. True infections will usually cause symptoms that can mask cervical fluid. For this reason, you should abstain from intercourse during an infection, since the signs may be too ambiguous to be reliable. Regardless, you should abstain anyway to allow your body a chance to heal and to avoid passing the infection back and forth. (For a more detailed description of true vaginal infections, see page 199.)

## *A Word About Your Cervical Position*

As discussed in Chapter 5, the changes in your cervix can also help you determine if you are fertile. However, it is considered an optional sign, since it is generally only used to confirm the changes in temperature and cervical fluid. For this reason, there are no specific rules about the changes in your cervix presented in this book. But I do encourage you to observe your cervix if you want one more fertility sign to corroborate the others.

## ৯ PUTTING IT ALL TOGETHER

You should be aware that the Peak Day of cervical fluid typically occurs a couple of days before the rise in temperature. This pattern has an advantage in that cervical fluid usually dries up quickly the day after the Peak Day, and thus most women can predict their temperature rise the day before it appears.

In addition, note that *before* ovulation, the cervical fluid is the critical fertility sign to observe, because it is the one that reflects the high estrogen levels indicating the impending release of the egg. But *after* ovulation, the temperature is the critical fertility sign, because it confirms that ovulation has indeed occurred.

The rules that apply to after ovulation will often work in harmony with each other, so that the third evening of high temperatures will coincide with the fourth evening after the Peak Day. However:

1. If there is a discrepancy between the two postovulatory rules, *always wait until both signs indicate infertility* to be most conservative (i.e., until the evening after the vertical line farthest to the right). This assures that all the signs have coincided before you consider yourself infertile.
2. *If in doubt, don't take a risk!* If your fertility signs don't make sense in any given cycle, it's not worth risking unprotected intercourse if it's critical that you avoid pregnancy.

The next two pages summarize the rules that you have learned in this chapter, as well as show you how they would typically appear on your chart.

## ❧ A SUMMARY OF THE FOUR FAM RULES ❧

The basic biological principles are italicized below each respective rule.

### 1. FIRST 5 DAYS RULE
**You are safe *the first 5 days* of the menstrual cycle *if* you had an obvious temperature shift 12 to 16 days before.**

*For most women, the combined risk of ovulation occurring on Day 10 or earlier and sperm living long enough to fertilize the egg is extremely remote.*

### 2. DRY DAY RULE
**Before ovulation, you are safe the evening of a dry day.**

*Sperm cannot survive in a dry vaginal environment, and the lack of cervical fluid indicates that estrogen levels are too low for ovulation to occur.*

### 3. TEMPERATURE SHIFT RULE
**You are safe the evening of the 3rd consecutive day your temperature is above the coverline.**

*The rise in temperature due to the release of progesterone indicates that ovulation has occurred, and waiting three days allows for the remote possibility of two or more eggs being released over a 24-hour period, with each one living a full day.*

### 4. PEAK DAY RULE
**You are safe the evening of the 4th consecutive day after your Peak Day.**

*The last day of wet cervical fluid or vaginal sensation indicates the imminence of ovulation, while allowing 4 days for drying up assures that any eggs released are already gone, and that the return of a dry vaginal environment is inhospitable to sperm survival.*

### A CAUTIONARY NOTE

While this box is a useful summary, you must clearly understand all the guidelines for each rule described in this chapter before using FAM for birth control. It is also critical that you don't consider yourself safe unless *all* the rules indicate that you're infertile. If you have any doubts, don't take the risk.

Finally, you should know that these rules are a highly effective form of contraception if they are consistently and correctly followed. However, the relative risks of natural birth control should be understood by the user. I therefore urge you to read Appendix D before relying on what you have learned in these last few pages.

NATURAL BIRTH CONTROL AT YOUR FINGERTIPS . . .

| Cycle Day | 1 | 2 | 3 | 4 | 5 | 6 | 7 | 8 | 9 | 10 | 11 | 12 | 13 | 14 | 15 | 16 | 17 | 18 | 19 | 20 | 21 | 22 | 23 | 24 | 25 | 26 | 27 | 28 | 29 | 30 | 31 | 32 | 33 | 34 | 35 | 36 | 37 | 38 | 39 | 40 |
|---|---|---|---|---|---|---|---|---|---|---|---|---|---|---|---|---|---|---|---|---|---|---|---|---|---|---|---|---|---|---|---|---|---|---|---|---|---|---|---|---|
| Date | | | | | | | | | | | | | | | | | | | | | | | | | | | | | | | | | | | | | | | | |
| Day of Week | | | | | | | | | | | | | | | | | | | | | | | | | | | | | | | | | | | | | | | | |

*Preovulatory Infertile Phase*    *Fertile Phase*    *Postovulatory Infertile Phase*

Temp Count: 1 2 3

**Waking Temperature**

| Cervical Fluid | ✱ | ✱ | ✱ | ✱ | (✱) | — | — | — | — | — | — | S | S | C | C | E | E | — | — | — | — | — | — | — | — | — | — | — | — | — | — | ✱ |
| Peak Day | | | | | | | | | | | | | | | | | PK | 1 | 2 | 3 | 4 |

*First 5 Days Rule*   *Dry Day Rule*    *Temperature Shift and Peak Day Rules*

**Chart 9.8. The fertile and infertile phases as defined by the four standard FAM rules.**

# CHAPTER 10

# Shortcuts:
# Minimum Charting with
# Maximum Reliability

For those of you who just skipped ahead to this page, don't even *think* of using the rules in this chapter until you've charted several complete cycles.

lthough the Fertility Awareness Method is really very simple once you've learned it, even experienced users don't necessarily want to chart every day to achieve maximum reliability. With a little experience under your belt, you can restrict charting to only about a third of the cycle and still attain all the information necessary to apply this method, without compromising contraceptive efficacy.

The reason you can have peace of mind using the shortcuts explained on these pages is that once you have ovulated, your body won't release an egg again until the following cycle. So once you've identified when the egg is dead and gone, it's unnecessary to continue charting until your next period.

It is my recommendation, though, that you chart without using shortcuts. I personally think it's easier to do it every day than to have to think about where you are in your cycle. As you've seen, charting is also about much more than just detecting when you can and can't get pregnant. And finally, by charting your complete cycle, you will often benefit from one of its most practical aspects: being warned often hours before you get your period by the drop in temperature that most women experience on the first day of the flow.

**Chart 10.1. Temperature Shift Rule with minimum charting.** Once she had her third high temperature above the coverline by Day 15, she no longer needed to chart her temperature until the next cycle because she had already established that ovulation had passed.

But if you still prefer to take shortcuts, you can use the modified guidelines discussed below. Contraceptive efficacy won't be compromised, as long as your fertility signs have confirmed that ovulation has already occurred for that particular cycle.

## 🌺 WAKING TEMPERATURE

It's unnecessary to take your temperature during your period, since these temperatures tend to be somewhat high or erratic anyway. In addition, once you've established the occurrence of a thermal shift by counting at least three high temperatures above the coverline, you needn't take your temperature again until your period from the next cycle is over. (Chart 10.1, above.)

## 🌺 CERVICAL FLUID

You never have to check your cervical fluid during your period. In fact, there is no point in checking while menstruating since the bleeding will mask it. And once you've established the first safe day under the Peak Day Rule, you needn't chart your cervical fluid again until your next cycle.

| Cycle Day | 1 | 2 | 3 | 4 | 5 | 6 | 7 | 8 | 9 | 10 | 11 | 12 | 13 | 14 | 15 | 16 | 17 | 18 | 19 | 20 | 21 | 22 | 23 | 24 | 25 | 26 | 27 | 28 | 29 | 30 | 31 | 32 | 33 | 34 | 35 | 36 | 37 | 38 | 39 | 40 |
|---|---|---|---|---|---|---|---|---|---|---|---|---|---|---|---|---|---|---|---|---|---|---|---|---|---|---|---|---|---|---|---|---|---|---|---|---|---|---|---|---|
| Cervical Fluid | ✳ | ✳ | ✳ | ✳ | ✳ | – | – | s | © | © | © | s | – | – | – | | | | | | | | | | | | ✳ | | | | | | | | | | | | | |
| Peak Day | | | | | | | | | | | PK | 1 | 2 | 3 | 4 | | | | | | | | | | | | | | | | | | | | | | | | | |

**Chart 10.2. The Peak Day Rule with minimum charting.** She started to check her cervical fluid as soon as her period stopped, in this case on Day 6. Once she established that she was 4 days past her Peak Day on Day 15, she could be fairly certain that she had already ovulated and would therefore not have to continue charting her cervical fluid until the next cycle. (However, in order to rely on this shortcut, it is imperative that she confirm ovulation through the Temperature Shift Rule.)

A cautionary note: *If you intend to rely on the shortcut version of the Peak Day Rule, it is critical that you establish that ovulation has passed by observing three high temperatures above the coverline.* This is because you may have a delayed ovulation in which your cervical fluid could mislead you into thinking you had already ovulated. If you were no longer charting that cycle, you would perhaps not notice the return of fertile cervical fluid. By observing a clear thermal shift, your chances of being misled in this way are virtually eliminated. Still, you should continue to check your cervical fluid throughout the cycle if the accuracy of your temperatures could have been compromised due to illness or other factors. As always, be conservative. (Chart 10.2, above.)

## ❧ CERVICAL POSITION

The position of the cervix is considered an optional fertility sign. This means that it's not necessary to check the cervix in order for the method to be effective. However, the cervical position is an excellent sign to cross-check the other two signs if there is ever a discrepancy between them.

| Cycle Day | 1 | 2 | 3 | 4 | 5 | 6 | 7 | 8 | 9 | 10 | 11 | 12 | 13 | 14 | 15 | 16 | 17 | 18 | 19 | 20 | 21 | 22 | 23 | 24 | 25 | 26 | 27 | 28 | 29 | 30 | 31 | 32 | 33 | 34 | 35 | 36 | 37 | 38 | 39 | 40 |
|---|---|---|---|---|---|---|---|---|---|---|---|---|---|---|---|---|---|---|---|---|---|---|---|---|---|---|---|---|---|---|---|---|---|---|---|---|---|---|---|---|
| Cervical Fluid | ✳ | | | | | | | | | | | | | | | | | | | | | | | | | | ✳ | | | | | | | | | | | | | |
| Peak Day | | | | | | | | | | | | | | | | | | | | | | | | | | | | | | | | | | | | | | | | |
| Vaginal Sensation | | | | | | | | | | | | | | | | | | | | | | | | | | | | | | | | | | | | | | | | |
| Cervix | | | | | | • | • | o | o | O | O | • | • | • | • | | | | | | | | | | | | | | | | | | | | | | | | | |
| | | | | | | F | F | M | M | S | S | F | F | F | F | | | | | | | | | | | | | | | | | | | | | | | | | |

**Chart 10.3. Observing the cervix with minimum charting.** Because she wanted to chart the minimal number of days necessary while still being as conservative as possible, she recorded her cervical position to verify that ovulation had passed.

Since checking the cervix is not altogether necessary, there are two shortcuts you could take at this point. You could choose not to observe the cervix at all, or you could merely check the cervix about a week per cycle. The time to start checking it would be at the first notice of wet-quality cervical fluid, continuing to check through to the third day after the cervix has begun to revert back to becoming firm, low, and closed. However, to use this shortcut, you may need to chart the cervix for several cycles to be able to detect the subtle changes that occur with it. (Chart 10.3, opposite below.)

## 🕸 A NOTE ON THE PREOVULATORY RULES

It should be obvious that if you choose to use these shortcuts, the preovulatory rules still apply. Thus, you can only assume you're infertile during the first 5 days of your cycle if you meet the criteria of the First 5 Days Rule. In addition, you must always follow the Dry Day Rule, and therefore must begin to chart no later than Day 6.

**Chart 10.4. The basic short-cut chart with the three primary fertility signs.**

## ꙮ THE FALLACY OF THE
## I-JUST-KNOW-WHEN-I'M-FERTILE MENTALITY

One word of warning about taking shortcuts: Once you decide not to chart every day, it can be very tempting to slack off and either chart even less than recommended, or stop altogether, convincing yourself that you just *know* when you're fertile. I cringe when women claim they don't need to record because they always know when they're fertile. Ironically, experienced women who have charted for years often feel they, too, can become lax in charting because they "just know." But even if your cycles have always been regular and your charts easy to interpret, there's always the chance that the next cycle will be different from all others. Like any other birth control method that "fails" because of improper use—such as leaving the diaphragm in the drawer—FAM must be used correctly to work.

Simply intuiting when you are or aren't fertile is not a reliable method of birth control. In fact, it's no method at all. You need to chart your temperature and cervical fluid, even if it's for just a third of your cycle. Otherwise, it can be too easy to forget what transpired on any given day. In the end, you may find that charting becomes so second nature that you won't even be tempted to take the shortcuts described above.

# PART FOUR

# PREGNANCY ACHIEVEMENT

# CHAPTER 11

# Maximizing Your Chances of Getting Pregnant

*Literature is mostly about having sex and not much about having children; life's the other way round.*
—DAVID LODGE (1935), British author

*I*f you're like most people trying to get pregnant, you probably remember the years of hassling with birth control and all that entailed—the diaphragms that flew across the room when you attempted to insert them, the condoms that broke at the peak of lovemaking or the Pill that caused you to balloon in weight. In fact, you may have even experienced sleepless nights worrying about whether you had accidentally become pregnant, even though you used birth control consistently.

Yet here you are, years later, perhaps bemoaning the fact that you spent so much time and energy trying to *avoid* pregnancy, only to discover that it may not have been so easy to get pregnant, after all. For some couples, getting pregnant may indeed be difficult. But for many, it can be as simple as learning how to optimize your chances of conception by identifying when your combined fertility is at its greatest. Surprisingly, the chances of a typical couple of proven fertility conceiving in any one menstrual cycle is no higher than about 25%. But you can increase the chances dramatically by identifying the optimal time to try.

While most would acknowledge the great benefits derived from advances in medical technology, there are drawbacks. One is that people are often led to believe that the most efficient and only way they will be able to get pregnant is through invasive procedures. Not only is this often untrue, it can also be counterproductive. Modern methods can ironically impede or delay the very pregnancy they were designed to aid. (For example, Clomid tends to dry up

**131**

cervical fluid, and artificial insemination may be inappropriately timed.) Today, there are countless ways to diagnose and treat so-called infertility. But if you think you might face a fertility problem, FAM should always be the *first* step in the pursuit of pregnancy.

When trying to get pregnant, dispense with all the misinformation well-meaning friends and clinicians seem to perpetuate. If you've read this book in sequence, and didn't sneak a peak at this chapter first, you should already know that there are a number of truths about fertility which differ from the myths you've heard.

*One of my couples illustrated the benefit of knowing you are still fertile even though it would appear that you are well beyond the day of ovulation. Carrie and Jake were extremely demoralized when I met them. They had been trying to get pregnant for nearly 2 years since the tragic death of their baby. Since they didn't have any trouble conceiving the first time, they were perplexed by why it was taking so long to get pregnant again.*

*In their particular case, what helped them to conceive again after those 2 years was the realization that if Carrie's temperature hadn't shifted yet, they were still considered fertile. She said that she was almost relieved when her temperature was still low on Day 22, because it meant they still had an opportunity to get pregnant that cycle. So rather than feeling anxious, she felt much more in control. They knew to continue having sex each day that she had wet cervical fluid and the temperature remained low. They had intercourse and conceived on Day 22. Sure enough, her temperature rose the next day, confirming that they had timed it just right.*

## Fertility Truths

1. A normal cycle is not necessarily 28 days; it ranges from about 24 to 36 days. It varies from woman to woman as well as within individuals.
2. You can ovulate as early as Day 8, and as late as Day 22 or beyond. The point is that women do not necessarily ovulate on Day 14.
3. Your most fertile day cannot be determined by your temperature. In fact, most women don't even experience the "temperature dip" that they've often been told to look for.
4. You are *not* most fertile the day of the rise in temperature, either. In fact, by the time the temperature rises, it's usually too late—the egg is already gone.

5. The key to identifying your most fertile phase is through cervical fluid, and not waking temperatures.

6. You don't need to stand on your head for half an hour after making love in order to get pregnant! If you are timing intercourse at the most fertile time, the sperm will swim up through the cervical fluid rapidly, regardless of what position you are in.

7. How often you should have intercourse during your fertile phase (i.e., every day or every other day) is a function of the combination of your partner's sperm count and your cervical fluid. It's not a hard-and-fast rule that applies to all couples alike.

8. Both men and women are equally likely to have a fertility problem. In other words, if a couple has trouble getting pregnant, one cannot assume it's automatically the woman's problem.

## Why Some Women Are More Fertile Than Others

Even being armed with accurate knowledge doesn't necessarily guarantee a timely pregnancy. If it is taking longer than you had anticipated, probably the last thing you want to hear are the annoying clichés of well-meaning women about themselves:

"They just call me Fertile Myrtle."

"He just has to look at me and I get pregnant."

"I've gotten pregnant on every method of birth control (giggle, giggle). I guess I was just destined to be a mom."

Actually, there are several reasons why such women do indeed tend to be more fertile than others. In addition to the obvious fact that their reproductive organs are healthy, they may have a long phase of extremely fertile-quality cervical fluid, providing them more opportunities to get pregnant. Also, women with short cycles tend to ovulate more often, which means that they have more fertile days in a given year. But even though these women have a biological head start, you can certainly level the playing field by charting your cycle.

*Vanessa and Max were a charming couple who had taken my class initially to avoid pregnancy. After 2 years of using FAM successfully, they decided it was time to try to get pregnant. But a trip to Mexico delayed their plans by several months while they allowed the malaria medications to dissipate from their bodies. So the first month in which they were able to try was March. Then a little detail looked like it was going to interfere. Max had just had major surgery on a shoulder that had eroded from years of playing basketball. He spent several days in the hospital after the operation.*

*His first night back home he was in a lot of pain, and was completely drugged to help him handle it. Vanessa walked in and proudly announced "Tonight's the night." The eggwhite was too obvious to miss. As Max recounted: "Trust me, sex was the furthest thing from my mind. Here I was, with my shoulder and arm taped to my torso to immobilize it, flat on my back, pumped with painkillers, and my wife walks in and says: 'It's time. I'm fertile.' Needless to say, I explained to her that I was hardly in a position, so to speak, to have sex, when she reminded me that she could take care of everything herself. So with me half out of it, she proceeded to do what was necessary to allow conception to occur. Sure enough, from that one single act of sex that cycle, we conceived our little boy Don."*

You may take a lot longer to get pregnant, of course. The point is that knowing when you are most fertile will expedite the process. If, after 4 to 6 cycles of timing intercourse on your most fertile days, you still haven't gotten pregnant, you should probably pursue diagnostic testing or fertility treatments. (Some couples may want to get a semen analysis even earlier, given how easy it is to have done.)

## A Word About Ovulation Predictor Kits

Before getting to the crux of how FAM can help you get pregnant, I want to say a few words about ovulation predictor kits, since so many of you will no doubt be tempted to use them. While they can in fact be quite useful, you should know by now that your own body usually provides you with as much valuable information as the kits, with less hassle and certainly at less cost. Still, if you do choose to use them (either exclusively or with Fertility Awareness), you should be aware that they can be misleading for the following reasons:

**1.** The kits only test for the occurrence of the luteinizing hormone (LH) surge that precedes ovulation. They don't indicate whether the woman has definitively ovulated afterward. In fact, a woman may occasionally experience a condition called LUFS (Luteinized Unruptured Follicle Syndrome) in which they have an LH surge but the egg never actually pops out of the ovary.

**2.** A woman may experience false LH surges in which she has mini-peaks of LH before the real one, causing her to potentially time intercourse too early for the sperm to survive long enough for the release of the egg.

**3.** The kit does not indicate whether the woman has suitable cervical fluid to allow sperm a medium in which to travel to the egg. In addition, by the time the kit does show a surge, the cervical fluid could already be starting to dry up.

**4.** The kits are only as accurate as the individual using them. There are typically many steps involved, any one of which can be performed improperly, rendering the test invalid. In addition, their accuracy can be compromised if exposed to excessive heat during delivery and storage.

**5.** The kits are only accurate if they test a woman's fertility right around the time of ovulation. This is a very significant point, because often the type of woman who purchases them is one who, by definition, has irregular cycles. Therefore, the typical kit, which has only 5 to 9 days' worth of tests, will often not have enough to cover the range necessary for her to determine ovulation.

For example, if Mary has cycles that are between 29 and 42 days, then her ovulation will generally vary between Days 15 and 28, which is a range of 13 days. The kits only provide 5 to 9 days' worth of tests, so it could be quite a challenge for the woman with irregular cycles to know on what day of the cycle to begin testing. What this means is that women with irregular or long cycles should not start testing their urine until they notice their cervical fluid start to get wet, so as to test at the most appropriate time around ovulation.

**6.** Some fertility drugs such as Pergonal, Danocrine, or injections containing HCG (e.g., P.A.P.L. or Profasi) can invalidate the results of these kits. Clomid does not have this effect.

**7.** Women over 40 and approaching menopause can have elevated levels of luteinizing hormone that are not indicative of ovulation. A kit should only show a surge of one day. If it shows more than one day, it is very likely invalid.

**8.** Finally, you should be aware that if you happen to be pregnant already, the kit will simply imply that you aren't ovulating. Of course, this is true, but this tells you nothing of your real condition (whereas charting would, as you'll soon learn).

## ❧ THE ROLE OF FAM IN PREGNANCY ACHIEVEMENT

I wish getting pregnant were always as easy as making love when the mood strikes. Yet for many people, it requires more knowledge than we were typically taught while growing up. And unfortunately, people can be incredibly educated and well-read and still require high-tech procedures to get pregnant. But for a lot of people presumed to have a fertility problem, FAM can help fulfill their desire to get pregnant in many ways.

Infertility can have many causes. FAM allows couples to hone in on them more quickly, thus helping their doctor determine if they require medical intervention. Conventional medical wisdom is for a couple to have intercourse for a full year before seeking help for pregnancy achievement. What an unnecessary waste of time and emotional energy that is for most people! Using FAM, couples often discover that getting pregnant simply involves optimizing their chances with newfound knowledge about their combined fertility, rather than simply trying haphazardly. In timing intercourse precisely with the most appropriate frequency, one should be able to tell if there is a problem within only a few months of trying.

*Anne is a 36-year-old woman who almost never menstruated from the age of 28 on. Naturally, she suspected that it would be a real challenge to get pregnant. A fertility doctor prescribed the ovulatory drug Clomid for 6 months. During that time, although she ovulated, she experienced a number of unpleasant side effects, the most serious being vision problems so severe that they caused her to see in quadruple. In addition, the Clomid exacerbated her problem of poor cervical-fluid production. So after several months of frustration on the drug, she decided to discontinue it. In fact, she and her husband, Jay, a physician, were so discouraged with the experience that they welcomed the break from feeling obligated to get pregnant.*

*One morning, about 4 months after stopping Clomid, she woke up "swimming in eggwhite," as she says. Since she hardly ever ovulated, she rarely experienced such fertile cervical fluid. They knew that if they had any hope of getting pregnant, they had to take advantage of that moment. Sure enough, she conceived that day, without the aid of anything but the knowledge of Fertility Awareness that they both possessed. Little Lena was born at home 9 months later.*

## Fertility Factors You Can Detect Through Waking Temperatures

As you saw from the couple above, cervical fluid is the critical fertility sign to chart when trying to get pregnant. But basal temperatures can be equally beneficial, for altogether different reasons. One of the most common mistakes couples make is trying to time intercourse by the waking temperature. Remember, temperatures are useful to determine *if* you are ovulating, and how long your luteal phase is. But they are not helpful for identifying impending ovulation, which is the most fertile phase of the cycle. So waiting for either the dip or rise in temperature is virtually useless for timing sex. The dip only occurs in a very small percentage of cycles, and by the time the temperature rises, it's usually too late.

However, I want to reiterate that taking your waking temperature is very useful for several reasons besides timing intercourse. Using the typical cycle in Chart 11.1 as a standard of comparison, you can see how temperatures can reflect numerous things about your fertility (see page 138).

Your waking temperatures show whether:

- you are ovulating at all (Chart 11.2)
- your luteal phase is long enough for implantation (at least 10 days), thereby preventing the need for painful and unnecessary diagnostic tests such as an endometrial biopsy. Note that a luteal phase is determined by the number of days between the rise in temperature and the first day of true menstruation, and not premenstrual spotting (Chart 11.3; also see box on page 141).
- your progesterone levels are high enough in your luteal phase (Chart 11.4)
- you are still fertile any given cycle as reflected by low temperatures (Chart 11.5)
- you may have gotten pregnant, as reflected by more than 18 high temperatures (Chart 11.6)
- you are in danger of having a miscarriage, as determined by a sudden drop in temperatures (miscarriages occur as often as one in three pregnancies) (Chart 11.7)
- you were pregnant before having what seemed to be just a "late period." (Chart 11.8)

**Chart 11.1. A typical ovulatory temperature pattern.** Note that ovulation had almost certainly occurred by the thermal shift on Day 17. Her luteal phase was 15 days, determined by counting the high temperatures from Day 17 through to the last day before her period on Day 32.

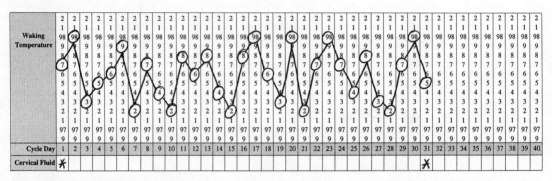

**Chart 11.2. An anovulatory temperature pattern.** Her temperatures indicate that she didn't ovulate because there was no thermal shift from a range of lows to a range of highs.

**Chart 11.3. A short luteal phase.** Note that while her 29-day cycle length is normal, her nine postovulatory high temperatures indicate a short luteal phase (counting Days 21–29). In order for implantation to successfully occur, it is believed that a woman should have a postovulatory phase of at least 10 days.

**Chart 11.4. Low postovulatory progesterone.** Note that her high temperatures do not remain above the coverline following ovulation. This could be an indication of low progesterone levels.

**Chart 11.5. A delayed ovulation.** Sabrina was able to determine that she was still fertile as late as Day 21, because her temperature had not yet risen and her cervical fluid was still wet. Therefore, she timed intercourse accordingly and got pregnant.

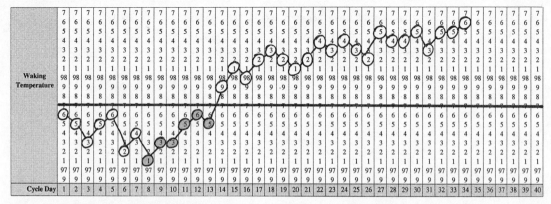

**Chart 11.6. A pregnancy chart.** Sandy could tell she got pregnant by Day 31, because she then had 18 high temperatures after ovulation. (The postovulatory phase is rarely more than 16 days if a woman is not pregnant.)

**Chart 11.7. Pregnancy followed by a miscarriage.** This woman was almost certainly pregnant, as seen by the fact that she had her 18th high temperature on Day 33, but she then got a warning that she was about to miscarry by the pattern of falling temperatures starting about Day 36.

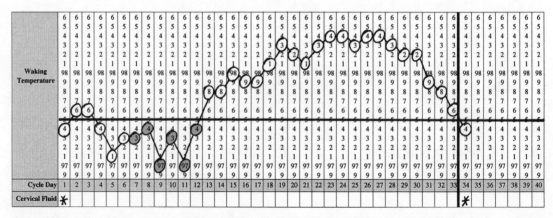

**Chart 11.8. Miscarriage that would have seemed like a late period.** Note that if she had not been charting, she wouldn't have been able to observe the 18 high temperatures, and thus she might have thought that her bleeding on Day 34 was simply a late menstruation rather than a miscarriage.

# Fertility Cycle # _____

Last 12 Cycles:    Shortest _____    Longest _____    Month _____    Year _____    This cycle length: _____

| Cycle Day | 1 | 2 | 3 | 4 | 5 | 6 | 7 | 8 | 9 | 10 | 11 | 12 | 13 | 14 | 15 | 16 | 17 | 18 | 19 | 20 | 21 | 22 | 23 | 24 | 25 | 26 | 27 | 28 | 29 | 30 | 31 | 32 | 33 | 34 | 35 | 36 | 37 | 38 | 39 | 40 |
|---|---|---|---|---|---|---|---|---|---|---|---|---|---|---|---|---|---|---|---|---|---|---|---|---|---|---|---|---|---|---|---|---|---|---|---|---|---|---|---|---|
| Date | | | | | | | | | | | | | | | | | | | | | | | | | | | | | | | | | | | | | | | | |
| Day of Week | | | | | | | | | | | | | | | | | | | | | | | | | | | | | | | | | | | | | | | | |
| Intercourse | | | | | | | | | | | | | | | | | | | | | | | | | | | | | | | | | | | | | | | | |
| Birth Control Method Used | | | | | | | | | | | | | | | | | | | | | | | | | | | | | | | | | | | | | | | | |
| Time Temp Taken | | | | | | | | | | | | | | | | | | | | | | | | | | | | | | | | | | | | | | | | |
| Temp Count | | | | | | | | | | | | | | | | | | | | | | | | | | | | | | | | | | | | | | | | |

Waking Temperature (scale 99 down to 97 repeated across all cycle days)

| Cycle Day | 1 | 2 | 3 | 4 | 5 | 6 | 7 | 8 | 9 | 10 | 11 | 12 | 13 | 14 | 15 | 16 | 17 | 18 | 19 | 20 | 21 | 22 | 23 | 24 | 25 | 26 | 27 | 28 | 29 | 30 | 31 | 32 | 33 | 34 | 35 | 36 | 37 | 38 | 39 | 40 |
|---|---|---|---|---|---|---|---|---|---|---|---|---|---|---|---|---|---|---|---|---|---|---|---|---|---|---|---|---|---|---|---|---|---|---|---|---|---|---|---|---|
| Cervical Fluid | | | | | | | | | | | | | | | | | | | | | | | | | | | | | | | | | | | | | | | | |
| Peak Day | | | | | | | | | | | | | | | | | | | | | | | | | | | | | | | | | | | | | | | | |
| Vaginal Sensation | | | | | | | | | | | | | | | | | | | | | | | | | | | | | | | | | | | | | | | | |
| Cervix | | | | | | | | | | | | | | | | | | | | | | | | | | | | | | | | | | | | | | | | |

Cervical Fluid Description

Miscellaneous
Ovulatory Pain
PMS
Illness
Stress
Travel
Exercise
Breast Exam (BSE)

## Legend

| Cervical Fluid Symbols | ✳ Menses | (✳) Spotting | — No Cervical Fluid | S Sticky | Ⓒ Creamy | Ⓔ Eggwhite |
|---|---|---|---|---|---|---|
| | Bright Red | Pink or Brown | Nothing | Sticky, Crumbly, Gummy, or Rubbery Yellow or White | Creamy, Lotiony, Milky, or Smooth Yellow or White | Slippery and Usually Stretchy Clear, Streaked or Opaque |
| Vaginal Sensation | Moist or Dry | Dry | | Dry or Sticky | Wet and/or Cold | Lubricative and Very Wet, May Feel Humid |

Cervix Symbols: • o O

| F | M | S |
|---|---|---|

F = Firm   M = Medium   S = Soft

• = Closed   o = Partly Open   O = Open

**Master Chart**

**HOW TO DETERMINE THE LENGTH OF YOUR LUTEAL PHASE**

Technically, the luteal phase is defined as the time from ovulation until your next period. The most practical way to determine how many days that comprises is by counting the high temperatures above the coverline. Do not include the day of the new period. There are two situations in which you might need to modify this slightly:

1. If your temperature drops below the coverline a day or two before you start your period, you simply include those low temperatures in the count.
2. If your thermal shift consistently occurs more than 2 days after the Peak Day, it probably means that your body reacts slowly to the heat-inducing progesterone released after ovulation. In such a case, it may be more accurate to count the second day after the Peak as the first day of the luteal phase rather than waiting for a thermal shift.

## How Charting Temperatures Can Prevent Unnecessary Interventions During Pregnancy and Delivery

As you can see, one of the most practical benefits of recording your temperature is to determine if and *when* you got pregnant. Probably the most important reason to know the date of conception is to determine when the true due date will be, and not the one based on the pregnancy wheel's assumption of a Day 14 ovulation. Knowing this will prevent inappropriately timed tests such as amniocentesis. In addition, it may allow you to avoid an unnecessarily induced labor due to a miscalculation of the due date. (This is especially problematic in women who tend to have long cycles.) While it's true that ultrasound clarifies many of these ambiguities, many couples still prefer to avoid such procedures.

If you are charting and prefer not to use ultrasound, there is a simple mathematical formula for calculating your approximate due date. Simply add 9 months to the day of your thermal shift and then subtract 7 days from that date. Thus for example, if your temperature shift was on January 20, you would jump ahead to October 20, and then subtract back 7 days, for an approximate due date of October 13. If you ovulated about Day 14, the estimated due date will be about the same for both the formula and pregnancy wheel. But if you ovulated well after Day 14, the formula will be substantially more accurate. (Regardless how you calculate the due date, remember that they are still, at best, approximations.)

### More on How to Use Your Temperatures to Determine If You Are Pregnant

*One of the couples who took my class had been trying to become pregnant for exactly a year when they heard about my seminars. They returned for their follow-up consultation the succeeding month after "completing" one full cycle. I use "completing" loosely here, because the day they came in, something seemed suspiciously different. As I welcomed them into my office and set Zoey's chart on the desk, my heart skipped a beat. Rather than seeing the typical 12-to-16-day luteal phase most women experience, I noticed that Zoey's was awfully long. After observing charts for over 13 years, I can usually spot such things immediately, without needing to count. But not wanting to give either of them a false sense of hope, I tried to discreetly look at the chart and count in my head . . . 12, 13, 14, 15, 16, 17, 18 . . . Yes, sure enough, she was pregnant. Today was the eighteenth day of her luteal phase.*

*When I finally looked up, my eyes caught Zoey's, and both of us started laughing. Alex just didn't get it. He said, "Toni, are you laughing for the reason I think you're laughing?" I said, "Well, do you have any other explanation for today's eighteenth high temp?" The light bulb finally went off, and he understood. At last, after a year of trying, they got pregnant the first cycle they charted.*

As you've seen, a general rule is that 18 high temperatures means you are pregnant (see Chart 11.6). And you can determine this without spending a dime on a pregnancy test (though it is advisable to confirm it with a clinician). In addition, you can usually tell even *before* 18 high temperatures whether you are pregnant by two means:

**1.** You can be fairly confident you are pregnant if your temperatures remain high 3 days beyond your longest luteal phase to date. For example, if your luteal phases are typically 12 days, and if your longest one has been 13 days, but one time it is 16 days, it is likely that you conceived that cycle. (Charts 11.9a and 11.9b)

**2.** If you notice a *third* level of temperatures beyond the typical biphasic pattern you experience every cycle, you are almost certainly pregnant. This third level of high temperatures is thought to be due to the extra progesterone circulating in pregnant women. (Unfortunately, not all women experience such a clear-cut triphasic pattern.) (Chart 11.10)

**Chart 11.9a. A typical 13-day luteal phase.** Sara has been charting as a method of birth control for about a year. Her luteal phases have always been 12 or 13 days, never more.

**Chart 11.9b. A pregnancy chart.** The first cycle Sara tried to get pregnant, she was able to tell she succeeded as soon as her 16th postovulatory high temperature (by Day 31), because she knew that her normal luteal phase never extended beyond 13 days.

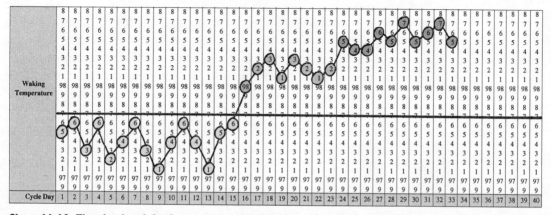

**Chart 11.10. The classic triphasic pregnancy pattern.** Note that Jenny was able to predict as early as Day 24 that she was pregnant because she was starting to observe a third level of high temperatures reflecting additional progesterone at the time of implantation. The fertilized egg burrows into the uterine lining about a week after ovulation.

## ❧ USING A COVERLINE

In order to interpret your chart, you'll want to draw a coverline to help you differentiate between low and high temperatures. You should review page 73 if you have not already internalized how to draw one. While the coverline is not as critical for pregnancy achievement as it is for contraceptive purposes, it is still a useful tool that will allow you to see more easily when you ovulated in any given cycle.

## ❧ MALE FERTILITY

You now understand why basal temperatures are so revealing for pregnancy achievement. And of course you already learned how critical cervical fluid is for conception to occur. But before you combine this information into an efficient strategy to use with FAM, you should at least know some basic information about male fertility and the standard semen analysis.

It's important to remember that in determining sperm count, the analysis of your partner's semen must do more than simply measure the number of sperm per ejaculate. It should also tell you what percentage of those sperm are of normal shape and size (morphology) and what percentage are rapidly moving forward (motility). It is a complete analysis of these three factors that actually tells you whether your partner's count is normal, low, or infertile, thus allowing you to strategize accordingly. In reality this is quite intuitive, for what ultimately defines male fertility is the number of sperm that have the capacity to fertilize an ovum.

As of this writing, his sperm count would probably be considered low if the total number of sperm per ejaculate fell below 50 million. It would also be considered low if less than 60% of the sperm were of normal morphology, or if less than 60% were of normal motility. In addition, a concentration of less than 20 million sperm per milliliter is considered low, regardless of the total ejaculatory volume.

I must caution, however, that the standards by which sperm counts are judged continue to evolve. Therefore, if your partner decides to get a sperm analysis, you should insist that his physician answer two questions as clearly as possible:

1. Is his sperm count considered normal, low, or infertile?
2. How did the lab reach this conclusion?

# THE THREE PRIMARY FERTILITY SIGNS

## WAKING TEMPERATURE

| 5 | 5 | 5 | 5 | 5 | 5 | 5 | 5 | 5 | 5 | 5 | 5 | 5 | 5 | 5 | 5 | 5 | 5 | 5 | 5 | 5 | 5 | 5 | 5 | 5 | 5 | 5 | 5 | 5 | 5 | 5 |
|---|---|---|---|---|---|---|---|---|---|---|---|---|---|---|---|---|---|---|---|---|---|---|---|---|---|---|---|---|---|---|
| 4 | 4 | 4 | 4 | 4 | 4 | 4 | 4 | 4 | 4 | 4 | 4 | 4 | 4 | 4 | 4 | 4 | 4 | 4 | 4 | 4 | 4 | 4 | 4 | 4 | 4 | 4 | 4 | 4 | 4 | 4 |
| 3 | 3 | 3 | 3 | 3 | 3 | 3 | 3 | 3 | 3 | 3 | 3 | 3 | 3 | 3 | 3 | 3 | 3 | 3 | 3 | 3 | 3 | 3 | 3 | 3 | 3 | 3 | 3 | 3 | 3 | 3 |
| 2 | 2 | 2 | 2 | 2 | 2 | 2 | 2 | 2 | 2 | 2 | 2 | 2 | 2 | 2 | 2 | 2 | 2 | 2 | 2 | 2 | 2 | 2 | 2 | 2 | 2 | 2 | 2 | 2 | 2 | 2 |
| 1 | 1 | 1 | 1 | 1 | 1 | 1 | 1 | 1 | 1 | 1 | 1 | 1 | 1 | 1 | 1 | 1 | 1 | 1 | 1 | 1 | 1 | 1 | 1 | 1 | 1 | 1 | 1 | 1 | 1 | 1 |
| 98 | 98 | 98 | 98 | 98 | 98 | 98 | 98 | 98 | 98 | 98 | 98 | 98 | 98 | 98 | 98 | 98 | 98 | 98 | 98 | 98 | 98 | 98 | 98 | 98 | 98 | 98 | 98 | 98 | 98 | 98 |
| 9 | 9 | 9 | 9 | 9 | 9 | 9 | 9 | 9 | 9 | 9 | 9 | 9 | 9 | 9 | 9 | 9 | 9 | 9 | 9 | 9 | 9 | 9 | 9 | 9 | 9 | 9 | 9 | 9 | 9 | 9 |
| 8 | 8 | 8 | 8 | 8 | 8 | 8 | 8 | 8 | 8 | 8 | 8 | 8 | 8 | 8 | 8 | 8 | 8 | 8 | 8 | 8 | 8 | 8 | 8 | 8 | 8 | 8 | 8 | 8 | 8 | 8 |
| 7 | 7 | 7 | 7 | 7 | 7 | 7 | 7 | 7 | 7 | 7 | 7 | 7 | 7 | 7 | 7 | 7 | 7 | 7 | 7 | 7 | 7 | 7 | 7 | 7 | 7 | 7 | 7 | 7 | 7 | 7 |
| 6 | 6 | 6 | 6 | 6 | 6 | 6 | 6 | 6 | 6 | 6 | 6 | 6 | 6 | 6 | 6 | 6 | 6 | 6 | 6 | 6 | 6 | 6 | 6 | 6 | 6 | 6 | 6 | 6 | 6 | 6 |
| 5 | 5 | 5 | 5 | 5 | 5 | 5 | 5 | 5 | 5 | 5 | 5 | 5 | 5 | 5 | 5 | 5 | 5 | 5 | 5 | 5 | 5 | 5 | 5 | 5 | 5 | 5 | 5 | 5 | 5 | 5 |
| 4 | 4 | 4 | 4 | 4 | 4 | 4 | 4 | 4 | 4 | 4 | 4 | 4 | 4 | 4 | 4 | 4 | 4 | 4 | 4 | 4 | 4 | 4 | 4 | 4 | 4 | 4 | 4 | 4 | 4 | 4 |
| 3 | 3 | 3 | 3 | 3 | 3 | 3 | 3 | 3 | 3 | 3 | 3 | 3 | 3 | 3 | 3 | 3 | 3 | 3 | 3 | 3 | 3 | 3 | 3 | 3 | 3 | 3 | 3 | 3 | 3 | 3 |
| 2 | 2 | 2 | 2 | 2 | 2 | 2 | 2 | 2 | 2 | 2 | 2 | 2 | 2 | 2 | 2 | 2 | 2 | 2 | 2 | 2 | 2 | 2 | 2 | 2 | 2 | 2 | 2 | 2 | 2 | 2 |
| 1 | 1 | 1 | 1 | 1 | 1 | 1 | 1 | 1 | 1 | 1 | 1 | 1 | 1 | 1 | 1 | 1 | 1 | 1 | 1 | 1 | 1 | 1 | 1 | 1 | 1 | 1 | 1 | 1 | 1 | 1 |
| 97 | 97 | 97 | 97 | 97 | 97 | 97 | 97 | 97 | 97 | 97 | 97 | 97 | 97 | 97 | 97 | 97 | 97 | 97 | 97 | 97 | 97 | 97 | 97 | 97 | 97 | 97 | 97 | 97 | 97 | 97 |
| 9 | 9 | 9 | 9 | 9 | 9 | 9 | 9 | 9 | 9 | 9 | 9 | 9 | 9 | 9 | 9 | 9 | 9 | 9 | 9 | 9 | 9 | 9 | 9 | 9 | 9 | 9 | 9 | 9 | 9 | 9 |
| 1 | 2 | 3 | 4 | 5 | 6 | 7 | 8 | 9 | 10 | 11 | 12 | 13 | 14 | 15 | 16 | 17 | 18 | 19 | 20 | 21 | 22 | 23 | 24 | 25 | 26 | 27 | 28 | 29 | 30 | 31 |

## CERVICAL FLUID

## CERVICAL POSITION

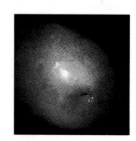

The chart and pictures above reflect the three primary fertility signs of one woman's cycle, which in this case was 30 days in length. These photos were taken on Days 12, 17, and 20. As she approaches ovulation around Day 17, increasing levels of estrogen cause her cervical fluid to become progressively wetter, developing into a pattern similar to the top photographs on the back of this page. In addition, her cervix becomes soft, high, and dramatically open. But quickly after ovulation, the strong effects of progesterone replace the influence of estrogen. Thus, her temperature shifts upward, her cervical fluid dries up, and her cervix reverts back to firm, low, and closed. (For the bottom pictures, her cervical fluid was removed so as not to obscure the opening. Also, note that the photos are unable to reflect the height of the cervix within the body, although they do reveal an obvious difference in its angle after ovulation.)

# TYPES OF CERVICAL FLUID

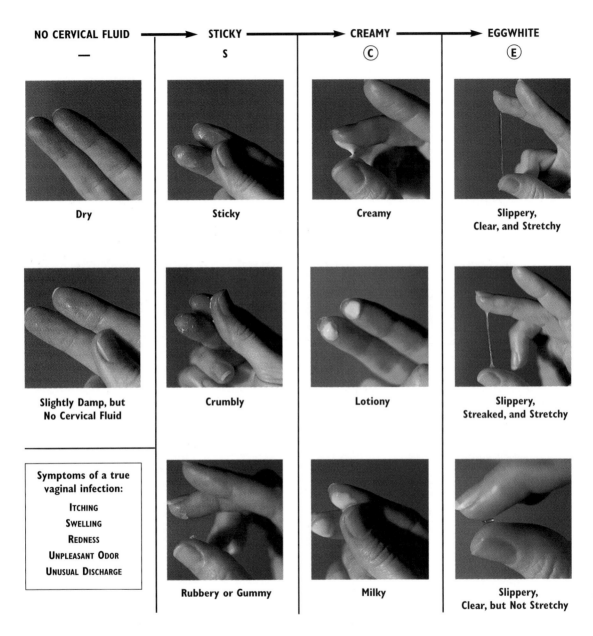

| NO CERVICAL FLUID → | STICKY → | CREAMY → | EGGWHITE |
|---|---|---|---|
| — | S | Ⓒ | Ⓔ |
| Dry | Sticky | Creamy | Slippery, Clear, and Stretchy |
| Slightly Damp, but No Cervical Fluid | Crumbly | Lotiony | Slippery, Streaked, and Stretchy |
| **Symptoms of a true vaginal infection:** ITCHING SWELLING REDNESS UNPLEASANT ODOR UNUSUAL DISCHARGE | Rubbery or Gummy | Milky | Slippery, Clear, but Not Stretchy |

Most women tend to be dry for a few days after menstruation, but as they approach ovulation their cervical fluid becomes increasingly wetter. The above photographs show healthy variations in what women may experience. Symptoms of a true vaginal infection are shown in the box to the bottom left. A woman's Peak Day of fertility is the last day of a slippery, lubricative-quality cervical fluid or vaginal sensation.

### Seeing the Forest Through the Trees

Note the obvious pattern of thermal shifts indicating ovulation in three of the author's charts, placed side by side. Even though there are a few temperatures that appear out-of-line or even missing, you can clearly see a pattern of lows before ovulation (blue) and highs after ovulation (pink).

### The Ferning of Fertile Cervical Fluid

When viewed under a microscope, the stretchy-type cervical fluid in the pictures on the opposite page look like a beautiful ferning pattern conducive to sperm motility (*left, above*). The drier, sticky types of cervical fluid do not have such a magical appearance (*right, above*).

### The Most Fertile-Quality Cervical Fluid

Fertile eggwhite-type cervical fluid exudes from this woman's open cervix right before ovulation.

# THE BEAUTY OF REPRODUCTIVE BIOLOGY

### The Drama of Ovulation
In the top photograph, the egg is just beginning to burrow through the ovarian wall. By the bottom the ovulatory process is almost complete.

### The Life of an Ovum
In the illustration above, a tiny egg within the ovary slowly develops its own follicle (red). After completely maturing, it bursts out of the follicle and through the ovarian wall, in the most significant event of the menstrual cycle: ovulation. In most cases, the just-released egg (blue) will continue on its journey, moving forward through the waiting fallopian tube.

The follicular material left behind in the ovary will soon form the corpus luteum (yellow), which emits progesterone. If fertilization does not occur, it will die within 12 to 16 days, causing progesterone levels to plummet and menstruation to follow.

If intercourse occurs in the short fertile phase surrounding ovulation, the sperm can meet the newly released egg within the tube, where fertilization takes place. The fertilized egg then continues the journey, implanting in the lining of the uterus about a week later.

# YOUR BODY, YOUR CYCLE: OVULATION IN PERSPECTIVE

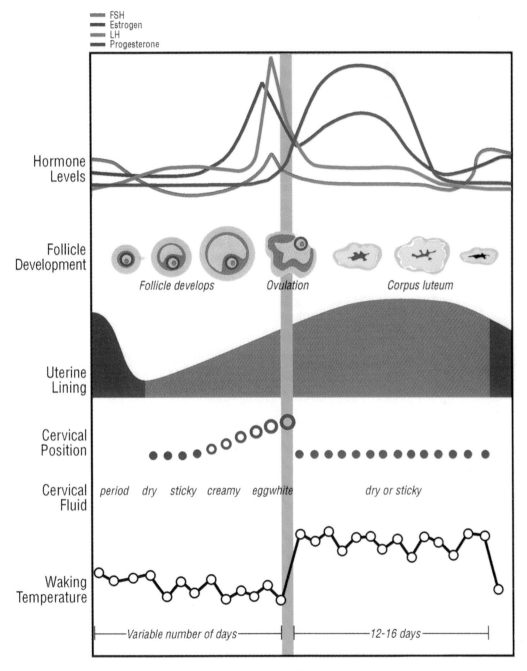

Note that the length of the phase before ovulation can vary widely, but the phase after ovulation is almost always 12 to 16 days. Within *individual* women, the postovulatory phase is remarkably consistent, usually not varying more than a day or so.

## The Journey Continues

The newly released egg begins its voyage down the fallopian tube. Fertilization must occur within the egg's short life-span, which may be up to 24 hours, though 6 to 12 hours is more likely for any given egg. It is for this reason that the vast majority of conceptions are assumed to result from *preovulatory* intercourse. Unlike the egg, sperm can survive several days, but only if fertile-quality cervical fluid is initially present to serve as a medium.

**Stretching the Concept of Perfect Timing**
To see how the cervical fluid (*far left*) led to the conception of this little guy, see page 17.

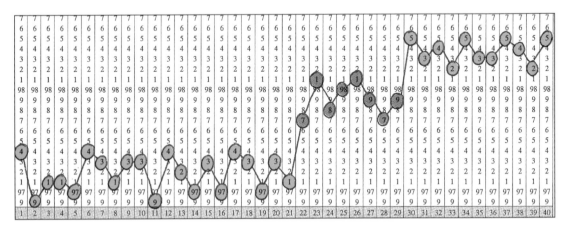

## A Triphasic Pregnancy Chart

When a woman becomes pregnant, her temperature pattern often evolves into three levels, as can be seen by the three colors above. The second level is the result of the progesterone released after ovulation, while the third level is thought to be the result of the pregnancy hormone HCG, which circulates after implantation. Note that this woman ovulated about Day 21, not Day 14, as seen by the fact that her thermal shift didn't occur until Day 22.

## A Typical Pregnancy Wheel

The calculating device to the left is considered indispensable in determining a woman's due date. However, it is often inaccurate since it assumes that all women ovulate on Day 14, regardless of when they really do. This wheel is set for a woman whose first cycle day was February 1st, and thus ovulation was assumed to have occurred on February 14th. In reality, she could have easily ovulated a week or more later, as is seen in the chart on the opposite page. Also note how the due date is referred to as the "Expected Date of Confinement," one of many curious terms discussed in Appendix L.

## Alternative Chart for Recording Exercise and Secondary Signs Such as PMS and Ovulatory Pain

Charting your cycle can be beneficial for reasons beyond merely identifying your fertility. In the chart to the right, the woman records when she exercises as well as various secondary signs such as cramps and headaches, using colors to make her chart more graphic. This woman is able to track pre-menstrual and menstrual cramps as well as pain after intercourse, two possible symptoms of endometriosis. Color-coding this way will help her doctor better diagnose her condition. Additionally, she circles BSE for the breast self-exam she does on Day 7 of every cycle. A master copy of this chart with 6 blank rows for color-coding can be found in Appendix J.

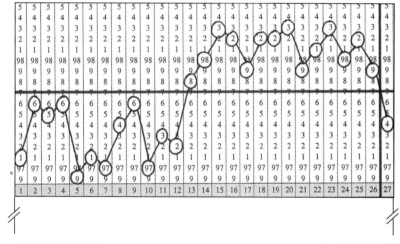

# JANE RESPONSIBLE'S CHART

## Fertility Cycle # 7

Last 12 Cycles: Shortest **27** Longest **32** Month **August - September** Year **'94** This cycle length: **30**

A blank master of this chart is on the last page of the book. The following key reflects this particular cycle's fertile days. Of course, cycles will vary, which is why consistently charting is so important.

Fertile phase   Infertile phase   Most fertile days

If a man's sperm count is subfertile, the analysis will be repeated at least one or two more times within a few weeks of each other. This is because different factors may impact sperm, and an occasional low sperm count may be an inaccurate reflection of his normal sperm.*

## OPTIMIZING YOUR CHANCES OF GETTING PREGNANT

If you are just starting to try to get pregnant, there's no particular reason for your partner to rush out and have a semen analysis. *Unless you have reason to think otherwise, you should tentatively consider his sperm count normal and follow the guidelines listed below for normal counts.* However, for those who have been trying at random for a year, or have been timing intercourse by charting for about four cycles, I would encourage you to have a sperm analysis as soon as possible. Sperm tests are a simple enough procedure and it's worth doing soon, since its results will help you know how to best time intercourse. Remember, fertility problems are equally divided between men and women.

Now you are ready for the nuts and bolts of maximizing your chances of pregnancy. This is the most practical part of the chapter on getting pregnant. The bottom line is that when deciding how to best time intercourse, the frequency with which you make love should be a function of your combined fertility. That is, it should be determined by your partner's sperm count and the timing of your fertile cervical fluid.†

### *If the Man's Sperm Count Is Normal*

Under these circumstances, you should have intercourse every day that you have wet cervical fluid or vaginal sensation, through to and including the day of the first rise in temperature. Of course, the closer you time intercourse to your Peak Day (the last day of wetness, as described on page 83), the more likely you are to conceive.

---

* One of the troubling realities of contemporary life is that men's sperm counts have plunged by about 50% since the 1930s. It's unclear what is causing this, but some theorize that it may be due to modern environmental toxins.

† Reread Chapters 5 and 6 if you don't remember how to identify the fertile cervical fluid necessary for conception to occur.

**Chart 11.11. When to time intercourse with normal sperm count.** Note that this couple started timing intercourse the first day she noticed wet (creamy) cervical fluid on Day 17, and continued every day through to the morning of the rise in temperature on Day 20. They were able to confirm that they succeeded 18 high temperatures later, by Day 37.

## If the Man's Sperm Count Is Low

You should have intercourse every *other* day that you have eggwhite cervical fluid *or* a wet vaginal sensation, through to and including the day of the first rise in temperature (if you don't have eggwhite, follow this guideline with the wettest cervical fluid you have). The reason you should have intercourse less frequently is because men with low sperm counts need the extra day to build up to higher, more fertile levels. (Chart 11.12)

Another way to increase your chances even more if the man's sperm count is low is the following: If you can, try to observe how many days you tend to have the most fertile-quality cervical fluid each cycle. For example, if you notice that you tend to have only two days of creamy cervical fluid (with no eggwhite) and your partner's sperm count is low, wait until the *second* day of creamy to have intercourse. This optimizes your chances the most, because the last day of creamy is considered the most fertile day of your particular cycle. By waiting until that day, you have allowed the sperm count to build up enough to maximize your chances of a pregnancy. (Chart 11.13)

**Chart 11.12. When to time intercourse with low sperm count.** Note that this couple started having intercourse the first day she noticed eggwhite on Day 12, but then had sex only every other day through to the morning of the rise in temperature on Day 16. This allowed the sperm count to build up on the "off days." They were able to confirm that they succeeded 18 high temperatures later, by Day 33.

**Chart 11.13. Maximizing your chances of conception when your partner's sperm count is low and you have minimal fertile cervical fluid.** Note that she only has about 2 days of creamy cervical fluid per cycle. Since his sperm count is low, they chose to time intercourse on the second and last day of her creamy cervical fluid, optimizing their chances of pregnancy by reserving the highest number of sperm for her Peak Day of fertility. They were able to confirm that they succeeded 18 high temperatures later, by Day 30.

The following table will summarize the best strategy for getting pregnant assuming two conditions:

a. You tend to observe a fairly consistent number of fertile days each cycle (i.e., creamy or eggwhite cervical fluid or lubricative vaginal sensation).
b. Your partner has a low sperm count.

| BEST STRATEGY FOR GETTING PREGNANT IF YOUR PARTNER HAS LOW SPERM COUNT | |
| --- | --- |
| **Typical Number of Fertile Days You Have Each Cycle (i.e., creamy, eggwhite, or lubricative vaginal sensation)** | **Strategy** |
| 1 fertile day | Only day—Have intercourse |
| 2 fertile days | 1st day—Abstain<br>2nd day—Have intercourse |
| 3 fertile days | 1st day—Have intercourse<br>2nd day—Abstain<br>3rd day—Have intercourse |
| 4 fertile days | 1st day—Abstain<br>2nd day—Have intercourse<br>3rd day—Abstain<br>4th day—Have intercourse |

It requires a certain amount of discipline to be able to pass up an opportunity to have sex on a day of eggwhite, knowing full well that eggwhite is the most fertile-quality cervical fluid on the continuum. But the principle is to consider the combined fertility of the two of you. If your partner's sperm count is low, you'll want to increase your chances by making sure that it is high enough on the *last* day of the most fertile cervical fluid or vaginal sensation, since that day is the closest fertile day to ovulation.

## If the Man's Sperm Count Reveals That He Is Infertile

The good news is that with today's advanced technologies, there is still hope for a pregnancy. See Chapter 14 for high-tech treatments.

## *Tips That Apply to Men with Both Normal or Marginal Sperm Quality*

A tip that may help men with either type of sperm count is to abstain from any ejaculation for at least a few days just before your cervical fluid begins to appear fertile. Of course, you may think this is like telling your mate to get off the bus at the stop before you. How would he know ahead of time when that is? But if you are really in tune with your body, you will be able to anticipate when it just begins to become slightly fertile. He should try to abstain from any type of ejaculation for those few "barely fertile" sticky days to build up a high enough count to take advantage of your ideal cervical fluid.

If you still haven't gotten pregnant after several months of trying this strategy, you may want to modify it slightly. In other words, those who had intercourse every day should try having intercourse every *other* day during your fertile cervical fluid. And those who had intercourse every 48 hours may want to try it every 36 hours instead.

Finally, most of the sperm is in the first spurt of ejaculate. Therefore, the man should try to penetrate deeply and remain still while ejaculating so that the majority of sperm will be deposited at the cervix, allowing easy access to the cervical opening.

## *A Note About the Semen Emitting Technique (Kegels)*

In order to time intercourse most effectively, you should eliminate residual semen so that it won't mask your cervical fluid in the following days. This is easily done by doing Kegels a few hours after sex. Those sperm with potential to fertilize will then have had all the time they need to get beyond the cervix.

## *Why to Include the Day of the Rise in Temperatures for Intercourse*

Given that you have already learned it is generally too late to conceive after the thermal shift has occurred, you may be wondering why I still suggest intercourse up through that very day. This is because there is still a small chance of conception due to several factors. A multiple ovulation may allow for another egg to still be viable, and there is even a slight possibility of a single ovulation occurring right after the shift. There is also a decent chance that the egg is still alive if ovulation occurred within the previous 12 hours. While odds are not good, it's still worth trying, particularly if you have intercourse the *morning* of the rise.

*Sexual Frequency: Maximizing Your Odds*

The number of days per cycle that you should have intercourse will be a function of your combined fertility. A woman will generally have fertile cervical fluid for 2 to 4 days. Depending on the man's fertility, you should take advantage of each of those days or just every other one. *The critical point is to include the Peak Day, which is the last day of eggwhite or lubricative vaginal sensation.* This day is considered the most fertile because it generally occurs either on the day you ovulate or the day before. Note that if you don't observe eggwhite, you should try for the last day of the wettest-quality cervical fluid you do have.

What that means, practically speaking, is the following: if you see eggwhite on Monday and take advantage of it by having intercourse that day—great. But, if you still see eggwhite that following Wednesday, have intercourse again, because the ovum has probably not yet been released, and you are still extremely fertile. (Of course, Tuesday would have also been a good day to try, assuming your partner's sperm count is normal.)

**Chart 11.14. Going for the gold . . . got it!**

## ✺ WHEN THE LONG-AWAITED PREGNANCY OCCURS

Once your temperatures remain above the coverline for at least 18 days and you have not gotten your period, you are almost certainly pregnant.*

### *Pregnancy Symptoms*

Beside the obvious 18 high temperatures above the coverline, there are often other signs of pregnancy, including:

- tender breasts or nipples
- nausea
- fatigue
- excessive urination
- light bleeding about 8 days after ovulation and/or around the time of your expected period, usually referred to as implantation spotting. It's typically caused by the fertilized egg burrowing into the endometrial lining.

---

* The one rare exception when 18 high temperatures may not reflect a pregnancy is in the case of a corpus luteum cyst, as discussed on page 280.

*False-Negative Pregnancy Tests*

Pregnant women may occasionally have a false-negative pregnancy test, meaning that they are in fact pregnant, but the test indicates they aren't. The most common reason for false-negative pregnancy tests is that they are performed too early, before the egg has had a chance to implant and start producing the pregnancy hormone HCG. In some cases, implantation may have occurred, but it may still be too early for the HCG to be detected. In either case, if your temperatures continue to remain above the coverline beyond 18 days, simply repeat the pregnancy test a week later, and it will almost certainly reflect a positive result.

## ❧ CONCLUDING REMARKS ON GETTING PREGNANT

As you've read, couples are usually told to see a physician if they haven't gotten pregnant within a year of trying. By now you should realize how unnecessary it is to wait a full year *if* you've been timing intercourse precisely. So if you have not gotten pregnant after 4 to 6 cycles of intercourse during your most fertile days, you should carefully read Chapter 14 to see what diagnostic tests and treatments to consider.

If, however, this chapter helps you to attain your dream of a healthy pregnancy, then congratulations! The joy that you'll receive will no doubt bring you bittersweet rewards to last a lifetime. As Elizabeth Stone once said, "Making the decision to have a child . . . is to decide forever to have your heart go walking around outside your body."

### SUMMARY OF WAYS TO OPTIMIZE CHANCES OF GETTING PREGNANT

1. The most important tip for getting pregnant is to have intercourse on the Peak Day, which is the *last day* of eggwhite cervical fluid or lubricative vaginal sensation. (If you don't observe eggwhite, try for the last day of the wettest cervical fluid you have.)
2. If your partner's sperm count is normal, have intercourse every day you have fertile cervical fluid. If his sperm count is low, have intercourse every *other* day that you have fertile cervical fluid. In either case, try to have sex through to and including the first morning of your rise in temperature.

# CHAPTER 12

# Practical Tips Beyond Fertility Awareness

eyond using the principles of Fertility Awareness to time intercourse most efficiently, there are a number of tricks that can help you conceive. Most are things to avoid, but some are positive things you can do. All of them should be considered in light of your own personal situation. Because so many of the tips deal with the interplay between diet and conception, you may want to explore this topic more thoroughly in Marilyn Shannon's book *Fertility, Cycles and Nutrition* (Couple to Couple League International, Inc., 1992).

## 〰 LUBRICANTS

Avoid artificial lubricants or vegetable oils when having intercourse, because these products often contain chemicals that kill sperm. Don't use petroleum jelly because it isn't water soluble. Even plain glycerin, once touted to be the only harmless lubricant, can kill sperm. Surprisingly, even saliva can act as a spermicide. The only product that *seems* to provide necessary lubrication without harming sperm is *real* eggwhite, as in "eggs over easy." Unfortunately, even this tends to obscure your cervical fluid, making it difficult to identify when you are at your peak fertility. Ideally you should take it slowly, so you can take advantage of your own natural sexual lubrication.

## 〰 POSITIONS DURING INTERCOURSE

Although no definitive studies appear to have been done, there is considerable speculation that if the man has a marginal sperm count, the best position for intercourse is the traditional missionary position. This allows for deepest penetration, and will thus deposit the sperm closest to the cervix. Some clinicians also believe that if your cervical fluid is not that fertile, or the sperm quality is marginal, it may be advantageous for you to remain lying down for up to half an hour in the basic position in which you had intercourse. The theory is that this will help assure the sperm time to travel up.

## ॐ HEALTHY DIET, WEIGHT, AND EXERCISE

You've probably heard it a million times before, but I'll repeat it again. When trying to get pregnant, your body should be as healthy as possible. This may mean limiting consumption of refined foods, excess sugar, caffeine, and products with additives. All of these can impede the liver's ability to metabolize hormones. Eating a well-balanced diet of wholesome foods can eliminate such potential problems. In addition, there is some speculation that heavy milk consumption may adversely affect fertility.

In order to ovulate, most women need at least 18% body fat. But just as being underweight can prevent ovulation altogether, being overweight can also alter your cycles by causing excessive production of estrogen, which interferes with the normal feedback system of the hormonal cycle. Some of the signs of excessive estrogen are prolonged periods of fertile cervical fluid buildup, delayed ovulation, and irregular cycles. To eliminate hormonal imbalances due to being under- or overweight, you should try to attain a normal weight through wholesome foods and exercise.

## ॐ CAFFEINE, NICOTINE, DRUGS, AND ALCOHOL

If you have unexplainable infertility, you and your partner should both seriously consider reducing or even eliminating caffeine, nicotine, drugs, and alcohol from your diet. In women, tobacco may decrease fertility, and caffeine seems to affect the ability to both conceive and nurture an embryo. Marijuana has been shown to disrupt a woman's ovulatory cycle. And as seen on page 336, antihistamines can dry up cervical fluid and thus interfere with sperm survival. Finally, alcohol is notorious for potentially causing fetal alcohol syndrome in the offspring of mothers who drink while pregnant.

In men, the following products may suppress sperm production: marijuana, tobacco, alcohol, antimalarial drugs, steroids, and ulcer medications.

## ✌ DOUCHES, VAGINAL SPRAYS, AND SCENTED TAMPONS

As you've read in previous pages, douching alters the normal acidity of the vagina and is not necessary for most women. It adversely changes the normal pH balance and can ironically lead to vaginal infections and PID (pelvic inflammatory disease). It can also alter the vaginal environment to such an extent that sperm can't survive. It may cause inflammations or allergic reactions that can kill sperm or impair sperm survival. And finally, it may wash away the very cervical fluid that sperm need to get through the cervix to the egg. Other than that, douching's no problem!

Vaginal sprays and scented tampons can also cause a pH imbalance as well as an allergic reaction to the chemicals used in the products. As you would expect, the resulting imbalance can impede sperm survival.

## ✌ ANTIBIOTICS

If you've ever had to take antibiotics for an extended period of time, you may have the unpleasant memory of battling yeast infections that might have resulted from the regimen. This is because antibiotics are notorious for killing the good bacteria along with the bad, often producing an overgrowth of Candida, a type of yeast that renders the vaginal environment inhospitable to sperm. One of the ways to counter the affects of antibiotics is to eat yogurt with acidophilus or ingest acidophilus tablets, because this replaces the good bacteria killed by the antibiotics. Many clinicians believe that inserting plain yogurt directly into the vagina is the most effective way to fight this type of infection, but women who are trying to get pregnant should never vaginally insert anything that may potentially introduce bacteria.

## ✌ FOR MEN: HOT TUBS, SAUNAS, BICYCLES, AND TIGHT CLOTHING

As you know, sperm are very sensitive to heat. While it's not clear how much is too much, it is wise if you're having problems conceiving to avoid anything that may expose the testes to excess heat. Hot tubs and saunas can be enjoyable, but from the sperm's perspective, it's basically like saying "life's a fish and then you fry."

Bicycling is another activity that may affect sperm counts. The constant bumping of the testes, combined with the added heat generated from sweating in the scrotal area may contribute to diminished sperm counts. If the man's sperm analysis is fine, then by all means, enjoy the daily bike rides. But if the sperm count is marginal, it's one more practical thing you might consider changing.

Even hot work environments may have a harmful effect on sperm production. It should come as no surprise that standing in front of a pizza oven 8 hours a day may not be the most efficient way to build up a sperm count. And finally, as far as the common wisdom to avoid tight underwear and pants—it certainly can't hurt. Obviously, if you find bikini briefs sexier and your partner wants to wear them occasionally to seduce you, more power to him! But he would be wise not to wear them every day.

The bottom line is that until you achieve the pregnancy you desire, you may want to avoid anything that causes the sperm to get too hot. And remember that it may take as long as 2 to 3 months after reducing such exposure for a new generation of healthy sperm to mature.

## ℘ CONDITIONS THAT MAY BE AMENABLE TO NONINVASIVE REMEDIES

There are a number of remedies you may want to try for fertility problems you detect through the Fertility Awareness Method. Many of them involve consulting with a qualified nutritionist, naturopathic doctor, or herbalist for best results.

### Limited Fertile-Quality Cervical Fluid

My professional experience is that one of the most commonly overlooked causes of subfertility is the lack of lubricative, slippery cervical fluid produced during a woman's cycle. Of course, the more days you produce it the more likely you'll be able to get pregnant. Women coming off the Pill are particularly susceptible to this problem. If charting has confirmed that your cervical fluid doesn't seem wet enough, or isn't wet for at least 2 days, there may be a simple remedy available. Before resorting to estrogen supplements or even more involved medical therapies, you might want to try any of the following remedies:

• Avoid drugs that may dry up cervical fluid, such as antihistamines, atropine, belladonna, Clomid (clomiphene citrate), cough mixtures

containing antihistamines, dicyclomine, progesterone, propanthe-
line, and tamoxifen.

- In order to increase the wetness of cervical fluid, you may want to consider using any of the drugs listed in Appendix J. But most of them should only be used with a doctor's prescription and for very specific conditions.

- Consider taking an expectorant found in cough syrups such as Robitussin, which has the active ingredient *guafenesin*. Along with helping to liquefy mucus in the lungs, it also has the added benefit of making your cervical fluid wetter.

- Take 10,000 to 20,000 IU of vitamin A daily. The Couple to Couple League (an NFP organization) has found that some women develop wetter and more fertile fluid with such a regimen. However, you should definitely consult with a qualified nutritionist before taking the vitamins, since an excessive amount is considered toxic (side effects may include such conditions as nausea, skin irritations, and lack of menses).

- Take 10 drops of potassium iodide daily. Dr. Landrum Shettles, the renowned obstetrician and professor, claims that this can dramatically increase the fertility of your cervical fluid. Of course, you'll want to verify with your physician that this is appropriate for you.

- Real eggwhites can be used as a lubricant in cases where the woman herself doesn't produce much fertile-quality cervical fluid; it should be room temperature. While no studies have yet shown that you can actually use it as a substitute, several articles do make clear that it is compatible with sperm viability. This is because both sperm and real eggwhites are made of protein. Of course, you shouldn't try this if you are allergic to eggs.

If these don't work, your doctor may prescribe estrogen supplements to increase the amount and quality of the cervical fluid that you have.

## Short Luteal Phases

If you discover that you have short luteal phases, there are a few steps you may want to take before relying on the traditional medical remedies of Clomid and progesterone prescriptions. Chapter 18 on PMS offers general dietary guidelines that have been shown to be helpful in treating both short luteal phases as well as the symptoms of PMS. Marilyn Shannon suggests that 200 to 600 milligrams a day of vitamin B6 may also help, but I encourage you to consult with a qualified nutritionist first.

### Anovulation Caused by Being Underweight

As mentioned earlier, women who are considered underweight by general nutritional guidelines may not be producing the estrogen required to trigger ovulation. These women may be able to end their anovulatory (and infertile) condition, whether it is caused by excessive exercise or simple undereating. The simplest and best advice is that they gradually gain weight by a combination of healthful diet and moderate exercise.

### Irregular Menstrual Cycles

There are many alternative health practitioners who believe that certain cycle irregularities are easily resolved through the use of herbs. You should consult with a qualified nutritionist or health care provider who has expertise in herbs and their impact on various bodily functions.

### Long Infertile Cycles (Hypothyroidism)

If you are one of those women who suffer from unusually long cycles in which you have extended periods of fertile-quality cervical fluid, you should also observe whether you have low basal-body temperatures. This is because the combination of these three symptoms often indicates low thyroid function (hypothyroidism), a condition that you may be able to treat by simple nutritional supplements. Marilyn Shannon suggests adding iodized salt to your diet, as well as lots of ocean fish, which is an excellent source of the iodine needed to treat the thyroid. She also recommends supplements of vitamins A, B, C, and E, in addition to zinc and selenium. Again, I would encourage you to see a qualified nutritionist before relying on these supplements.

### Repeat Miscarriages

Miscarriages occur at a surprisingly high rate of about one in three pregnancies. If you discover that what you thought was an inability to conceive is in fact a problem of repeated miscarriages, there may be certain steps you can take at home before consulting a physician. To start, you should immediately eliminate smoking, and alcohol and drug consumption, including caffeine. Ideally, all of that should be achieved a few months before a planned conception, as should the attainment of your ideal body weight. If charting reveals that you have short luteal phases (10 days or less), you may consider the general dietary guidelines discussed in the chapter on PMS (page 231).

While miscarriage problems may be remedied by dietary changes, I do not mean to minimize the importance of seeking a physician's diagnosis in dealing with this issue, especially if it occurs more than once. In learning to chart and recognize the miscarriages when they occur, you have already gone far in helping the doctor guide you to a healthy pregnancy (see page 189 for more on miscarriages).

## 🕉 FOR MEN

### *Low Sperm Count*

Unless clearly dealing with a case of blockage only treatable by surgery, there are several noninvasive treatments that men with subfertile sperm counts may want to consider before moving on to more serious medical procedures. Just remember that most everything a man tries on his own will probably not be detected in the ejaculate for 2 to 3 months. This is because it takes that long for newly created sperm to reach maturity.

Mild cases of zinc deficiency have been implicated in some low sperm counts. This is because the highest concentrations of zinc in the body are found in sperm and the prostate gland. Studies also suggest that a deficiency in Vitamin A or B, and even selenium, can similarly affect male fertility. Almost half of the man's supply of selenium is located in the testicles and seminal ducts next to the prostate. For recommendations on dosages, consult a nutritionist.

Arginine is considered a nonessential amino acid, yet it seems to help a number of men with this problem. Specifically, studies have shown that taking an oral dose of 4 grams a day of pure, powdered arginine dissolved in water can markedly increase sperm count and motility in some men.

Finally, low sperm count may be remedied by making some simple changes. As mentioned earlier, Jacuzzis, tight clothes, or anything else that may cause excess testicular heat should be avoided as much as possible. And perhaps the most obvious but overlooked change is to simply make sure that ejaculations are kept to a maximum frequency of once every 48 hours. For men with marginal counts, this may be all that is necessary to bring it up to normal.

## Sperm Agglutination

One of the most dramatic results of a fertility study was that of men with a condition called sperm agglutination (or clumping of sperm). Twenty-seven men who had this problem were divided into two groups. One group of 20 men each received 1,000 mg a day of a Vitamin C pill containing calcium, magnesium, and manganese. Every single man in that group got his wife pregnant during the study! By contrast, not one of the men in the control group was able to impregnate his spouse. Although the study was small, the results were striking. So if your partner is diagnosed with sperm agglutination, you'll certainly want to discuss this potential remedy with his doctor.

## 🌿 OTHER FACTORS TO CONSIDER

### Age

One of the most important reasons for the prevalence of subfertility is the relatively late age at which many people today attempt to start having children. The unfortunate biological reality is that as women reach their mid-30s, their infertility risk increases dramatically.

There are several reasons why couples in their 30s face a greater possibility of lower fertility. Some factors are easily remedied through simple education, while others are a regrettable function of biology. One of the most fundamental and easily rectified reasons for impaired fertility is that as couples age together, they tend to have intercourse less frequently, thus decreasing their odds of conception. While the average pair in their mid-20s may have sex up to three times a week, it's believed that typical couples in their mid-30s have intercourse twice weekly or less. Of course, charting would help them time their lovemaking to fully compensate for their possible decline in sexual frequency. Two acts of intercourse on perfectly timed days easily beat a dozen randomly performed acts throughout the entire cycle.

There are physiological changes that also affect overall fertility rates. As women age, the quantity and quality of fertile cervical fluid tends to decline. I've noticed that women in their 20s will generally have 2 to 4 days of eggwhite, while women approaching their late 30s will often have a day or less. This decline can lead to impaired fertility if intercourse is not timed properly. In addition, as women enter their late 30s, they tend to have more anovulatory cycles, and often those in which the egg is released have shorter luteal phases.

Unfortunately, what may be the most important age factor is not the ability of older women to conceive, but rather the odds of the fertilized egg surviving implantation. Research now shows that as women grow older, the percent of conceptions that end in miscarriage rises dramatically. This is certainly true for those pregnancies of which the woman is aware. But perhaps more significantly, there is strong evidence that as women approach 35, extremely early miscarriages occur more and more frequently. By her 40s, the average woman may face a 50% miscarriage rate, most of which are not detected.

What is not clear is the exact cause of this increase in miscarriages as women get older. There is some speculation that the mother's ability to nurture the egg is compromised as she ages. What appears more likely is that the older eggs themselves become increasingly less able to survive after fertilization. There is also the possibility that as men age, their sperm contribute to the increased risk of fetal loss. Whatever the precise reason, couples who delay having children until their 30s will unfortunately face a progressively greater risk of reproductive difficulties. And while both FAM and various high-tech strategies may help shift the odds back in your favor, you should know that it's definitely easier to conceive a child and carry it to term in your 20s than it is in your mid-30s or later.

## Stress

One of the most damaging reproductive myths is that stress leads to infertility. While there is no doubt that stress is associated with diminished fertility, the opposite appears to be more accurate—that is, infertility leads to stress. So the old adage "Just relax and you'll get pregnant" is well meaning but generally misguided.

There are several ways, though, in which stress can indirectly influence fertility. One is simply that leading a busy life and all the stress that entails may leave little time or energy for a couple to actually have intercourse frequently enough to achieve pregnancy. (Of course, as you now know, intercourse doesn't need to be frequent as long as it is well timed.)

A second way is that stress itself may affect when ovulation occurs. In fact, one of the most common causes of delayed ovulation is both physiological and psychological stress. This is because stress can dramatically affect the functioning of the hypothalamus, that gland in the brain responsible for so much of the reproductive system. It is the hypothalamus that is responsible for the regulation of appetite, temperature, and most important, emotions. It also regulates the pituitary gland, which in turn is responsible for the release of FSH and LH. When stress affects the hypothalamus, the end result can be delayed emission of these reproductive hormones, which are necessary for the release of a mature ovum. (It is not known what triggers an early ovulation, but stress does not appear to play a role.)

As you know, the timing of ovulation will determine the length of the cycle—the later it occurs, the longer the cycle will be. Occasionally, if stress is severe, it can actually prevent ovulation from occurring altogether. If stress were to affect your cycle, then one of two things would probably happen:

**1.** You would have a longer-than-average cycle, with ovulation occurring later than usual and menstruation following 12 to 16 days beyond, if pregnancy did not occur. (Chart 12.1)

**2.** You would have a long cycle, but wouldn't release an egg (an anovulatory cycle). If this were the case, the cycle could theoretically

**Chart 12.1. A long cycle due to stress.** With her in-laws arriving for a week, is it any wonder that Shelly had a delayed ovulation leading to a long cycle? Note that she started to prepare to ovulate about the time they arrived, but didn't actually do so until after they left, about Day 22.

**Chart 12.2. Anovulatory cycle due to stress.** Note that Talia's body started to prepare to ovulate about Day 15, but then she broke her leg skiing. A couple of weeks later, as she was finally starting to recover and prepare again to ovulate, her basement flooded. At this point, her body decided to throw in the towel and not release an egg at all. On Day 40, she had anovulatory bleeding rather than a true menstrual period.

extend for months. Or you would have a long cycle followed by anovulatory bleeding, which is the result of a drop in estrogen (as opposed to progesterone). Remember that in an ovulatory cycle, the corpus luteum dies, and the sudden drop in progesterone causes the uterine lining to shed. But with anovulatory cycles, it is the drop in estrogen that usually causes the bleeding. (Chart 12.2)

While it is true that stress can prevent ovulation, it more commonly delays it. For this reason, it is especially important to learn to focus on the signs that indicate *approaching* ovulation. That way, if stress is causing delayed ovulation, you can at least take control by identifying when you are about to ovulate, and thus take advantage of the most fertile time. Of course, the sign that indicates impending ovulation is the wet cervical fluid (especially eggwhite quality) that develops just before you release an egg.

One of the ironies of how stress and the desire to get pregnant can interact is that couples may inadvertently prevent pregnancy by focusing on the mythical Day 14. For example, in women who usually have average-length cycles, a vicious circle can develop in which the stress of continually not achieving pregnancy may only delay ovulation. This in itself wouldn't be a problem, if the couple were taught how to identify when the woman was about to ovulate.

In women who typically have longer cycles, stress may not be delaying ovulation at all. However, if the couple is unaware of when the woman does ovulate, they may be having intercourse too early for conception to occur, thus subjecting themselves to the needless anxiety of misperceived infertility. With both examples, the most constructive advice is not a well-meaning admonition to "just relax." Rather, it would be to tell them to chart their cycles, and then time their lovemaking accordingly. (Chart 12.3)

Stress is also notorious for causing cervical-fluid patches of wetness interspersed with drier days. It's as if the body keeps making attempts to ovulate, but the stress continues to delay it. If this should happen, remember that the temperature will ultimately indicate when you have finally ovulated. So if you

**Chart 12.3. Mistimed intercourse during a long cycle.** Note that ovulation didn't occur until about Day 20. Whether caused by stress or just typical of this woman's cycles, the end result is that intercourse the week before could not result in the conception they sought.

observe patches of slippery- or eggwhite-quality cervical fluid, take advantage of those days until you see the confirmation that ovulation has indeed taken place by a rise in temperature.

You should understand that stress may not necessarily affect a cycle at all, and that it will affect individual women differently. In addition, continual stress may tend to normalize over time, so that the woman's body eventually stops perceiving it as stress, and thus cycles may revert back to the way they were before.

## Synthetic Hormones

Certain synthetic hormones have left a disastrous legacy of reproductive abnormalities on both the women who took them and their offspring. The most notorious of the group is DES, which was taken by pregnant women from the 1940s to 1970s to prevent miscarriages. Many of the daughters of these women have suffered a range of reproductive problems, from malformed uteri to a rare form of vaginal cancer. The sons of these women often have lowered sperm counts and other anomalies. If you are having trouble conceiving and suspect that your mother may have taken DES while pregnant with you, you should consult a doctor who is experienced with the treatment of DES offspring.

Even the Pill occasionally has been implicated in infertility for the simple reason that ovulation may be delayed for months or even years following its use. Charting your cycle will help you determine when your fertility is finally starting to resume again.

## The Jewish Practice of Niddah

As you already know if you are a Jew who observes Niddah, this custom forbids you from having intercourse for 7 days following the last day of your period. If you are an observant Jew who practices Niddah and meet any of the following three conditions, it may be affecting your ability to conceive.

- Your cycles tend to be fairly short (i.e., less than 25 days or so)
- Your cycles are average length but you bleed for at least 7 days
- You have midcycle spotting

The reason the practice may be impeding your ability to get pregnant is that it forbids you from having intercourse during what may be your most fertile phase. For example, if you have cycles of about 24 days, you are probably ovulating about Day 10, but not allowed to resume intercourse again until about Day 13. And even if you have average-length cycles but your periods last 7 days or more, you would again find yourself abstaining until about Day 14 or so, possibly a bit too late for your particular ovulation. Finally, if you happen to be a woman who has occasional midcycle spotting, the Niddah would again require you to abstain at the time you are most likely ovulating.

Needless to say, if you practice Niddah and you would like to conceive, I would highly recommend charting to determine whether this may be the reason you aren't getting pregnant. Then discuss it with your rabbi to see what modifications are acceptable according to Jewish law.

# Lovemaking Versus Babymaking

*Just at the time when you are probably feeling the need for greater closeness with your spouse, the demands of trying to conceive interfere with the pleasure of your physical relationship. The intimacy and enjoyment of sex could help you escape the strain of infertility, but sex serves only as a reminder of the pain. It becomes a revolving door: you end up feeling anxious and frustrated, which is how you felt when you started.*

—LINDA P. SALZER
from *Infertility: How Couples Can Cope*

*D*oes this sound familiar? If you've been trying to get pregnant for a while, it's very likely that you have experienced some of the emotions Linda Salzer communicates above. But so much of the anxiety associated with trying to achieve a pregnancy every cycle could be eliminated if couples were taught exactly when the woman can and cannot get pregnant. Knowing that women can only get pregnant a few days per cycle can actually be a liberating feeling for many couples, in that it leaves the rest of the cycle free for either:

- pure lovemaking, without the pressure of feeling that the entire cycle must be utilized to avoid missing an opportunity to conceive,

or

- choosing not to make love but take a break from the routine of "babymaking."

Sexual problems often arise between couples touched by infertility because sex has taken on one main function: a means of reproduction. What is often lost is the emotional expression of lovemaking—the tenderness, passion, and joy. Charting the woman's cycle can free you once again to be spontaneous and tender for most of the cycle, knowing that you are in control.

Of course, some couples' fertility problems will require high-tech treatment, but ironically, these procedures may actually free them to enjoy lovemaking for what it is—and *not* as a means of conceiving. In essence, the frustration of trying to conceive is no longer theirs to endure, in much the same way that FAM relieves couples of this burden for most of the cycle.

Although a person's sexuality is separate from his or her fertility, society often equates them, leaving many people dealing with infertility to feel that they are somehow less sexual. This is extremely unfortunate since the two are quite different. When couples have sexual problems as a result of their quest to get pregnant, they may experience emotions ranging from unresolved anger and fear to anxiety or guilt. Even worse, communication between them often deteriorates.

## 🖗 MAINTAINING A SENSE OF HUMOR

It may reassure a couple to know that what they are experiencing is absolutely normal. Many endure similar feelings. Having a sense of humor about the stresses on your love life can help pull you through the rough times, as the following illustrates:

*Diana had very irregular cycles, only having ovulated about eight times in the prior 4 years. Because she had excessively high levels of prolactin (the hormone normally present in breastfeeding women), she was prescribed Parlodel and Clomid to regulate her cycles. Along with the drugs and FSH shots, she had several ultrasounds taken. In addition, she would put her legs up on the wall for about an hour after intercourse. After about 6 months of trying, nothing worked. On the advice of her gynecologist, Diana and Steve tried using fresh eggwhites to simulate fertile-quality cervical fluid.*

*Before making love, they removed an egg from the refrigerator, separated it, and inserted the eggwhite into a pastry decorating bag. After Diana comfortably positioned herself, Steve blew the ice-cold eggwhite into her vagina through the pastry bag nozzle. Diana laughed so hard she "farted" from her vagina and all the eggwhite squirted out in one fell swoop. So much for that cycle.*

*During the next cycle they decided to try things a little differently. Having learned their lesson from the first time, they let the egg sit at room temperature first. Then they used an applicator (the type typically used for vaginal cream) to insert the eggwhite. They conceived that day—Mother's Day. Today they have a precious daughter, Tessa.*

Admittedly, it can be hard to maintain a sense of humor amid the pain of infertility. But so many who have survived such frustration often say that it was their sense of humor that pulled them through.

## ❧ SEXUAL PROBLEMS THAT MAY ARISE DURING ATTEMPTS TO CONCEIVE

*When I had my baby, I screamed and screamed. And that was just during conception.*

—JOAN RIVERS

### The Woman

Probably the most common sexual problem women experience while struggling with infertility is a lack of lubrication, which can make intercourse very painful. Just as men may have problems with erections, women may not feel sexual when lovemaking becomes less an expression of affection than a means to attain a goal.

As discussed in the preceding chapter, it is imperative that couples not use artificial sexual lubricants or saliva, since these can actually kill sperm. If they need to, they should only use eggwhites for lubrication. But the ideal would be to make time to tenderly take care of each other with lingering foreplay, allowing your natural lubrication to flow.

### The Man

The impact of a couple's sexual difficulties can strongly affect the man. After all, the pressure is usually on him to achieve an erection and ejaculate during intercourse if conception is to occur, and thus it is not surprising that impotence is the most common problem men face when dealing with infertility.

Impotence is often related to general stress and fatigue, and thus to the extent that infertility brings new stress to life, it is commonly exacerbated during attempts to get pregnant. Of course, the importance of charting in this context is that once men realize that they don't need to perform throughout the cycle, it can take the pressure off during the few days their partner is fertile.

### The Couple

It is ironic but well known that the biggest problem a couple dealing with infertility may have is simple lack of sexual desire. Needless to say, waning sexual interest can be especially problematic when trying to get pregnant. Unfortunately, it can result from the entire range of emotional and physical anxieties that often accompany fertility problems.

If sexual apathy becomes an issue, I would recommend seeing a therapist who can help work through the sexual facets of infertility. I would also highly encourage you to contact your local RESOLVE chapter. It is an excellent organization devoted to meeting the needs of couples struggling with fertility issues. (See Appendix M for the address.)

## 🙠 RECAPTURING THE ESSENCE OF LOVEMAKING

Infertility doesn't have to damage a couple's sexual relationship. In fact, it can have a positive influence and strengthen a couple by drawing them closer through the intimate sharing of their frustrations. Couples often develop a profound respect for each other's strength during such a trying time. Therapists suggest that the first step to revitalize your sexual relationship is to determine when your sexual relationship *was* fulfilling.

Were you more aroused during vacations? Did you feel more attracted to your partner after an intimate talk? A sexy movie? A relaxing dinner? Did you find your sexual relationship more exciting in the beginning of your relationship when you made more conscious efforts to be sexy for your partner?

The key to rekindling sexual desire for your spouse is to try to remember what sparked your passion initially, and purposefully seek to repeat those wonderful moments. One means of doing this is to communicate your desires and frustrations so that you can be sensitive to each other's needs—and move on toward renewing your former sexual relationship.

If you are like most couples struggling with getting pregnant, you may need to work at keeping your relationship alive and stimulating. Find exciting new places to make love. Work at making yourself sexually enticing for your partner. Notice and comment on your partner's attractiveness. And plan special times together—away from the stresses of everyday life.

Perhaps most important, you now have the knowledge to realize that the very notion of babymaking, with all its pressures and implications, need only concern you in the few select days leading up to ovulation. For the rest of the time, you should be able to forget your fertility-related concerns and return to the carefree lovemaking that was, and should always be, a healthy part of your relationship.

# CHAPTER 14

# What Next?
# Tests and Treatments
# That *May* Be Necessary to
# Achieve Pregnancy

*The world is moving so fast these days that the man who says it can't be done is generally interrupted by someone doing it.*
—Elbert Hubbard (1856–1915)

T he most important advice for a couple trying to get pregnant is to chart the woman's cycle as the *first* step. It's astounding how something so fundamental is routinely ignored. Of course, there will be individuals for whom FAM won't be enough to get pregnant. Even then, charting will help determine what testing or treatment is needed, often bypassing inappropriate or unnecessary interventions.

## ❧ FACTORS NECESSARY FOR ACHIEVING PREGNANCY WITHOUT USING HIGH-TECH AIDS

In order to discuss what medical procedures you may need to get pregnant, you should first understand what is required for pregnancy to happen through intercourse alone:

- a woman who is ovulating
- a man who has sufficient sperm production (number, motility, and shape)
- intercourse with ejaculation

- adequate sperm transport and fertilization
- efficient embryo transport and appropriate environment for implantation

Practically speaking, this means that if you have any obvious impediments, such as chronic anovulation or blocked fallopian tubes, I'm afraid the Fertility Awareness Method will not be able to help you. But there are some fertility problems that are still amenable to natural treatments. Believers in holistic remedies would encourage you to consider seeking help through those channels if you feel more comfortable doing so.

When first beginning to chart, you should verify that there are no obstacles to pregnancy that you can clearly identify. This would include anovulation, lack of fertile-quality cervical fluid, and excessively short luteal phases, as well as recurrent miscarriages. If your charting reveals nothing wrong, but you are still unable to get pregnant after *optimally timing* intercourse for 4 to 6 cycles, your partner should get a semen analysis. If his sperm count is subfertile, try timing intercourse by the FAM guidelines discussed on page 148 for another few cycles. If, however, his count is normal, you yourself should be given a comprehensive fertility workup to determine the problem.

## ❧ THE MAN'S FERTILITY WORKUP

As mentioned earlier, when people think of fertility problems, they tend to think of them as primarily a woman's issue. But, as you know by now, fertility problems affect men and women equally. The reason a man should be tested first is that his own workup is fairly simple, cheap, and hardly uncomfortable! The foundation is the semen analysis, which is easily obtained by having the man ejaculate into a cup.

Remember that even though the analysis is usually referred to as a "sperm count," the expression is somewhat misleading. The count is only one facet of the whole analysis. As discussed in Chapter 11, the key to judging a man's fertility is not so much to look at the total number of sperm per ejaculate, but rather the total number of those sperm released that are of normal shape and motility.

Based on that analysis, a physician will be able to tell you whether your partner's sperm count is considered normal or subfertile. You should be aware that if the analysis shows a subfertile count, he would be expected to have at least two more analyses performed with at least 2 to 4 weeks in between in order to verify the results.

One additional investigation that is often routinely done with the sperm sample is called the sperm penetration assay, or the hamster egg penetration test. It is the best test currently available to determine the fertilizing capabilities of a man's sperm. As the name implies, the sperm is placed immediately next to hamster eggs to see whether they can penetrate them, since such penetration generally correlates with how well sperm can penetrate human eggs. Like any test, though, it's not perfect; 5 to 10% of men whose sperm do not "pass the test" are still able to eventually impregnate their partners. Likewise, some men whose sperm do fine in the test are still unable to fertilize their partner's eggs. However, it is considered fairly standard in a fertility workup, and should be taken for what it's worth.

Depending on the results of the semen analysis, the physician may perform a variety of other procedures. These include a physical exam to look for varicoceles, prostate problems, or testicular anomalies and blood tests to ascertain hormonal levels. In addition, the doctor may need to take semen cultures to determine the presence of sperm clumping (agglutination) or genital tract infections, as well as X rays of his sperm-producing tissues. Once the source of the problem is identified, there may be a variety of treatments possible (see page 178).

## ❧ THE WOMAN'S FERTILITY WORKUP

You'll now see why it is much more logical for the man's fertility workup to be performed first. The woman's is clearly a substantially more extensive undertaking, usually involving several stages.

### 1. Preliminary Fact-Finding
The clinician should take a comprehensive medical history and review any previous fertility tests before performing a standard pelvic exam. The exam is to rule out any obvious physical problems of the uterus, ovaries, or cervix, such as fibroids, cysts, or infections.

### 2. Diagnostic Analyses
There are a number of fairly noninvasive means of determining potential problems. In women, the four general areas of concern in the reproductive system are:

- Uterine and fallopian tube abnormalities
- Cervical problems

- Dysfunctional ovulatory cycles
- Endometriosis

The tests and procedures discussed below are used to detect problems in any of the above areas. They are listed in order of least invasiveness.

### A. Waking (Basal Body) Temperature Charting

As you know, this is the sign that is easiest to ascertain and puts control in your hands. Taking your waking temperature will help you determine whether:

- you are ovulating
- your luteal phase is long enough for implantation (at least 10 days)
- your progesterone levels are high enough in your luteal phase
- you may have a thyroid problem (either hypo- or hyperthyroid)
- you are still fertile any given cycle as reflected by low temperatures
- you may have gotten pregnant, as reflected by more than 18 high temperatures
- you are in danger of having a miscarriage, as determined by a sudden drop in temperatures after an apparent conception
- you were pregnant before having what seemed to be just a "late period"

### B. Hormone Blood Tests

Blood tests are one of the most fundamental means of determining if the woman is producing normal reproductive hormones or has a hormonal imbalance. They can determine levels of FSH, LH, estrogen, and progesterone. The progesterone serum in particular detects if ovulation has occurred, and if there is an adequate amount of progesterone after ovulation. The importance of progesterone in the latter phase of the cycle is to maintain the lining for implantation to occur. Progesterone serums are usually taken about a week after ovulation, when it is typically at its highest level.

### C. Cervical-Fluid Ferning Test

This is a test in which cervical fluid is removed from the woman's vagina and observed under a microscope to determine if it has the characteristic fertile ferning pattern. In order for the test to be valid, though, it is imperative that it is done *when the woman's cervical fluid exhibits its most fertile characteristics* (i.e., her wettest, most slippery days), and not necessarily on Day 14, as is commonly done. If the cervical fluid is indeed fertile, it will form a beautiful ferning pattern on the slide (see photograph on page 3 of color insert).

### D. Postcoital Test

This test is done to determine whether the couple's sperm and cervical fluid are compatible. In other words, can the man's sperm survive inside the woman's cervical fluid? In order to determine this, a sample of cervical fluid is taken from the woman's vagina within 2 hours of intercourse. Again, in order for the test to be valid, it is imperative that it be done when the woman has fertile-quality cervical fluid, and not necessarily on Day 14, as it often is. If the two are compatible, the clinician will be able to observe live sperm swimming forward in the cervical fluid.

### E. Ultrasound

The only way to determine definitively if ovulation has occurred is with ultrasound. This procedure offers a means of being able to actually observe if and when ovulation occurs. It's especially useful in detecting the condition LUFS (Luteinized Unruptured Follicle Syndrome), in which the woman's body produces all the signs of ovulation, but without actually releasing an egg (see page 185).

Ultrasound can also be helpful in detecting ectopic pregnancies—those which develop outside of the uterine lining. Its main disadvantage is that it is not practical on a daily basis since it requires a doctor's appointment.

### F. Endometrial Biopsy

The endometrial biopsy sounds ominous, but is fairly simple. We tend to associate the word "biopsy" with cancer, but the test has nothing to do with that. Its purpose is to determine if the uterine lining (endometrium) is sufficiently developed during the luteal phase of the cycle. The lining must be mature enough to be able to sustain the implantation of a fertilized egg.

The test is usually done a couple of days before the woman's expected period. A tiny piece of the uterine lining is removed and biopsied. Unlike the tests listed above, it can be uncomfortable because it may cause cramping or a sharp pain from partially dilating the cervix. The timing of this test is critical, because if it's done too soon after the egg is released (especially in the case of delayed ovulations) it can deceptively appear as if the woman has an undeveloped endometrium. Likewise, if it's done too late after ovulation, the woman may start her period before the test has been completed. Charting is thus strongly recommended in order to time this test appropriately.

### G. HSG (Hysterosalpingogram)

The purpose of an HSG is to determine if the woman's fallopian tubes are open. It involves shooting dye through the cervix and uterus to see whether it spills out the fallopian tubes into the pelvic cavity. Although the test can be quite useful, it does have its limitations. For one thing, the tubes occasionally spasm during the procedure, giving the appearance of being blocked, when in reality it may have been the test itself that caused the tubes to appear closed.

Another potential problem is that if the tubes are only scarred but not blocked, the HSG would not necessarily reveal that. The concern with scarring is that it could lead to a tubal pregnancy, in which the fertilized egg begins to burrow into the tube rather than the uterine lining.

### 3. Surgical Investigation

If the tests in section 2 above fail to identify a problem, there are two primary surgical diagnostic procedures that can be very helpful in pinpointing potential impediments to pregnancy.

### A. Laparoscopy

The best way to have a "window into the womb" is through a laparoscopy —exploratory surgery that is used to view the internal pelvic area, especially the ovaries and fallopian tubes. The procedure is most commonly used to detect endometriosis. It usually involves a tiny incision in the navel through which a lighted tube is inserted to view the pelvic region. Although the procedure is fairly routine, it is usually done with general anesthesia.

### B. Hysteroscopy

The least performed exploratory surgery is a hysteroscopy—a procedure to view the inside of the uterus. It is primarily done to determine if the woman's uterus has fibroids or other conditions that may affect the ability to carry a pregnancy to term.

### 4. Chromosome Analysis (if necessary)

Some people are born with congenital problems that aren't evident until they try to get pregnant. Chromosome analysis can reveal the nature of the problem, which may be related to sexually dysfunctional anatomy.

### 5. *Genetic Counseling (if necessary)*

Some families may carry a recessive gene for certain birth defects. If you or your partner has such a family history, you may wish to get genetic counseling to determine what your chances are of giving it to your offspring.

## ૭ WAYS OF RESOLVING INFERTILITY: AN OVERVIEW

Once you've identified a fertility problem, you can often resolve it through one of the following treatments:

1. Optimizing the chances of getting pregnant by using FAM to time intercourse when you are the most fertile.
2. Correcting the basic underlying problem.
3. Bypassing steps in reproduction through assisted reproductive technologies.

The following is a brief synopsis of the fertility treatments listed above.

### I. OPTIMIZE CHANCES OF GETTING PREGNANT BY TIMING INTERCOURSE AT THE MOST FERTILE TIME

As discussed in detail in Chapter 11, the most fertile time in a woman's cycle is the *last day* of the most fertile-quality cervical fluid or vaginal sensation. If a man's sperm count is normal, the couple should have intercourse every day that the woman has wet cervical fluid through to the first morning of the rise in temperature. If a man's sperm count is low, the couple should have intercourse every *other* day of wet cervical fluid through to the first morning of the rise in temperature.

### IIA. CORRECT THE MAN'S BASIC UNDERLYING PROBLEM

As with women, the man's fertility may be improved simply by changing diet and eliminating coffee, tobacco, recreational drugs, and alcohol. Some people believe that homeopathic and naturopathic treatments as well as nutritional supplements may also be useful. Still, men facing infertility problems usually have a variety of overlapping symptoms that require medical intervention. While fertility specialists generally view male infertility as easier to detect but more difficult to cure than the female counterpart, it is also true that some of the more prevalent problems can be successfully treated. Male infertility may be due to problems relating to any combination of the following:

- Low sperm count
- Varicoceles
- Damaged sperm ducts
- Hormonal deficiency
- Testicular failure
- Sperm antibodies

## A. Low Sperm Count

The most common cause of male subfertility is low sperm count, believed to be due to a variety of causes. Among these are hormonal insufficiency, bacterial infections, and varicoceles, all of which may be treated by standard medical procedures discussed below. Success rates vary depending on the cause. Unfortunately, low sperm count often has no detectable source, though abnormal testicular maturation dating back to embryonic development is suspected. In these cases, there is currently no known treatment to increase the sperm count. However, such couples may still be able to utilize a variety of high-tech procedures to take advantage of the sperm that exist (see page 185).

## B. Varicoceles

The most likely cause of diminished sperm counts are varicoceles in the scrotal sac. About 30 to 40% of infertile men have them, though often they have no impact on fertility. They almost always occur in the left testicle, since the spermatic vein enters the renal vein at a right angle on that side, allowing pressure to build. The most plausible reason why this would affect sperm is that the pooled venous blood overheats the sperm production centers of the testicles. And, as you know, heat can kill sperm.

Either general or local anesthesia can be used to operate on them. The effective sperm count improves in about 80% of infertile men after surgery, but only half of these men typically go on to impregnate their partners. This would suggest that male infertility is often caused by a series of overlapping problems.

### C. Damaged Sperm Ducts

Blocked sperm ducts may account for about 10 to 15% of all male infertility. Scarring in the vas deferens may prevent the sperm from reaching the cervical fluid as it flows through the urethra. This is often caused by an infection that is the result of an STD. The vas deferens may also be blocked by a varicocele which is pressing against it. Some of these cases can be corrected without surgery, but most would require a minor operation to eliminate the blockage or scarring. Microsurgery is generally extremely effective in restoring fertility to men whose only problem is obstruction of sperm outflow.

### D. Hormonal Deficiency

The next most common cause of male subfertility is hormonal deficiency. It is usually due to an insufficient or erratic release of FSH and LH, the sex hormones that are necessary for sperm production (these hormones, discussed extensively throughout this book, are also produced by the male reproductive system). If hormonal deficiency is causing low sperm count, it may be possible to treat the problem with GnRH analogs or gonadotropins. Male hormonal problems are generally complex and difficult to cure, though the chances of success are much greater when the problem results in marginal sperm count, as opposed to the complete cessation of sperm production.

### E. Testicular Failure

Another fairly common problem is testicular failure, in which the amount of reproductive hormones being released from the pituitary is sufficient, but the testes fail to respond appropriately and therefore do not produce sperm. The causes for this condition range from illnesses such as mumps and various STDs to physical traumas caused by surgery, tumors, and drugs. It may even be caused by a sports injury, in which a sudden blow to the testes may lead to reduction in the flow of oxygen to the spermatogenia, thus causing the cells to die. Unfortunately, there appears to be no effective treatment that will improve sperm production in cases where no sperm are present. If there are some sperm, however, fertility drugs may be able to increase the numbers.

### F. Sperm Antibodies

In some men, the problem is caused by production of antibodies to their own sperm, so that the immune system effectively destroys the sperm as soon as they are produced. This occurs in about 10% of infertile men, though the numbers may be higher among those who underwent a vasectomy and then reversed it. If a man has developed antibodies against his own sperm, he may be prescribed steroids, which are potent drugs that suppress the immune system (clearly such treatment has its disadvantages). There is also some evidence that adrenal hormones may restore fertility in certain cases.*

Another option is to have the sperm washed. This is a procedure in which the semen is mixed with culture media in a test tube and then rapidly spun. Although it doesn't dislodge antibodies, it does permit separation of the best swimmers, allowing for artificial insemination high in the woman's reproductive tract. In fact, intrauterine insemination (IUI) is the most common treatment for sperm antibodies. If IUI is unsuccessful, then the couple can try one of the assisted reproductive technologies such as IVF or GIFT.

Many of the above-mentioned conditions as well as some less common fertility-related problems can clearly be treated by new advances in medicine. But the fact remains that many men will not be able to father their own children. As the revolution in advanced reproductive medicine continues, there may one day be hope even for those men who produce no sperm at all. In the meantime, the most reasonable course of action for a couple facing this dilemma may be to use a donor for artificial insemination.

## IIB. CORRECT THE WOMAN'S BASIC UNDERLYING PROBLEM THROUGH THE FOLLOWING

### A. Change in Diet or Nutritional Status

As discussed in Chapter 12, being either too thin or too heavy can compromise a woman's fertility. If a woman is too thin, she may cease ovulating altogether. And if she is too heavy, her extra fat can excrete excess estrogen that paradoxically suppresses the normal hormonal feedback system.

---

* It is also possible that the woman may develop antibodies against her partner's sperm. If this happens, there are a number of treatments that can be used. If her cervical fluid is incompatible with his sperm, hormones can be prescribed to change its composition, or she can use normally unnecessary douches to change its acidity. If she has antibodies in her cervical fluid, she may be prescribed steroid treatments (such as Prednisone) or, interestingly enough, condom therapy. Condom therapy to get pregnant? Actually, the principle is that the couple should use condoms during intercourse for a period of 6 months in hopes of weakening the antibodies in the woman's immune system that attack her partner's sperm. When the couple does resume unprotected intercourse, it needs to be timed precisely for conception, lest she once again start building antibodies against his sperm.

Additionally, some women are more sensitive than others to unbalanced diets or diets lacking in necessary vitamins and nutrients. Because the discussion of appropriate nutrients for optimal fertility is a book in itself, I would recommend *Fertility, Cycles, and Nutrition* by Marilyn Shannon.

### B. Naturopathic and Homeopathic Treatments

Naturopathy is a system of medicine that treats health conditions by utilizing the body's inherent ability to heal. Homeopathy is a system of medicine in which minute amounts of natural substances from plants, minerals, and animals are used to treat chronic conditions that fail to respond to standard Western medicine. Both systems have devoted adherents, including those who believe various infertility problems may be successfully treated through their practice.

For those determined to exhaust all natural possibilities before moving on to more conventional approaches, I have recommended a couple of books that deal with various other forms of alternative medicine, including herbal treatments and acupuncture (see page 348).

### C. Drug Therapy

The following is a list of the most commonly prescribed drugs used in treating subfertility. Whenever any drug is prescribed, you should always verify with your physician precisely what the drug is for and what the potential side effects are.

*1. Drugs to Induce Ovulation (Clomid and Pergonal)*

Two of the most commonly prescribed drugs to induce ovulation are Clomid and Pergonal. Clomid is considered the least invasive of the two, and in principle, is prescribed when a woman is either not ovulating at all or only sporadically. It is also used when she has a short luteal phase. In reality, Clomid is often prescribed as a matter of routine even when the woman's fertility problem is not known. Pergonal, on the other hand, is an extremely potent drug and is usually prescribed only when Clomid doesn't work. Pergonal is also used for the assisted technologies of IVF, GIFT, and ZIFT.

*2. Drugs to Suppress Ovulation (Lupron and Danazol)*

Occasionally, it is necessary to suppress ovulation in order to abate conditions such as endometriosis. Women are typically prescribed anovulatory drugs for about 6 months or longer, after which they are then instructed to try and get pregnant. These drugs are also used in conjunction with high-technology treatments.

### 3. Drugs to Reduce Hormones (Parlodel and Prednisone)
Some women have an excessively high level of hormones that may disrupt their normal ovulatory cycle. Parlodel is used to reduce prolactin, the hormone that normally circulates in women who are breastfeeding. Prednisone is used to reduce excessively high levels of testosterone in women.

### 4. Drugs to Support the Ovulatory Cycle (Estrogen and Progesterone)
Estrogen is critical for the development of fertile cervical fluid. Often, when women are prescribed Clomid to induce ovulation, it has the unfortunate side effect of drying up the necessary cervical fluid. In these cases, estrogen can be prescribed along with the Clomid to counteract its drying effects.

Progesterone is usually given to support a short or insufficient luteal phase. It's typically given either by injections, suppositories, or oral tablets. It acts to prevent a newly pregnant woman from menstruating before the egg has had a chance to implant, thus decreasing the odds of a miscarriage.

### 5. Drugs Used in Conjunction with Assisted Technologies
There are a few drugs that are not used alone, but are considered effective when prescribed in conjunction with the high-technology procedures discussed below. The most common among these are GnRH agonists, HCG, and Metrodin, all of which promote ovulation in order to maximize the chances of an assisted conception.

### 6. Antibiotics to Treat Infections
Pelvic inflammatory disease as well as a variety of genital tract infections may be responsible for subfertility. Most of these conditions can be successfully treated with various antibiotics if treatment is given early enough.

## D. Surgery
Nowadays, surgery means not only traditional cutting with a scalpel, but perhaps just using a simple laser beam. It may be performed to correct obstructions such as tubal scarring and cervical polyps. In addition, surgery can remove adhesions such as those caused by endometriosis and scarring from pelvic inflammatory disease. Finally, it can be used to remove growths such as fibroids in the uterus. While the prospect of under-

going an operation is admittedly not pleasant, advances in technology do mean that many procedures can now be done on an outpatient basis.

## &phi; A SPECIAL NOTE ON TWO KEY FERTILITY PROBLEMS

Before discussing possible high-tech treatments, there are two conditions of which you should be aware. The first one, endometriosis, is one of the most widely diagnosed fertility problems. The second, Luteinized Unruptured Follicle Syndrome (LUFS), is rarely detected but has recently emerged as a prime suspect in inexplicable infertility cases.

### Endometriosis

One of the most peculiar causes of infertility is endometriosis, a surprisingly prevalent disorder in which normal endometrial tissue like that which lines the uterus grows outside the uterus. The misplaced tissue may develop anywhere within the abdominal cavity, growing in small superficial patches, in thicker, penetrating nodules, or within cysts in the ovary. The condition is highly unpredictable in that it may remain in a few very small areas or spread invasively throughout the pelvis. One of the most puzzling aspects of endometriosis is that the degree of pain it causes is not a valid indicator of the severity of the condition. It may cause absolutely no symptoms even though it has spread extensively, or cause excruciating pain even though there is minimal spreading.

A paradox of endometriosis is that pregnancy is one of the few natural conditions that seems to cause the disease to regress temporarily. Yet it is the condition itself which often causes infertility. There are basically two types of treatment: hormones or surgery.

The goal of hormonal treatment is to simulate pregnancy or menopause, the two natural conditions known to inhibit the disease. Women are prescribed either birth control pills, synthetic progesterones called progestins, analogs of GnRH called Lupron, or the drug Danazol. The latter is the most commonly prescribed, and is usually taken for at least 6 months in order to be most effective. While less invasive than surgery, hormonal therapy has its limitations. It only works in mild cases, has many side effects, and requires much more time to diminish the disease.

Surgery, on the other hand, can remove adhesions, implants, or blood-filled cysts. Laparoscopy can often be used to drain fluid and remove small patches through laser or electrical current. But not all cases can be treated through the laparoscope. Occasionally more extensive surgery is necessary when scar tissue is thick or involves delicate structures.

Finally, some patients need a combination of both medical and surgical therapy. But if a woman doesn't respond to any of the above, she still may be able to achieve pregnancy through one of the assisted technologies such as IVF.

## Luteinized Unruptured Follicle Syndrome (LUFS)

You should be aware that even if you have all the classic signs of ovulation, including fertile cervical fluid and clear biphasic temperature patterns, it is still possible that you may not actually be ovulating. This is because some women suffer on rare occasions from a condition called LUFS. In these cases, the woman has no physical symptoms other than infertility itself, but ultrasound reveals that the ovum remains stuck within the luteinized follicle, unable to pass through the ovarian wall to a possible conception. It is now estimated that up to 30% of unexplained infertility is due to this condition. If ultrasound did reveal that you have LUFS, it's still possible that one of the assisted reproductive technologies could help you conceive.

## III. BYPASS STEPS IN REPRODUCTION THROUGH ASSISTED REPRODUCTIVE TECHNOLOGIES

The procedures below are listed in approximate order of invasiveness, from least to most. IVF, GIFT, and ZIFT are all variations of the same thing. They all involve optimizing your chances of pregnancy through actively intervening with the natural reproductive process and uniting the sperm and egg together. The differences are a function of where fertilization occurs (in or out of the body), and where the egg and sperm are returned to the body (uterus or fallopian tubes).

### A. Artificial Insemination (AI)

This is the simplest and least technologically complex of the assisted reproductive technologies. It is usually performed when the man has a low sperm count, when the woman's cervical fluid is not considered fertile enough, or when there is simply unexplained infertility. In addition, of course, it is often used by women without male partners. AI typically involves using a catheter to gently insert the man's sperm just outside the cervix, or directly into the uterus (thus the expression intrauterine insemination, or IUI). The sperm may be that of your partner or a donor.

Nowadays, AI usually involves "sperm washing," a process that dramatically increases the motility of the sperm by mixing it with a culture media and then placing it in a centrifuge. In addition, it is considered much more effective if the woman's ovulation is artificially stimulated through ovulatory drugs, most notably, Pergonal.

### B. IVF (In Vitro Fertilization)

IVF is a procedure that is most commonly done on women whose fallopian tubes are blocked. It involves removing several eggs from the woman's ovaries and fertilizing them with her partner's sperm in a petri dish outside her body, then placing the 2-day-old embryo in her *uterus*. The challenge with IVF is not fertilization, but implantation.

### C. GIFT (Gamete Intra-Fallopian Transfer)

This procedure solves the implantation problem of IVF, but requires that the woman's fallopian tubes be open. As with IVF, the eggs are removed, but the sperm and eggs are inserted into the *fallopian tube* and left to fertilize on their own. GIFT is considered two to three times more successful than IVF because the placement of the sperm and egg into the tubes (rather than the uterus) re-creates the more natural conditions necessary for a successful implantation.

### D. ZIFT (Zygote Intra-Fallopian Transfer)

This procedure is a logical answer to the situation where the man's sperm quality is marginal, but the woman's tubes are still open. With ZIFT, the egg is first fertilized in a petri dish, and the resulting zygote is returned to the *fallopian tube,* after which it continues to naturally travel down to implant in the uterus.

### E. Micromanipulation

This is one of the most exciting techniques developed for those conditions in which sperm appear unable to penetrate the egg. It is a procedure in which a single sperm is inserted directly into the ova through the assistance of high-tech instruments. After the fertilization, which occurs in a petri dish, the newly created embryo is placed in the woman's uterus.

### F. Ovum Transfer

One of the most dramatic advances in fertility technology allows a post-menopausal women to carry and deliver a child. Using a petri dish, her partner's sperm are used to fertilize the eggs from a younger donor. The embryo is then transplanted into the uterus of the woman desiring pregnancy. Of course, the embryo is not biologically related to her, but is still related to the man.

## The Difference Between IVF, GIFT, and ZIFT

|  | **IVF** | **GIFT** | **ZIFT** |
|---|---|---|---|
| Fallopian Tubes Need to Be Open | No | Yes | Yes |
| Where Fertilization Takes Place | Petri dish outside the uterus | Fallopian Tube | Petri dish outside the uterus |
| Where Egg and Sperm (or the Fertilized Egg) Are Returned To | Uterus | Fallopian Tube | Fallopian Tube |
| Good Option for Poor Sperm Quality | Yes, if tubes closed | No | Yes, if tubes open |
| Surgery and Hospitalization Required | No | Yes | Yes |

I have chosen not to list an estimated success rate per cycle because the data available in the medical literature and from the infertility clinics is extremely inconsistent and confusing. For example, a straight pregnancy rate is often claimed (whether a miscarriage results or not), when it is the "take home baby rate" that is obviously more relevant for intelligently analyzing your options. The bottom line is that the technology continues to improve, but success is never assured. And even for those who eventually succeed, it often takes at least several cycles before a healthy pregnancy results.

What is generally accepted is that GIFT and ZIFT have dramatically greater success rates than IVF. Still, many couples choose to try IVF because it is a simpler and less costly procedure that can be performed on an outpatient basis. And obviously in certain cases, such as when the woman's fallopian tubes are blocked, GIFT and ZIFT are not even options. It should also be noted that IVF allows clinicians to verify that fertilization has indeed occurred (this is not possible with GIFT). This is especially helpful for couples where the man's sperm quality is poor because it's uncertain whether his sperm can fertilize the woman's eggs.

## The Steps Necessary for IVF, GIFT, or ZIFT

Before you seriously consider any of these technologies, you should be aware that they all involve a series of procedures that can be both physically and emotionally uncomfortable. In general, IVF, GIFT, and ZIFT will all involve variations of the following:

1. The woman is prescribed a series of hormones throughout her cycle (usually in the form of injections), which include any combination of:

   - **Pergonal** * (a purified preparation of FSH)
   - **Lupron** (a drug that prevents a premature LH surge)
   - **HCG** (Human Chorionic Gonadotropin, a hormone that acts like luteinizing hormone when injected)
   - **Progesterone** (the hormone you normally make in the latter

* If you've heard some outlandish story about how Pergonal has been harvested from the urine of postmenopausal nuns in Italy—for once, 'tis true! One of the paradoxical effects of menopause on a woman's body is to produce massive quantities of FSH as a way of trying to trigger the ovaries to continue to ovulate. Since FSH is needed to induce ovulation in clinically stimulated cycles, such as those prepared for insemination, IVF, GIFT, and ZIFT, isn't it logical to use nuns' urine? You're probably thinking, "Why didn't I think of that? Nuns' urine. It's so obvious." (For an even more bizarre hormonal source, see page 242.)

phase of your cycle, but which may cease being released as an effect of Pergonal)

2. The man's sperm are "washed" to improve their quality, maximizing the chances of success.
3. In the final step, a dozen or so of the woman's matured eggs are aspirated from her artificially stimulated ovaries. Then, depending on the procedure chosen, fertilization will be attempted in either a petri dish (ZIFT or IVF) or her fallopian tubes (GIFT). If the eggs are fertilized in the petri dish, several will be returned to either her tubes (ZIFT) or her uterus (IVF).

## ✎ DEALING WITH MISCARRIAGES

Unfortunately, all the high-tech procedures discussed above will probably not help if you are experiencing repeated miscarriages. For unlike any other infertility issue, this is not a problem in achieving pregnancy, but rather in keeping the embryo viable after conception has occurred. It is also unfortunate, but true, that as women age into their 30s, miscarriages become the most prevalent cause of infertility, with undetected ones probably composing the vast majority of fetal loss.

While the assisted reproductive technologies have little role to play in the miscarriage problem, there are hopeful medical advances being made. Of course, before you can begin seeking treatment, you must first be aware that you have the problem. As you have already learned, charting can play a critical role in this area. FAM can both identify miscarriages as they occur (as seen by 18 or more high temps followed by bleeding), or identify the abnormally short luteal phases that would make a successful implantation highly improbable.

If you do discover that you are in fact getting pregnant but losing the embryo, you should at least know that the majority of women in your situation will still be able to go on and have healthy babies. But aside from the obvious steps you should take to make sure you are in the healthiest condition possible, I urge you to consult a qualified fertility specialist. Better yet, you should bring the doctor your Fertility Awareness charts. By doing so, you will not only feel more in control, but you may very well be expediting the process that leads to a healthy baby.

*Deborah and Burt used FAM to get pregnant, but the pregnancy sadly ended in a miscarriage due to a blighted ovum (a strange phenomenon in which a sac develops, but an embryo never does). Because they had no problem initially getting pregnant, they decided not to resume charting when they were ready to try again.*

*Deborah had one normal cycle following her miscarriage, but the cycle after that was extremely long and confusing to them. When she had spotting on Day 54, she didn't know whether it was ovulatory spotting, implantation bleeding due to pregnancy, or the signs of a possible miscarriage. She only realized then how frustrating it was to not have charted that cycle, because it left her completely in the dark. She got a pregnancy test, which came back negative. Of course, she still wasn't sure if the test was accurate, because she might have ovulated so late that the test could have indicated a false negative if her body had not yet had a chance to produce enough HCG to be detected.*

*As it turned out, Deborah was not pregnant. Either she didn't ovulate that cycle, or she simply had an extremely delayed ovulation. In any event, all of their confusion could have been eliminated had they simply charted. Needless to say, they learned from this experience how valuable charting is, even for those who seemingly have no problem getting pregnant. After waiting a few cycles they tried again; this time they charted, and were thrilled to discover they were pregnant through temperatures that remained above the coverline beyond 18 days. As I write this, she is 7 months pregnant with a baby boy.*

## Causes of Miscarriages

### Infections

One of the surprising things about the role of infections in miscarriages is that the more common ones are not considered responsible. So having a bad cold, the flu, or a fever during pregnancy is *not* likely to harm your fetus. But there are certain infections that may, including mycoplasma, toxoplasmosis, chlamydia, listeria, malaria, and monilia (this last one only when an IUD is in place at the time of accidental conception).

In addition, there are infections associated with certain procedures that may cause a miscarriage, including those from a cervical stitch used to tighten a weak cervix, an IUD, an organism called campylobacter, and prostaglandins in semen during intercourse itself (which is only of concern to women who have previously miscarried). If a cervical or semen sample reveals an infection, you and your partner will most likely be prescribed antibiotics.

Finally, there are certain viruses that are known to be dangerous during pregnancy, including the most notorious, German measles (rubella), and herpes (if the initial viral attack occurred during the first 20 weeks of pregnancy). Other viruses may also cause miscarriages, including mumps, measles, hepatitis A and B, and parvovirus.

### Endocrine Problems (Hormonal)

The most common cause of hormonal problems leading to early miscarriages is that of an abnormal luteal phase. As you've read, in order for a fertilized egg to have a chance to implant and mature, the corpus luteum must maintain the latter phase of the cycle for at least 10 days. In addition, once pregnancy occurs, it must continue to live long enough for the developing placenta to take over the function of providing nutrition for the embryo. The corpus luteum should live about 10 weeks beyond conception, so if you had a miscarriage before then, one of the first things the doctor would suspect is a possible corpus luteum deficiency.

Of course, you yourself should suspect a potential problem if your basal temperatures reflect a luteal phase of 10 days or less.* If it does, your doctor will most likely perform a blood test and endometrial biopsy to confirm this. If you do indeed have a problem with progesterone production in the latter phase of your cycle, you will probably be prescribed a natural version of it. Many doctors will also prescribe Clomid in the first phase of the cycle, in the hope that it will promote an optimal ovulation and a healthy progesterone level afterward.

### Uterine Abnormalities

One of the most common causes of miscarriages in the second trimester is what is unfortunately referred to as an "incompetent cervix." As the name implies, it is a weak cervix that tends to dilate before the fetus has reached full term. Some women are born with congenital abnormalities of the uterus which are shaped in such a way that the baby can't grow big enough before it runs out of room and causes the cervix to dilate. Uterine anomalies are often the result of a woman's mother having taken DES while pregnant with her.

If your physician suspects that recurring miscarriages may be due to structural problems of your uterus, he or she will probably perform a hysterogram.

---

* While most of the medical literature suggests that a 10-day luteal phase should be sufficient for implantation, it's also true that 10- or even 11-day luteal phases could be a potential problem in certain cases.

This procedure is basically an X ray of the uterus using injected dye to determine its shape. Another diagnostic procedure often used to view the uterus is a laparoscopy, in which a narrow tube is inserted through the naval to view the uterus and tubes. Occasionally the doctor may perform a hysteroscopy, a relatively new technique that allows the inside of the uterus to be viewed.

One of the least-invasive treatments, especially in the case of a weak cervix, is to place a suture in it to prevent it from dilating prematurely. But if the uterus is malformed or has uterine adhesions, it can usually be successfully treated only through surgery.

Finally, if you have fibroids (or benign tumors) in or on your uterus, you are not alone. By age 40, about 40% of women have them. They generally don't require any treatment unless they grow exceedingly fast or cause severe bleeding or pelvic pressure. Your physician will often recommend doing nothing, in the hope that the fibroids themselves will not interfere with the pregnancy, since their removal is often more invasive than necessary.

### Genetics (Chromosomes)

A large percentage of early and first miscarriages are believed to be due to chromosomal damage. Fortunately, chromosomal miscarriages are not considered a recurring problem, and thus the chance of another one due to similar reasons is small.

### Antibodies

One of the more peculiar types of problems that leads to miscarriages is that of the mother producing antibodies that, in essence, reject her own fetus. It's now thought that up to a third of recurring miscarriages are due to this immunological phenomenon. The good news is that there is a new though admittedly controversial treatment available.

Through a blood test, a woman can determine if she is producing such antibodies. If it is discovered that she is, she is then injected with her partner's white blood cells to produce the necessary blocking factor that prevents her from rejecting his half of the fetus's tissue. Although the treatment is still somewhat experimental, the results have proven to be very encouraging.

In addition, some women develop another type of immunological problem involving what are called antipholipid antibodies, which promote blood clotting (coagulation). Their unfortunate effect is to inhibit the growth of the placenta and the transport of nutrients to the fetus. A special blood test will usually detect the problem. Usually the woman is prescribed a baby aspirin a day along with daily injections of the anticoagulant heparin.

**Medical Disorders**

Finally, miscarriages tend to occur more frequently in women who have medical conditions such as uncontrolled diabetes, thyroid disease, high blood pressure, or heart disease. If your physician diagnoses any of these, he or she will probably refer you to an internist for treatment before you attempt to get pregnant again.

## The Dilemma of Advanced Maternal Age

There is an unfortunate biological reality that all women wishing to be mothers should internalize as soon as they become adults. The fact is that women in their late 30s and older are at much greater risk of miscarriage, for the simple reason that as they age the eggs within their ovaries continue to age with them. It is not completely understood why older ova lose their ability to sustain a healthy pregnancy after they are fertilized, but it's clearly symptomatic of the same biological phenomenon causing the increased risk of birth defects in the babies of older women.

While medical advances continue to be made, solving the problem of miscarriage among women in their 40s continues to be one of the greatest reproductive challenges. I urge you to keep up to date, and of course if at all possible, try to have the children you want before the issue ever arises.

## Types of Pregnancy Loss Beyond Vaginal Miscarriages

In addition to regular miscarriages in which the fetus is expelled through the vagina, there are a few other types of failed pregnancies of which you should be aware.

**Ectopic Pregnancy:** A condition in which a fertilized ovum attaches itself *outside* of the uterus (usually in the fallopian tube) and begins to grow.

**Missed Abortion:** A most unfortunate term to describe a fetus that has miscarried, or died, but has not been expelled naturally.

**Blighted Ovum:** A pregnancy in which no fetus ever developed in the pregnancy sac.

**Molar Pregnancy:** A rare condition in which a normal pregnancy goes awry, becoming a benign tumor at about 10 weeks.

## ✌ FAM, INFERTILITY, AND MODERN MEDICINE

Reproductive medicine continues to make headline-capturing advances. While I believe that a low-tech option such as FAM is the preferred solution to infertility problems whenever possible, you should be aware of FAM's limits. Just as important, you should now know that even if you can't have a baby by completely natural means, charting will certainly help you identify the problem, and exploit the various solutions that the miracles of modern medicine increasingly offer.

# PART FIVE

# BEYOND FERTILITY: PRACTICAL BENEFITS OF CHARTING YOUR CYCLE

# CHAPTER 15

# Maintaining Your Gynecological Health

*Sex is a pleasurable exercise in plumbing, but be careful or you'll get yeast in your drain tap.*

—RITA MAE BROWN

Have you ever thought about how odd it is that intimate details about your body are filed in a medical office across town? Why shouldn't you have access to such records in your own home? Once women learn to chart, they take control of all facets of their health care—from annual exam results to the symptoms that may prompt them to seek medical help.

The form at the end of this chapter can be used as a master sheet for an annual exam. Make an enlarged duplicate of it, then copy it onto the back of the cycle in which you get your yearly physical, taking the chart with you when you go. You'll find it a practical way to keep track of your gynecological health, as well as such details as your weight and blood pressure, what tests you've had and what their results were (e.g., mammograms, Pap tests, etc.), and what your breast exam revealed regarding lumps or potential problems. You can use the back of the regular charts to record anything else worth remembering.

Most women have fairly common conditions that are considered medically normal, but may appear problematic simply because they are not taught about the healthy female body. As mentioned earlier, both normal gynecological conditions and potential problems can be more easily identified through charting, including:

- vaginal infections
- abnormal bleeding

- nabothian (cervical) cysts
- endometriosis
- premenstrual syndrome
- breast lumps

By now, the above list should be familiar to you. But I think it's important to repeat why charting is so beneficial for your gynecological health. One of the points I made in the beginning of this book is that charting enables a woman to understand her body in a practical way. As you'll recall, I said that a woman who charts every day is so aware of what is normal for her that she can help her clinician determine irregularities based on *her* symptoms rather than the average woman's symptoms. Charting her menstrual cycle allows a woman to actively contribute to her gynecological well-being by working with her health care provider. This concept cannot be stressed enough. The remainder of this chapter will discuss both normal and abnormal gynecological conditions and how FAM can be used to distinguish the two.

## ✌ NORMAL, HEALTHY CERVICAL FLUID VERSUS REAL VAGINAL INFECTIONS

### Normal, Healthy Cervical Fluid

From a health perspective, the obvious benefit of learning about your own pattern of cervical fluid is to be able to determine if and when you have a true vaginal infection.

*Marsha is an American FAM instructor teaching in Israel. While getting her master's degree in public health in the States, she had an annual Pap test. Since she was charting her cycles, and planned her appointment for midcycle, she happened to have a lot of slippery, stretchy cervical fluid. As the physician removed the speculum, he exclaimed, "My dear, you have an infection" to which she replied, "Excuse me? I feel fine and don't have any symptoms." He replied, "Look at this discharge!" showing her the Pap stick with the obvious cervical fluid on it. "Well, I know I'm in my fertile phase and these are just my fertile secretions." The nurse stood behind him, winking and nodding in agreement with her. He curtly and abruptly responded, "Well, we can't know for sure. I'm going to prepare these slides for STDs, including gonorrhea, syphilis, and chlamydia" and then proceeded to prescribe a week's antibiotics to take until the results came back. Needless to say, she didn't take the drugs. Nor did the results test positive for any infections. As she cynically sighed, "I knew this was normal for me. But what about the average woman who doesn't know FAM? What kind of message does this send her?"*

Is it any wonder that women grow up believing they are dirty all the time and need to douche and spray away the "discharge"? The continual advertising of douches and feminine sprays only acts to reinforce the confusion between healthy cervical fluid and what is, in fact, a true infection. Millions of dollars a year are spent promoting vaginal douches alone.

If you think this is harmless, consider a well-known talk show whose topic one day was gynecology. No sooner had the two OB/GYNs finished explaining why douches and sprays were unnecessary and potentially infection-producing, when the show cut to a commercial. And what was the commercial about? You guessed it—vaginal sprays! Only a minute earlier, one of the gynecologists cynically commented that the income he generated from treating women who had developed infections from using these products was enough to send all his children to college. And nowadays, with over-the-counter products readily available for yeast infections, how many women buy them every month to try to eliminate the supposed infection that keeps recurring?

Realistically, though, there are going to be times when you really do have a vaginal infection. Obviously, knowing your own pattern will enable you to detect the onset of infection almost immediately, treating it before you become uncomfortable. One of the reasons women are often misdiagnosed, as was the instructor above, is that a "symptom" during one time in a woman's cycle may be nothing more than a fertility sign in another. So, for example, wet secretions midcycle are absolutely normal, but may be an indication of infection if they occur in the latter phase. (One exception to this is explained on page 288.) Of course, the sooner you detect a potential infection, the sooner you can treat and eliminate it.

## Symptoms of Vaginal Infections That Can Be Distinguished from Normal Cervical Fluid

Fortunately, once you know your own cervical-fluid pattern, you'll be able to clearly see that true infections almost always appear with any number of unpleasant symptoms that distinguish them. Vaginal infections can range from STDs such as chlamydia and herpes to various forms of vaginitis and, of course, the generic yeast infection. While it is beyond the scope of this book to identify the individual symptoms and treatments for all these conditions, the following symptoms are definitely not part of healthy cervical-fluid secretions, and should therefore be seen by a qualified clinician:*

- Abnormal discharge
- Itching, stinging, swelling, and redness
- Unpleasant odor
- Blisters, warts, and chancre sores

## Avoiding Infections

There are certain precautions you should take to avoid contracting infections in the first place. Aside from the obvious consequences of douching, you should be aware that wearing clothing that is either damp or too tight may create an unhealthy vaginal environment. Also be sure to always wear cotton underwear and lingerie that allows your body to breathe.

## &#8450; NORMAL SPOTTING VERSUS ABNORMAL BLEEDING

## Normal Spotting

One of the most misunderstood facets of the woman's cycle is that of normal spotting. This type of light bleeding, which occurs between periods, has a number of causes. It is usually brownish because, unlike a normal menstrual flow, the blood barely trickles out of the body. A common mistake many women make is to assume that all bleeding episodes are periods. In reality, true menstruation is the bleeding that occurs about 12 to 16 days following the release of an egg. Any other type of bleeding is either anovulatory bleeding, normal spotting, or symptomatic of a problem.

### Ovulatory Spotting

Simply stated, some women have a day or two of light bleeding right around ovulation. Not only is this spotting normal, but it's another fertility sign that can help identify where they are in their cycle. It's usually the result of the sudden drop of estrogen just before ovulation, and tends to occur more often in long cycles.

---

* For a comprehensive discussion of various gynecological infections and conditions, I would encourage you to get a good, general women's health book such as *Understanding Your Body* by Felicia Stewart, MD, et al., or *Womancare* by Jane Patterson, MD.

**Chart 15.1. Ovulatory Spotting.** It is perfectly normal for women to have spotting around ovulation, in this case on Days 14 and 15. (Ovulation is clearly seen to have occurred by the thermal shift on Day 16.) Had the spotting occurred several days away from ovulation, it could have been a sign of abnormal bleeding.

> *Another FAM instructor describes her experience using a diaphragm before she learned a natural method of birth control. Every now and then, when she would remove it after making love, there would be a little blood and slippery cervical fluid mixed in with the spermicide. She would find it very confusing and wonder whether her partner had injured her cervix during intercourse. It wasn't until years later that she realized that the blood she had seen periodically was merely ovulatory spotting collected in the diaphragm.*

### Anovulatory Bleeding and Spotting

Occasionally women don't release an egg, for several reasons. One is that estrogen doesn't reach the threshold necessary for the egg to be released. When this happens, the drop in estrogen is enough to cause a slight shedding of the lining of the uterus. At other times, estrogen may continue to stimulate the growth of the uterine lining to such an extent that it can't support itself sufficiently, and breakthrough bleeding occurs. In women over 40, the cause of anovulatory bleeding is often the result of a decreased sensitivity to the hormones FSH and LH. The result is that the woman may not ovulate, and without progesterone to sustain the lining, spotting or bleeding may occur. In all these cases, though, the bleeding is not technically menstruation. The way to determine if a woman did indeed ovulate is through charting the temperature.

Remember, ovulatory cycles reflect a classic temperature pattern of low before ovulation, followed by high after.

### Implantation Spotting

Likewise, if a woman was trying to get pregnant and noticed spotting rather than bleeding anytime from about a week after her thermal shift, she should consider taking a pregnancy test because it may be "implantation spotting" rather than a period. When the egg burrows into the endometrial lining of the uterus, a little spotting may occur. She can also confirm if she is pregnant by noting if her temperatures continue to remain high beyond 18 days. This would indicate that the corpus luteum was staying alive to support a pregnancy.

### Breastfeeding Spotting

Women who have just delivered a child may find that after the initial lochia has stopped, they have an episode of spotting at about 6 weeks postpartum. It's usually due to the withdrawal of hormones that had been circulating at high levels when the woman was pregnant. In addition, while breastfeeding, hormone levels can fluctuate due to the varying needs of the baby. Because of this temporary hormonal imbalance, breastfeeding women may experience a number of anovulatory spottings. (See Appendices B and C on how to use FAM while breastfeeding.)

### Spotting After Office Procedures

Women will often spot after office procedures such as Pap tests, cervical biopsies, cryosurgery, cautery, laser surgery, pelvic exams, IUD insertions, and abortions. This is normal.

### Spotting with Birth Control Pills and Estrogen Replacement Therapy

In addition, women will usually experience withdrawal bleeding during the week in which they are not taking either the Pill or postmenopausal hormone replacement therapy.

## Abnormal Bleeding

As you now see, spotting can be absolutely normal. But it can also be an indication of a potential problem. If you note unexplainable bleeding on your chart, it should alert you to seek medical care. Fortunately, most cases of abnormal bleeding are also accompanied by other symptoms.

You should be particularly alert to such signs as cramping or abdominal back pain, abnormal vaginal discharge, and fevers and chills, as well as any kind of pain during urination or intercourse. Such symptoms when accompanied by abnormal bleeding could be symptomatic of a variety of conditions, from pelvic infections to various STDs. You should also consult a doctor if you have abnormal bleeding with persistent ulcers or growths on the cervix, since these could be symptomatic of cervical cancer. Fortunately though, most cervical polyps or other similar growths will be benign.

## ✌ NORMAL NABOTHIAN CYSTS ON THE CERVIX VERSUS ABNORMAL CERVICAL POLYPS

### *Normal Nabothian Cysts on the Cervix*

An example of a common female condition is nabothian cysts. As mentioned earlier, they are little bumps that women occasionally develop on their cervix. Women who haven't been taught about these cysts may panic the first time they feel one, not realizing they are completely harmless. Women often feel them for the first time while checking their cervix or inserting a diaphragm or cervical cap. They usually disappear on their own, but if they don't, you should probably have them checked by a clinician the first time you feel one to rule out anything else. Then simply draw them on your chart in the miscellaneous section and keep track of them. You can chart them as follows:

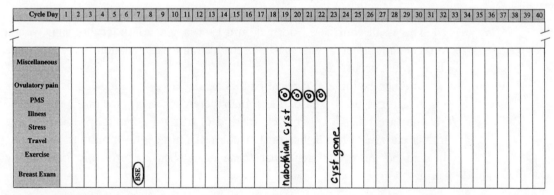

**Chart 15.2. Nabothian cyst on the cervix.** Note that the location of the cyst is recorded with a dot on the cervix drawing.

## Abnormal Cervical Polyps

Polyps are small, tubular or tear-shaped growths that protrude from the mucus membranes of the cervical canal. Unlike nabothian cysts, which are quite firm, these tend to be somewhat spongy. And even though they are considered abnormal, they're almost always benign. You may not even be aware you have one unless you checked your cervix or experienced one of their symptoms— unusual bleeding. This is due to their vulnerable position in the vagina, making them susceptible to being tapped, especially during intercourse. They are typically not painful, but may cause excess cervical fluid due to irritation of the mucus glands. If you think you may have one, you should consult a physician.

## 🜊 NORMAL CYCLE-RELATED PAIN VERSUS ABNORMAL PAIN

### Normal Cycle-Related Pain

Unfortunately, female pain can be a little tricky. Certain pains during a woman's cycle can be absolutely normal. For example, midcycle pain, which is often referred to as *mittelschmerz,* can be caused by a number of factors:

- the follicles swelling within the ovaries
- the egg passing through the ovarian wall
- a small amount of blood being released at ovulation, irritating the pelvic wall
- contraction of the fallopian tubes

This is all considered normal, and even a secondary fertility sign. When you feel *mittelschmerz,* you can be pretty certain that ovulation is about to take place or just occurred.

Another example of cyclical pain is headaches, which tend to occur in the postovulatory (luteal) phase. If a woman weren't charting, she might not realize that they are related to her cycle instead of being a potential problem. If she finds a pattern of headaches on her chart at only certain points in her cycle, she can be more confident that these headaches are probably hormonally based.

| Cycle Day | 1 | 2 | 3 | 4 | 5 | 6 | 7 | 8 | 9 | 10 | 11 | 12 | 13 | 14 | 15 | 16 | 17 | 18 | 19 | 20 | 21 | 22 | 23 | 24 | 25 | 26 | 27 | 28 | 29 | 30 | 31 | 32 | 33 | 34 | 35 | 36 | 37 | 38 | 39 | 40 |
|---|---|---|---|---|---|---|---|---|---|---|---|---|---|---|---|---|---|---|---|---|---|---|---|---|---|---|---|---|---|---|---|---|---|---|---|---|---|---|---|---|
| Cervical Fluid | ✳ | ✳ | ✳ | ✳ | ✳ | | | | | | | | | | | | | | | | | | | | | | | | | | ✳ | | | | | | | | | |

| Miscellaneous |
|---|

BSE

Cramps
Headache
Breasts tender

**Chart 15.3. Various pains throughout the cycle.** Colors can be used to keep track of cyclical pains or other symptoms. Note that you should fill in the specific symptoms you want to track in the far left column of the chart. The master chart with these color-coding rows can be found in Appendix K.

## Abnormal Pain

On the other hand, if you notice pelvic pain that is intense or occurs at other times in the cycle, it could be an indication of any number of conditions, including endometriosis. This is where the uterine lining (the endometrium) begins to grow outside of the uterus, often attaching to other parts of the internal reproductive system. It can result in adhesions and scarring, and potentially impede fertility. One of the classic symptoms of endometriosis is pelvic pain before and during menstruation, as well as during intercourse (see page 184).

By accurately tracking your symptoms on your chart, you can help your doctor determine if you need further testing to determine the cause of the pain. For this reason, women should learn to recognize what is considered normal, cyclical pain, as opposed to that which is more intense or occurs at unexpected times of the cycle. This is obviously because the latter cases are more likely to indicate a potential health problem. A simple but graphic way to keep track of symptoms during your cycle is through the use of colors as shown on page 7 of the color insert.

| Cycle Day | 1 | 2 | 3 | 4 | 5 | 6 | 7 | 8 | 9 | 10 | 11 | 12 | 13 | 14 | 15 | 16 | 17 | 18 | 19 | 20 | 21 | 22 | 23 | 24 | 25 | 26 | 27 | 28 | 29 | 30 | 31 | 32 | 33 | 34 | 35 | 36 | 37 | 38 | 39 | 40 |
|---|---|---|---|---|---|---|---|---|---|---|---|---|---|---|---|---|---|---|---|---|---|---|---|---|---|---|---|---|---|---|---|---|---|---|---|---|---|---|---|---|
| Miscellaneous | | | | | | | | | | | | | | | | | | | | | | | | | | | | | | | | | | | | | | | | |
| Ovulatory pain | | | | | | | | | | | | | | | | | | | | | | | | | | | | | | | | | | | | | | | | |
| PMS | | | | | | | | | | | | | | | | | | | | | | | | | | | | | | | | | | | | | | | | |
| Illness | | | | | | | | | | | | | | | | | | | | | | | | | | | | | | | | | | | | | | | | |
| Stress | | | | | | | | | | | | | | | | | | | | | | | | | | | | | | | | | | | | | | | | |
| Travel | | | | | | | | | | | | | | | | | | | | | | | | | | | | | | | | | | | | | | | | |
| Exercise | | | | | | | | | | | | | | | | | | | | | | | | | | | | | | | | | | | | | | | | |
| Breast Exam | | | | | | | (BSE) | | | | | | | | | | | | | | | | | | | | | | | | | | | | | | | | | |

**Chart 15.4. Charting breast self-exam.**

## 🙠 NORMAL CYSTIC BREASTS VERSUS CANCEROUS BREAST LUMPS

### Normal Cystic Breasts

Charting your cycle can help you differentiate between normal cyclic breast changes and abnormal breast lumps. The texture of breasts in women with fibrocystic breasts tends to be fairly lumpy, becoming more so in the postovulatory phase of their cycle. By knowing when they have begun that phase, they can determine if their lumps are normal and cyclical, and make the necessary lifestyle adjustments to try to lessen the discomfort of fibrocystic breasts. But if the lump(s) remain throughout the cycle, charting can be extremely beneficial in tracking whether further examination should be made by a health practitioner.

Charting is an excellent way to remind you to do a monthly breast self-exam on Day 7 of your cycle. (Note the BSE symbol in the Miscellaneous column at the bottom of the master chart.) The reason you should perform the exam on that day is because it is the hormonally optimal time since your breasts are least susceptible to lumps or tenderness caused by progesterone. After completing your self-exam, circle the notation on the chart.

### Cancerous Breast Lumps

The prospect of breast cancer is extremely frightening to all women. However, you should know that most lumps are benign and that cancers of the reproductive system are curable if detected and treated early. You, yourself, can directly

# PERFORMING A BREAST SELF-EXAM: DAY 7 OF EVERY CYCLE

Lift arms above shoulders and continue to look for any changes.

Stand in front of a mirror and observe breasts for any dimpling of the skin, changes in the nipple, or redness and swelling.

Put hands on hips and bend slightly.

Check breasts while showering, using the soap to help your hands glide over your breasts.

Lie on a bed with a pillow under one shoulder, placing your arm behind your head. Feel for lumps or thickening with the opposite hand.

affect your chances of finding cancer early if you maintain a healthy lifestyle, get annual pelvic exams and Pap tests, do monthly breast self-exams, and make a point to promptly attend to suspicious symptoms.

The following are warning signs to look for in your breasts. The important point is to notice whether they remain indefinitely, or disappear with the new cycle. Obviously, anything that persists should be examined by a clinician.

- Breast lump or thickening (firm, nonmovable lumps are especially important to watch for)
- Lump in underarm or above collarbone
- Swelling under the arm
- Puckering or dimpling in one area of the breast
- Persistent skin irritation, flaking, redness, or tenderness of breast
- Sudden change in nipple position (such as nipple inversion)
- Bloody nipple discharge

## SCHEDULING THE BEST TIME FOR PHYSICAL EXAMS, CONTRACEPTIVE FITTINGS, VACCINATIONS, AND SURGERY

Another benefit of charting is that it can help you identify the most effective time in your cycle to have physical exams, contraceptive fittings, vaccinations, and surgery. The best time to schedule a Pap test is about midcycle, when the cervix is naturally dilated. In the case of fitting for diaphragms or cervical caps, having it done at the wrong time can mean the difference between complete contraceptive protection and an unplanned pregnancy! Since the cervix clearly changes around ovulation, it only makes sense to get fitted at the time when the method *is most likely to fail.* Remember that when a woman is fertile, her cervix becomes soft, high, and open. That is the best time to do it.

A practical piece of advice would be to have a rubella vaccination performed just after your period. This would assure that you aren't pregnant at the time. This is critical for this particular vaccine, since the effects of the rubella virus on the fetus of pregnant women is potentially disastrous.

Of less significance but certainly interesting are the results of a study that found that postoperative nausea and vomiting is increased in women undergoing laparoscopic tubal sterilization during the first 8 days of their cycle. Of course, one study is hardly convincing, but it is worth noting that surgeries may be affected by when they're performed.

*A pelvic exam typically includes a bimanual and a pap test. The clinician inserts a finger into the vagina to be able to stabilize the uterus from the inside while gently pressing down on the abdomen to palpate the uterus and ovaries from the outside. The pap test is done primarily to detect the presence of pre-cancerous cells of the cervix.*

Some recent studies have suggested that having breast cancer surgery after ovulation may increase your chances of living longer without a recurrence of the disease. One theory for the difference in outcome is that estrogen in the first part of the cycle could stimulate the growth of cancer cells. You should be aware, however, that these findings are controversial and far from reflecting a general consensus.

Since further research may prove that timing surgeries to a particular phase of your cycle increases the odds of a positive outcome, you should ask your physician about it. If the surgery is not serious, it may not be so important. But if it involves something as profound as your survival, I would encourage you to do your homework, and research the latest studies with a discriminating eye.*

## 🐚 STAYING HEALTHY AND KEEPING INFORMED

The information in this chapter has been written to help you distinguish between what is normal and what may require medical attention. Ideally, you should also get an annual exam. The form on the opposite page can serve as a useful record of your overall health in much the same way your fertility charts track your cycles.

---

* The breast cancer studies found in the medical literature may have shown less than convincing results because all of them divided the survival rates of the women into groups based on what cycle day surgery was performed, and not on whether they were truly in their pre- or postovulatory phase. Indeed, the last major study I read in *The Lancet* (June 18, 1994, p. 1545) subdivided 1,175 patients into two groups, with those having allegedly undergone surgery in the postovulatory luteal phase comprising Days 15 to 36. Of course, any women who eventually had a cycle of 30 days or longer were almost certainly placed in the wrong group, since as you now know, such women most likely ovulated on Days 16 through 22, and not on Day 14, as was assumed.

None of the studies have structured the research to *truly* divide the women into pre- and postovulatory status. This is not surprising given the logistical hurdles involved in doing so. But if research along these lines could be done (working with women who do chart their temperatures), there is a greater chance of finding a definitive answer to this question.

## ANNUAL PHYSICAL EXAM

Date _____ Day of Cycle _____ Doctor _____

Weight _____ lbs.

Blood pressure _____/_____

Heart _____

Lungs _____

Urine test _____

Blood test _____ White blood cells _____

Cholesterol _____ Ratio _____ HDL _____

Pap test (class) _____ White blood cells _____ Yeast _____

Chlamydia test _____

Other tests _____ _____

_____ _____

_____ _____

Breast exam _____ _____

_____

Cervix
anomalies _____

_____

Uterus or
ovary anomalies _____

_____

_____

Miscellaneous _____

_____

_____

# CHAPTER 16

# Appreciating Your Sexuality and Nurturing Your Relationship

*"How is your sex life? How often do you have sex?" asked their respective therapists. Alvy Singer reflected. "Hardly ever, maybe three times a week," he whined. "Constantly . . . I'd say three times a week," Annie Hall complained. He felt deprived. She felt exhausted.*
—SCENE FROM WOODY ALLEN'S MOVIE *Annie Hall,* 1977

Does that sound familiar? A woman's sexuality doesn't have to be the mystery so many people think it is. In reality, there are a number of reasons why women and men differ sexually. Most women tend to view lovemaking as an emotional and intimate experience, not just a physical act. So women tend to get aroused if they feel trust and affection in the hours and even days leading up to intercourse. Men, on the other hand, tend to place more importance on the visual and other stimuli at the actual time of sexual interaction.

In addition, a woman's physical experience of sex is quite different from a man's simply because her clitoris is located outside of her vagina. This one fact can dramatically affect every aspect of her emotional and physical sexuality. Men need to realize this.

Finally, a woman's sexuality is often closely tied to her cycle. Many women themselves don't understand this. Is it any wonder, then, that men often find women somewhat confusing? But men who help their partners chart often maintain that they finally understand female sexuality in a way that often eluded them before. They describe the newfound wisdom that they've acquired in understanding an aspect of women that is so frequently misunderstood.

These next few pages will hopefully clarify the puzzle and make you appreciate the secret of your sexuality.

## Why Orgasms During Intercourse May Be Hard for You to Attain

> *In the case of some women, orgasms take quite a bit of time. Before signing on with such a partner, make sure you are willing to lay aside, say, the month of June . . .*
>
> —BRUCE JAY FRIEDMAN

As you probably know, the most sensitive part of the man's body is near the tip of the penis. On the woman, it is the clitoris. The problem is that because the clitoris is situated outside the vagina, intercourse is often not as intense for women as it is for men. In fact, studies indicate that a large majority of women are unable to achieve orgasm through penetration alone.* Internalizing this one physiological fact and really understanding how it can affect a woman's sexuality is critical for men to develop a truly loving, sexual relationship with their partner.

Because a lot of people don't really know basic human anatomy, misunderstandings result. For example, women often fake orgasms because they don't want to hurt their partner's feelings or they don't think it's worth the longer time and effort it would take to have one. This type of deception can poison an intimate relationship, which is unfortunate because it could so easily be resolved if both people understood the difference between male and female physiology. Needless to say, communication between partners is the key to developing a fulfilling and warm sexual relationship.

It's a good thing we don't live in the 1870s. John Davenport would have us believe that women shouldn't have orgasms at all. As he described it in *Curiositates Eroticae Physiolgiae* (1875), the result of orgasm in women was that:

> She burns and as it were, dries up the semen received by her from the male, and if by chance a child *is* conceived, it is ill-formed and does not remain 9 months in the mother's womb.

Indeed. In any case, it's over a century later, and we certainly don't believe that female orgasms are harmful anymore. But the length of time it takes for a

---

* This is pretty amazing in light of the brainwashing bestowed upon a whole generation of women by Sigmund Freud. His theory of female sexuality was rooted in the delusional belief that women who weren't able to attain a "vaginal orgasm" exclusively during intercourse were immature and in need of psychotherapy.

woman to climax can be frustrating if people don't understand how normal it is for women to take longer than men. Even if communication between a couple is completely open and healthy, women usually require more stimulation to reach an orgasm.

Many men assume that as soon as the woman has become lubricated, she is ready to be penetrated. For most women, this is not true. Vaginal lubrication is one of the *first* signs of arousal. It only signals that she is gradually becoming more interested in further love play. Most women still need considerable time and *sensual* (rather than sexual) touching to become fully aroused. In fact, one of the most common complaints women make about men as lovers is that they rush through the motions and are too narrowly focused on the genitals, rather than the whole body. You've probably heard it before, but in this context it's worth repeating the adage: "Women make love in order to touch, men touch in order to make love."

## What You Can Do to Increase Vaginal Feelings During Intercourse

For some women, being asked if she has had an orgasm during intercourse is a sign that her partner doesn't really understand what excites her. In his excellent book, *Sexual Solutions,* Michael Castleman asks men to develop a different sexual perspective:

> Imagine your own feelings if a woman climaxed courtesy of your oral-clitoral stimulation, then asked you: "Did you come?" Many men would resent the question: "How can you even ask if I've come? I've been stimulating you. You haven't touched me where it counts!" Women feel the same way.

Still, many women can increase their chances of having an orgasm during intercourse by learning what positions best stimulate their clitoris. Many women who can climax in this way say the optimal position is straddling on top of their partner, with one of them directly stimulating her clitoris. Most women agree that intercourse in the missionary position is simply not enough to lead to orgasm.*

---

* One of the most failproof ways for women to achieve an orgasm is through using a vibrator. Many couples include it as part of their lovemaking. If a woman has never had an orgasm, she may want to try using a vibrator by herself to learn what level of intensity works for her. The best type of vibrators are those that can easily stimulate the clitoris and *not* those that are shaped like a penis.

"It's a little disorienting when Louise tells
me that I can always be replaced by a
pulsating shower."

In addition, many people don't realize that the vagina is a muscle that can
be strengthened just like any other. Both men and women find that sex can be
more fulfilling when the woman has control over her vaginal muscle. The way
to strengthen it is through Kegels or vaginal contractions. By simply tightening
and releasing the vagina every day, you can increase sexual satisfaction for both
of you. You can do any combination of Kegels that's comfortable. A key advantage of these exercises is that they can be done any time, anywhere, without
others being aware of it. So, for example, you can do Kegels while talking to
your grocer or giving a presentation at a corporate meeting. The point is to do
them as often as necessary to maintain a healthy, strong vagina that promotes
sexual gratification for you and your partner (see page 85).

## Why You May Feel Sexier Midcycle

Juicy, luscious, delectable, succulent, and delicious . . . no, I'm not talking
about a pineapple. I'm referring to fertile cervical fluid as described by the
renowned childbirth educator, Sheila Kitzinger. As you know, women often
develop abundant amounts of slippery, wet cervical fluid as they approach
ovulation. Since it feels wet and lubricative, women are conditioned to associate
it with sexual excitement. Of course, arousal fluid tends to dissipate in a few

seconds when waved in the air. True fertile cervical fluid will remain on your finger.

Besides the similarity between fertile cervical fluid and sexual lubrication, something else is responsible for women often feeling more sexual midcycle. The high levels of estrogen around ovulation act to heighten sexuality in many women. They may also notice that their vaginal lips feel fuller and tend to blossom open. Again, this is related to the increased hormones before ovulation. These physical changes can make women feel especially sexual at this time.

This increased sexuality can admittedly be somewhat untimely for women who use FAM for natural birth control. They often feel that their fertile phase is the time they especially want to have intercourse. But many FAM users view the fertile phase as a time to be especially creative with other forms of lovemaking, knowing that in a few days they can resume intercourse again (of course, barriers can also be used).

## Why Intercourse Can Be Uncomfortable During Certain Phases of the Cycle

You may occasionally feel a deep pain during intercourse. Or perhaps you notice discomfort during certain sexual positions, especially if you straddle atop your partner. Remember that when your estrogen levels are low and you're outside your fertile phase, particularly after ovulation, your cervix tends to be low in your vagina. During these times, it is possible that your partner's penis can actually tap your cervix during intercourse.

The reason you may feel the discomfort only when you straddle him is that the cervix tends to drop lower in that position. This makes sense when you consider that the best way to check the cervix is by squatting, since this is the position that pushes the cervix to its lowest point. This doesn't mean that you can't ever enjoy sex in that position, but you should be aware of the fact that when you're not fertile, your cervix may be too low to be comfortable.

## How Birth Control Can Affect Your Sexuality

It should come as no surprise to you that birth control can be a source of tension between many couples. Because no method is perfect, there may be drawbacks that undermine a couple's intimacy by tending to place the burden on the woman. For example, if a woman feels resentful that she has to endure urinary tract infections from the diaphragm, or vaginal dryness from the Pill, she may not be as receptive to intercourse as the man would be.

But if her partner lovingly participates in her charting, she will probably be much more sexually responsive. In essence, through his actions he can show her how respectful he is of her body and comfort, and how much he wants to share in the responsibility of contraception. The fact is that birth control doesn't have to be a decisive issue in the bedroom.

> *Among my first clients was a charming couple, Erin and Nick. As we were reviewing Erin's charts, I realized the writing was barely legible. It said something about her menstrual cramps that day, but I couldn't decipher it. When I asked her what it said, she held it up to her eyes, squinted, then turned to Nick and said, "Honey, what did you write here? I can't read it either." As it turned out, the entire chart was in his writing, down to the most intimate details of her menstrual cycle.*

## How Your Partner Can Participate in Your Charting—and Why He Should

> *Men fear women.*
> *Men fear women period.*
> *Men fear women's periods.*
> *Men fear women not getting their periods.**

Men are often criticized for not taking a bigger role in birth control and even pregnancy achievement. But the truth is that many men are very caring and loving and would be happy to be more actively involved if only there were a way they could. As you've seen, with the Fertility Awareness Method, there is. The beauty of charting is that a man can be as involved as his partner— taking her temps, jotting down her fertility signs, determining when her fertile phase has begun and ended. And rather than perceiving it as work, most people agree that the minute or two a day is so enlightening that it can be fun rather than a chore. Men who help their partners chart find that they discover a lot about them in the process. Ultimately, FAM can draw couples together.

The reality is that aside from the condom, withdrawal, or a vasectomy, the Fertility Awareness Method is the contraceptive most conducive to male involvement. Remember that the FAM rules were designed for the combined fertility of the man and woman together. Men are fertile every single day, whereas women are only fertile a few days per cycle. The first part of the

---

* Adapted from *Beyond Putting the Toilet Seat Down* by Jack York and Brian Krueger.

| Cycle Day | 1 | 2 | 3 | 4 | 5 | 6 | 7 | 8 | 9 | 10 | 11 | 12 | 13 | 14 | 15 | 16 | 17 | 18 | 19 | 20 | 21 | 22 | 23 | 24 | 25 | 26 | 27 | 28 | 29 | 30 | 31 | 32 | 33 | 34 | 35 | 36 | 37 | 38 | 39 | 40 |
|---|---|---|---|---|---|---|---|---|---|---|---|---|---|---|---|---|---|---|---|---|---|---|---|---|---|---|---|---|---|---|---|---|---|---|---|---|---|---|---|---|
| Cervical Fluid | | | | | | | | | | | | | | | | | | | | | | | | | | | | | | | | | | | | | | | | |
| Peak Day | | | | | | | | | | | | | | | | | | | | | | | | | | | | | | | | | | | | | | | | |
| Vaginal Sensation | | | | | | | | | | | | | | | | | | | | | | | | | | | | | | | | | | | | | | | | |
| Cervix | | | | | | | | | | | | | | | | | | | | | | | | | | | | | | | | | | | | | | | | |

5-day sperm survival   1-day egg survival (2 days for possible multiple ovulation)

**Chart 16.1.** The woman's fertile phase is determined by egg *and* sperm viability.

woman's fertile phase is a reflection of the man's fertility (that is, the potential for sperm to survive 5 days in fertile cervical fluid). The second part is a reflection of the woman's fertility (that is, the potential for an egg to survive one day, with an additional day added for a possible double ovulation). More succinctly stated, then, a woman's fertile phase is a function of the respective fertility of both partners.

Many men who learn about the menstrual cycle are struck with the idea that the length of their partner's fertility is primarily determined by their own continuous fertility, and thus feel equally responsible for contraception. By being so aware of their partner's cycle, they are more understanding and cooperative because they can no longer feign ignorance. It's worth remembering that many accidental pregnancies result from a lack of communication between the two partners. FAM is a wonderful way to involve both individuals equally in such an important aspect of a couple's life.

The Fertility Awareness Method encourages couples to communicate, simply because it is more effective if both partners understand it together. As you've seen, men often choose to do the actual charting. In order to record the woman's fertility signs, he may ask her about all facets of her cycle—from what kind of cervical fluid she had, to whether she had breast tenderness or felt depressed during the day. In other words, the man can become intimately in tune with his partner's biology and emotions by simply recording her chart. The potential for furthering intimacy is obvious. As one of my male clients said, "If you can talk about cervical fluid, you can talk about anything!"

# CHAPTER 17

# Choosing the Sex of Your Baby

For those of you who just skipped ahead to this chapter, it is critical that you fully understand the information discussed in Chapters 5, 6, and 11 before attempting to follow the guidelines presented here.

*T*rying to choose the sex of the baby you conceive may strike many as unethical or just plain bizarre, but others find it exciting and even fun. Over the years, several theories have been posited to help people increase the chances of conceiving a boy or girl, yet they've contradicted each other, leading many to discount the possibility altogether. Indeed, such theories have been hypothesized since the Middle Ages, though one wonders how seriously they were taken at the time. The noted Italian physician Trotula wrote in 1059:

> If they wish to have a male child let the man take the womb and vulva of a hare and have it dried and pulverized; blend it with wine and let him drink it. Let the woman do the same with the testicles of the hare and let her be with her husband at the end of her menstrual period and she will conceive a male.

Fortunately, the gender selection techniques discussed in this chapter have eliminated the hare.

Since the 1970s, Dr. Landrum Shettles, M.D., Ph.D., has developed a scientifically based, fairly simple way in which to increase your chances of having a boy or girl. He has written an informative book called *How to Choose the Sex of Your Baby* (Doubleday, 1989). This chapter adapts many of the critical points in his book but emphasizes Fertility Awareness principles to help improve your odds. You may wish to read Dr. Shettles's own work for more thorough coverage of the topic.

While various studies have shown the Shettles method to be quite successful, I must emphasize here that its overall effectiveness is still widely disputed in the medical community. I do not profess to be an expert on this subject, but I discuss it in this book because once you know the fundamental principles of Fertility Awareness, this method of gender selection is relatively easy to apply. In addition, it is clear that of all the natural theories proposed, Shettles's method is the best supported by scientific studies.

Of course, even the method's most ardent supporters do not suggest it is anywhere near foolproof. Dr. Shettles himself claims that it is about 80–90% effective for choosing boys and 75–80% effective for choosing girls when the method rules are followed correctly. The reason for the lower rates for girls is that it is more difficult to appropriately time intercourse when trying for a female.

The most fundamental principle on which the Shettles method is based is that sperm determine what sex a baby will be. The male sperm (XY chromosomes) are smaller, lighter, faster, and more fragile than the female sperm (XX chromosomes).* The female sperm are generally bigger, heavier, slower, and heartier, and thus they tend to live longer than the male sperm. All of this means that if you desire a boy, you should time intercourse as close to ovulation as possible so that the fast, light, male sperm reach their prize first. Likewise, if you prefer a girl, you should time intercourse as far from ovulation as you can while still allowing conception to occur.

The primary evidence on which Shettles bases his method is that male sperm generally beat female sperm when put through a race course of alkaline, fertile-quality cervical fluid in laboratory containers. Sperm retrieved from the woman's reproductive tract also confirm that male sperm are faster than the female sperm, but that female sperm are more resilient.

### The Evidence that Indirectly or Partially Supports the Shettles Method Can Be Divided by Gender Outcome:

**Male**
- Artificial insemination (AI) results in a preponderance of male offspring, which makes sense, given that AI is always done as close to

---

* For simplicity's sake, for the remainder of this chapter, I will refer to sperm carrying male XY chromosomes as "male sperm," and sperm carrying female XX chromosomes as "female sperm."

ovulation as possible. The closer to ovulation, the more likely the male sperm will race up to the egg before the slower, heavier female sperm.

- Younger men and women tend to have more male conceptions than older individuals. It's hypothesized that the reason for this is that younger men generally have higher sperm counts and younger women tend to have more copious, alkaline quality cervical fluid—both of which favor male conceptions.

## Female

- More girls tend to be born to couples who use in vitro fertilization for achieving their desired pregnancies. Researchers speculate that more female sperm are capable of surviving the stresses imposed on them through the rigorous laboratory procedure.
- Men with low sperm counts tend to have more female sperm. (Shettles theorizes it may be because the same factors that would cause a low sperm count are likely to kill many of the more fragile male sperm, such as heat, certain drugs, and toxic substances.)
- Studies show that undersea divers in Australia and high-performance military aircraft pilots elsewhere have predominantly fathered daughters. Researchers theorize the reason may be due to the fact that both are subject to unusual environmental stresses, including shifting atmospheric pressures, varying oxygen tension, possible radiation, and excessive scrotal heat from tight-fitting wet suits and flight suits. It makes sense that the sperm that would survive such abuse are the hardier female sperm.
- Anesthesiologists tend to father more girls than boys. It's also known that they are exposed to many toxic substances in the course of their career, so it's understandable that the female sperm are the ones that are more likely to survive in greater numbers.
- A study of men with non-Hodgkin's lymphoma revealed that 154 out of 190 children born were girls, again revealing the resilient nature of female sperm.

## Both

- Fraternal twins (from two different eggs) are usually the same sex, which would support the idea that timing of intercourse is of critical importance in determining the sex of the baby. Since fraternal twins are conceived within 24 hours of each other, the conditions within the mother's reproductive tract are presumably the same for each conception.

Although the debate continues, it is true that many carefully controlled studies from Japan to Nigeria seem to clearly show what Shettles has now proposed for over 20 years: *The critical variable in terms of gender selection is the timing of intercourse in relation to ovulation.*

## ✿ FERTILITY AWARENESS AND GENDER SELECTION

Before seeing how Fertility Awareness specifically fits in with the Shettles method, you should chart at least three cycles before attempting gender selection in order to really know your own cycle well. If just starting to chart, it is best to either abstain or use condoms so as not to mask cervical fluid. This will help you to accurately identify its pattern while preventing a pregnancy that wasn't well-timed for the gender you want.

## ✿ TIMING INTERCOURSE FOR A BOY

> You should have intercourse on your Peak Day, as well as the following day.

If you desire, you can initially have intercourse in the first part of the cycle, but only on dry days. Once you start to have any cervical fluid, you should abstain in order to minimize the risk of conceiving a girl. *Then, have intercourse on what you perceive will be your Peak Day as well as the day after.* (In order to determine your Peak Day, review pages 83–84.)

Remember that, ideally, you are trying to time sex as close to ovulation as possible. Dr. Shettles says that you should try to time intercourse for the day of ovulation itself, but, in reality, it makes more sense to time for the Peak Day, which is often the day before. This is because by the time ovulation occurs, the cervical fluid will have frequently dried up already, thus dramatically reducing the possibility of conception for any gender. In any case, without the use of ultrasound, there is no practical way to truly know which precise day you are ovulating.

**Chart 17.1. Timing intercourse for a boy.** Note that when timing for a boy, the couple should try to have intercourse on the Peak Day as well as the following day. Here the Peak Day was on Day 15, and thus intercourse was timed accurately.

One of the reasons to chart a few cycles first is to *determine how many days of fertile cervical fluid you usually have.* Generally speaking, most women tend to have a fairly consistent number of eggwhite days each cycle. (Those who don't produce eggwhite will usually produce creamy, wet cervical fluid.) You can clearly see that the better you know your cervical-fluid pattern, the more likely you will time sex accurately, and thus conceive the baby boy you both desire.

## A Note on Basal Body Temperatures

For most women, temperature charting has little strategic value in gender selection. For predictive purposes, the only women to benefit from charting their temperature in this situation are those few who show a dip before the thermal shift. In those women, the dip usually does coincide with the day of ovulation, and thus it could be useful in timing for a boy. For all other women, temperatures are still practical, but only for identifying when ovulation occurred in retrospect, and thus for seeing how accurately you timed intercourse for either gender.

### Using Ovulation Predictor Kits for Choosing a Boy

I believe that cervical fluid is the most appropriate way to time intercourse for gender selection purposes. However, if you do decide to use ovulation predictor kits, Shettles recommends that you choose one that will allow you to test your urine any time of day, not just the first morning's urine. This is because a woman is most likely to detect an LH surge that indicates impending ovulation when she tests between 11 A.M. and 3 P.M. You should test again after 5 P.M. The two tests should be spaced about 10 hours apart, with noon and 10 P.M. considered ideal. Wait about 12 hours after you first detect the LH surge to have intercourse, since sex immediately after detection may increase the chance of conceiving a girl.

Finally, you should be aware that women with irregular or long cycles should not start testing until they notice their cervical fluid start to get wet. This will ensure that the kits are at least being used at the most appropriate time, as ovulation approaches.

## ≈ TIMING INTERCOURSE FOR A GIRL

> You should have intercourse several days *before* your Peak Day, but preferably not closer than 2 days before.

It may take a little more patience and perseverance to conceive a girl, because the timing is trickier. You'll want to have intercourse far enough away from ovulation to assure that mostly female sperm remain, but close enough to still allow a conception to occur. As with trying for a boy, the better you know your cervical-fluid pattern, the more likely you'll be able to time sex correctly.

The key is to time intercourse from *4 to 2 days before your Peak Day*. (In order to determine when that is, review pages 83–84.) What this means, practically speaking, is that you should first try 4 days before you anticipate the Peak Day. However, if that fourth day is no wetter than sticky, you should initially try the third day before. If that doesn't work, try a day closer the following cycle. But for the first few cycles, do not have sex any closer than 2 days before you expect your Peak Day.

**Chart 17.2. Timing intercourse for a girl.** Note that when timing for a girl, this couple has sex on Day 11, which they estimate to be 4 days before their Peak Day. If they fail to conceive, they may try in later cycles just 2 or 3 days before the estimated Peak Day (the equivalent of Days 13 and 14 in the sample above).

If you have gone several cycles without conceiving, you may decide to try intercourse on what you estimate to be only 1 day before your Peak Day. The fact is that doing this greatly increases the odds of conceiving, but the risk of having a boy also goes up. I personally suspect that a girl is still more likely because it appears that ovulation most often takes place the day after the Peak Day, or a full 2 days after you would have intercourse. However, it's also true that ovulation may occur on the Peak Day itself, in which case the Shettles method would predict a male conception. You now see why it's harder to time for a girl!

*Remember, the point is to try to have intercourse as far from ovulation as you can and still have conception occur.* After the cutoff date, you should abstain from intercourse or use barriers until you are outside your fertile phase. If you continued to have sex right up through ovulation, you would dramatically increase the risk of conceiving a boy.*

---

* Obviously, if you have any problems with infertility, it is probably not worth following the guidelines for having a girl.

*Why Basal Body Temperatures and Ovulation Predictor Kits Are Essentially Useless for Choosing a Girl*

Because gender timing for a girl involves having sex as far in advance of ovulation as possible while still allowing for conception, neither temperature charting nor ovulation kits are helpful. As you know, the temperature shift will generally only tell you that you've already ovulated, not that ovulation is approaching. Since you are trying to conceive several days before this shift will occur, the bottom line is that it has no strategic value.

Likewise, ovulation kits are almost as useless for timing intercourse to conceive a girl, since they only detect the LH surge, which itself only occurs a day or so before ovulation. If intercourse for a girl is truly well timed, it will have almost certainly occurred before either the temperature or kit could tell you where you are in your cycle.

## ❧ CONCLUDING REMARKS ON GENDER SELECTION

The guidelines presented in this chapter may greatly increase your odds of conceiving the gender of your choice. However, I should emphasize again that even the method's most ardent supporters do not claim that they are foolproof. Thus, if you are someone who would be greatly disappointed by the birth of your *second* choice, you should strongly reflect on the potential risk before trying to conceive. If you do choose to make the attempt, good luck!

## GUIDELINES FOR MAXIMIZING THE ODDS OF SUCCESSFUL GENDER SELECTION

|  | Boy | Girl |
|---|---|---|
| **Ideal Timing of Intercourse** | Day of ovulation, or the day before. | 4 to 2 days before ovulation. |
| **Timing Sex with Cervical Fluid** | Have sex on your Peak Day (the *last* day of eggwhite cervical fluid or lubricative vaginal sensation), as well as the following day. | Have sex several days *before* your Peak Day (the last day of egg-white cervical fluid or lubricative vaginal sensation), but not closer than 2 days before. Note that 1 day before increases the odds of conception, but also the risk of conceiving a boy. |
| **Timing Sex with Ovulation Predictor Kits** | Test two times a day. Have sex 12 to 24 hours *after* LH surge. | Not useful for girl gender selection. |
| **When to Stop Having Intercourse Before the Target Day** | Can have intercourse every preovulatory *dry* day, but then abstain until the target day. | Can have intercourse every day right up to the last target day. |

# CHAPTER 18

# Premenstrual Syndrome:
# It's Not All in My Head?

*A*h, yes. Premenstrual syndrome. The common condition whose cause eludes researchers and doctors alike. At times, it seems as if there are as many theories about PMS as there are symptoms. "It's a hormonal imbalance." "No, it's due to a vitamin deficiency." "Actually, it's related to prostaglandins." "Wrong. It's obviously due to an endorphin deficit."

The only thing that researchers and clinicians can agree on is the validity of the condition itself, and the fact that it can be debilitating for many women. So what is PMS? Basically, it is a condition that can cause a variety of unpleasant physical and emotional symptoms in the luteal (postovulatory) phase of the woman's cycle. Although most women tend to experience it in the week or so leading up to menstruation, it can happen any time from ovulation on. Yet the timing of the symptoms is often consistent within each woman, and thus charting may be able to give you the opportunity to deal with it constructively.

## ❧ THOSE DELIGHTFUL SYMPTOMS

It's been estimated that as many as nine out of ten women experience at least some form of PMS during their reproductive years. Since it is unclear what causes it, there are different theories as to how best to treat it. One of the better books on the subject is *Premenstrual Syndrome Self-Help Book* by Susan M. Lark, M.D. (Celestial Arts, 1984). If you are adversely affected by PMS, I would encourage you to read it, since it clearly explains practical ways in which you can alleviate many of your symptoms.

Even the way symptoms are categorized varies among clinicians, though most tend to classify them into the four different groupings below. Still, be aware that most women don't necessarily fit neatly into any single category:

| | |
|---|---|
| Type A | Anxiety<br>Irritability<br>Mood swings |
| Type B | Bloating<br>Weight gain<br>Breast tenderness |
| Type C | Cravings (especially for sweets)<br>Fatigue<br>Headaches |
| Type D | Depression<br>Memory loss<br>Moodiness* |

## ✒ DIAGNOSING AND CHARTING PMS

The most important point in diagnosing PMS is that you determine whether the symptoms are *cyclical* in nature. If you experience them periodically throughout your cycle, they would not be considered PMS. Of course, what makes it cyclical is the hormonal changes that occur in an ovulatory cycle. This means that technically women who don't ovulate shouldn't experience classic PMS. That would include preadolescent girls as well as those who are pregnant or postmenopausal. One would also expect women on the Pill to not experience PMS symptoms since they don't ovulate either, but for inexplicable reasons, they often have heightened symptoms.

When trying to determine if you even have PMS, the first step is to chart your symptoms along with your fertility signs. By recording both, you can verify the cyclical nature of the symptoms you have and what factors may trigger them. The best way to keep track of the various symptoms is to draw narrow rows in the Miscellaneous column of your chart, and write them in the margin (or use one of the master charts in Appendix K). Most women find that

---

* For some women, moodiness can actually be positive. As my friend Tanya describes it, PMSS stands for Premenstrual Sentimentality and Silliness.

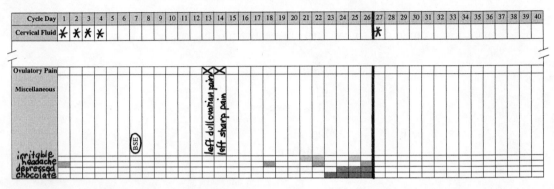

**Charting 18.1. Charting PMS signs.** Dana records various PMS signs using different colors near the bottom of the chart. This allows her to quickly determine whether her symptoms are cyclical or indicative of a problem requiring medical attention. (A special chart with the narrow lines already drawn is in Appendix K.)

color-coding is an excellent way to immediately visualize when they occur in the cycle. Use colors that you associate with the particular symptom.

For example:

| | |
|---|---|
| Headaches | Red |
| Chocolate cravings | Brown |
| Depression | Blue |
| Irritability | Fluorescent green (or some other irritating color) |

## ❧ TREATING PMS

Once you have determined the cyclical nature of your PMS symptoms, you can then decide on appropriate steps to take. Many women find that just being aware of their cyclical nature can help alleviate them. When you realize that your depression, irritability, or headache is only a sign that your period is a few days away, you should have less cause for concern. Often the symptoms themselves create needless anxiety as women wonder if they are "going crazy" or suffering from a serious illness. The knowledge and control that come with charting can be the first step in managing PMS.

There are many self-help therapies that seem to work well for women, but if you suffer severe symptoms, I would encourage you to get medically evaluated before attempting to treat yourself through change in diet, vitamins, or minerals. Severe PMS (such as depression or panic attacks) can be an indication that you have underlying problems that may require therapy before you decide to tackle the symptoms alone.

Treatments range from alternative health care to traditional medical therapy, with self-help approaches somewhere in the middle. Your goal should be to discover the best solution for your particular situation. I have listed self-help treatments first, since they tend to be the easiest and most accessible for most women.

## Self-Help Approaches

Self-help therapy is geared toward preventing PMS altogether, rather than just treating the symptoms. Of course, you may not always be able to do so, in which case you may want to take one of the nonprescription drugs discussed on page 233. If you are charting your cycle, be on the lookout for when your temperature rises so that you can be especially attentive to the following suggestions.

### Dietary Considerations
The fact is there is probably no better way to control PMS symptoms than proper diet. The nutritional guidelines that almost all experts recommend include the usual emphasis on a well-balanced diet of whole grains, fruits, and vegetables, including legumes. And as expected, PMS symptoms can be greatly alleviated by dramatically cutting back on everything you no doubt love, including all foods high in sugar, salt, and fat. Drugs such as alcohol, nicotine, and caffeine should also be avoided. Finally, you should know that many nutritionists believe that a variety of vitamins, minerals, and herbs can go a long way in alleviating various PMS symptoms. For a thorough treatment of this topic, I would again encourage you to read the *PMS Self-Help Book*.

### Exercise and Yoga
You just can't seem to get away from advice to exercise, can you? Whether your concern is weight loss, lowering cholesterol levels, maintaining cardiovascular fitness, or PMS, the bottom line is that exercise is an excellent therapy for numerous ailments. One reason is that it activates the production of endorphins, a naturally occurring stimulant in your body. This explains why people usually feel so good after exercising. The trick to using exercise to benefit you the most is to maintain a regular exercise program of at least three to five times a week, about 30 minutes each session.

In addition to vigorous exercise, yoga is an excellent source of relief for many PMS sufferers. Traditionally, the goal of yoga has been to promote balance and harmony in the practitioner. Adherents of yoga will tell you that there's nothing better for promoting health on all levels—physical, mental, emotional, and spiritual.

### Rest

Of course, once you've exercised, you have to rest sufficiently to maintain optimal health. The common wisdom is that people should get at least 7 to 8 hours of sleep per night. Some need more. Ultimately, your body will tell you what feels best. Some women find that something as simple as going to bed earlier while premenstrual helps lessen PMS symptoms.

### Stress Reduction

Who today doesn't experience stress at least occasionally? Of course, some stress is inevitable. Advice to reduce stress would seem hollow if there was nothing you could do about it. But stress can affect a woman so profoundly that it really is worth encouraging you to try whatever you can to eliminate at least some of it from your life. Do whatever works for you, whether it's yoga, meditation, dancing, or going to a movie. Whatever you do, at least be aware that stress in the postovulatory phase is going to exaggerate your PMS symptoms. This is especially the time to reduce it, if at all possible.

### Coping with Emotions

For many women, one of the most distressing aspects of PMS is the sense of feeling emotionally out of control every cycle. It's as if their emotions are exaggerated tenfold. It can be especially distressing to women who are used to thinking of themselves as caring, warm people. They often feel as if their anger, anxiety, or depression is out of character for them. But remember, women in our society are socialized to always be nice, always be the caretaker, always be giving, and never show dissatisfaction. Perhaps a better way to perceive your premenstrual emotions is to recognize that it is a time when you finally allow yourself to express the frustrations society expects you to suppress.

Of course, if you feel that the intensity of your emotions during this time is incapacitating or harmful to your relationships, then you should seek the help of a therapist in addition to a clinician. Because therapists are more objective, they can often help clarify your seemingly complex emotional state, even if the problem is hormonally based. Remember, PMS doesn't cause emotions, but it will exaggerate what is already there.

### Nonprescription Drugs

There are currently a variety of over-the-counter drugs that are designed to deal with specific PMS symptoms. These drugs, which include various analgesics, antihistamines, and diuretics, have proved effective against such symptoms as uterine cramps, headaches, and breast tenderness. Again, I suggest that you read the relevant sections of a more comprehensive woman's health book, such as *Understanding Your Body,* by Felicia Stewart, M.D., et al., or at minimum, talk to an informed pharmacist. Finally, it should be clear that while drugs such as Tylenol and Advil will certainly relieve many discomforts, a concerted regimen of healthy diet and vigorous exercise would do more by minimizing such symptoms in the first place.

## Alternative Health Care

Homeopathic and naturopathic treatments seem to be helpful for some women, but you need to consult a qualified practitioner who is trained to diagnose you as a whole, and not just examine your symptoms. Some find relief through either acupuncture or acupressure, both of which perceive PMS as the result of imbalance or blockage of vital energy, or "chi." Osteopathy, reflexology, and aromatherapy may be helpful as well. Of course, in all these cases, you need to consult a professional to determine if these might work for you. Many of the more specialized PMS books discuss the theory and practice of alternative treatments in more detail.

### Using Drugs and Alternative Therapies Together

You may prefer to try to eliminate PMS through the natural alternatives just discussed. However, your symptoms may be so severe that you might want the quick relief drugs can provide. The good news is that natural and medical therapies aren't mutually exclusive. You can use medication for severe symptoms while simultaneously changing your lifestyle to try to prevent PMS symptoms in the future. Eventually, then, you could go off the drugs altogether and rely strictly on natural means to control your symptoms.

## Traditional Medical Treatments

There are a number of standard medical therapies that you may want to try. But before consulting with your physician, it may help to have charted your symptoms for several cycles so that he can efficiently arrive at the most accurate diagnosis.

### Progesterone Therapy

The major hormonal therapy for PMS is progesterone. Until recently, it was unclear whether it worked at all. And again, it often had more side effects than it was worth. Luckily, a breakthrough occurred in the late 1980s with the formulation of an oral, micronized progesterone pill. Unlike the unpalatable methods of the past, which involved either injections or suppositories, the new oral pill is easy to take and has few side effects. And because it is derived from wild yams and soybeans, it is considered an absolutely natural substance. Today, progesterone therapy is starting to gain wide acceptance as a treatment with potentially great benefits for many women.

### Tranquilizers and Antidepressants

If you suffer serious postovulatory anxiety, mood swings, or depression, your doctor may prescribe any number of tranquilizers or antidepressants. Some work by elevating levels of neurotransmitters like serotonin and norepinephrine—chemicals in the brain that regulate personality, mood, sleep, and appetite.

### Antiprostaglandin Medication

Probably the most painful symptom of both PMS and menstruation is uterine cramps. We now know that they are caused by imbalances in prostaglandins—chemicals produced in the uterine lining that increase prior to menstruation. Luckily, there are effective drugs such as Motrin that eliminate the cramping.

### PMS, Conventional Medicine, and Long-Term Solutions

You should keep in mind that there are always potential side effects whenever you take any drugs. Remember that while medications can be extremely useful in eliminating PMS symptoms, they will only be effective as long as you are taking them. Since PMS is known to get worse with age (lucky us!), that could mean years on drugs for women who are severely affected. While the dietary and other natural alternatives can involve considerable sacrifice, you should at least know that you have various choices that offer much relief.

## &#x224;&#x240; KEEPING SANE ALL CYCLE LONG

The reality of womanhood is that PMS is an unfortunate fact of life for most, and even a fairly debilitating experience for some. Like menstruation, it is hardly an experience most women would choose to have. But treatments do exist, and you do have some influence in restricting its severity, if not achieving its complete prevention. Perhaps as important, you may have the ability through charting to pinpoint your own PMS pattern, allowing you to take preventative action in the days immediately prior to its usual arrival.

No small advantage of such warning may also be to educate your partner, who could be sensitized to the cyclical basis for your physical and emotional changes. By being attuned to your cycle, a man can understand why, for example, you may be feeling depressed or premenstrually unresponsive, sexually or otherwise. Such knowledge on his part won't make PMS go away, but with both of you sensitive to your cycle, it can help minimize its impact.

Peggy is driven to
the brink of
Madness

# CHAPTER 19

# Demystifying Menopause

*Perhaps with education and proper perspective, we can look forward to the day when people will stop viewing menopause as a crisis, or even as "the change," and see it more appropriately as "yet another change." For living is constant change. That is its essence and its promise.*

—DR. KATHRYN MCGOLDRICK, former editor-in-chief of the
*Journal of the American Medical Women's Association*

*M*enopause. The word itself evokes countless emotions in women—everything from dread and fear to excited anticipation and relief. But it wasn't until fairly recently that the word was even uttered aloud. For some reason, it was a stage in a woman's life that was simply not discussed in polite company. Perhaps a lot of the stigma formerly associated with menopause related to a woman's primary role being defined as a mother, since it is true that menopause signals the end of the biological potential to reproduce.

Luckily, things have changed considerably. Women's roles have expanded dramatically, and society no longer defines a woman simply by her capacity to give birth. Today, many women are making the decision not to have children altogether, yet they still feel feminine and fulfilled.

Needless to say, the topic of menopause is so big that I couldn't do it justice in just one chapter. I would encourage you to read about it more thoroughly in any number of good books available today. Much of the information contained in this chapter is adapted from an excellent book called *Natural Menopause* by Susan Perry and Katherine A. O'Hanlan, M.D. (Addison-Wesley, 1992). I specifically refer you to their work because they treat menopause for what it is—a natural biological transition, not a medical event.

## ✌ WHAT EXACTLY IS MENOPAUSE?

"I thought it was when women stopped having periods."
"Isn't it when women run out of eggs?"
"I think it's when women reach about 50."
"It's when a woman can finally enjoy sex without having to worry about getting pregnant."

Actually, all of the above have kernels of truth, but I should clarify a few terms. "Menopause," in the strict biological sense, refers only to the final menstrual period. The "climacteric" is the 10 to 15 years preceding the final period, during which the ovaries gradually stop maturing eggs and releasing large amounts of hormones. (Actually, there is disagreement as to whether post-menopausal women still have a few ova left that simply no longer respond to hormonal stimuli or in fact have completely run out of them.) Finally, the "change of life" is the somewhat euphemistic term used to include the emotional, intellectual, and obvious physical changes that a woman experiences during this transitional time.

In the end, menopause is a uniquely individual experience. Some women glide right through it, barely noticing any changes at all. Others have a harder time, often choosing medical help to cope with the challenges it presents. The only definitive statement that can be made is that menopause is when menstruation stops, which for most women is about age 50.

## ✌ CLASSIC SIGNS OF IMPENDING MENOPAUSE

The most obvious way to tell if you are nearing menopause is by noticing the three classic signs that most women experience to varying degrees:

- menstrual cycle irregularities
- hot flashes
- vaginal dryness

Medical professionals refer to the above as symptoms, but it makes more sense to refer to them as signs. After all, "symptoms" imply disease, and certainly menopause is nothing more than a natural passage of life. Many women are beginning to question the medicalization of menopause, just as they have insisted on natural approaches to birth control, pregnancy achievement, and childbirth. They want to perceive it as a healthful part of their lives—perhaps different, but with distinct advantages.

Gail Sheehy, author of the groundbreaking book *Menopause, The Silent Passage,* describes what it was like to educate people about this universal transition:

> As I traveled around the United States giving lectures and appearing on TV and radio talk shows, the conversation about menopause had to be started up from scratch in each city. . . . Reactions from male talk show hosts were sometimes comical.
>
> "Menopause," gulped a Cleveland man on the midday news. "Is that like—impotence?"
>
> "Um, no," I murmured lamely . . . "Baldness. Is that like Alzheimer's?"

## Changes and Irregularities in Your Menstrual Cycle

One of the first signs of impending menopause is a change in your menstrual cycle. About 80% of women experience some kind of cyclic change, often as early as 7 years before. Typically, women first find that their periods become heavier and more frequent as their cycles shorten. But eventually, their periods start to become lighter and less frequent as their cycles become longer, and ovulation becomes more sporadic. These latter changes are due to ever-decreasing levels of estrogen.

### A Word About Menopause and Ovulation Predictor Kits

A tempting way to detect if you are still ovulating is through one of the many ovulation predictor kits widely available. But you should be aware that these kits can be especially unreliable if you are indeed nearing menopause. The reason for this is that premenopausal women tend to have exceedingly high levels of LH that don't necessarily trigger ovulation.

In addition, using the kits to detect menopause is impractical since a woman may ovulate so sporadically during this time that it would be nearly impossible to pinpoint when to even use them. Because they only come in 5- or 9-day supplies and cost from $30 to $50 a kit, you would be spending a pretty penny to verify whether you're still ovulating. Charting is cheaper, easier, and simply more accurate.

### Confusing Irregular Cycles with a Pregnancy

Keep in mind that unless you chart your cycles, menopause may make you think you are pregnant when you are not. The reason for this is that you may seem to skip periods (which, as you should know by now, can just indicate very long cycles). In fact, "missed periods" may be normal during this transition, though it could also be a sign of pregnancy. If you are charting, there are two ways to tell the difference between the two:

- You are probably pregnant if you have more than 18 consecutive days of high temperatures, especially if you also experience tender breasts and nausea. (However, you'll need to confirm it with your doctor. Home pregnancy tests are unreliable during menopause due to fluctuating pituitary hormones.)

- You are probably *not* pregnant if your temperature pattern shows consistently low temperatures, or a delayed ovulation that indicates that you are merely having a long cycle. These extended cycles become increasingly likely if you are experiencing hot flashes and a dry vagina.

### Heavy Periods

During the years leading up to menopause, women may also find that their periods become either heavier or lighter, longer or shorter—all due to changing hormones. Of course, irregular bleeding can be symptomatic of a medical condition, so it's especially useful during this time to continue charting and report any conspicuous abnormality to your clinician.

If you do find that your periods are getting unusually heavy, there are some practical tips you may want to consider. Try to avoid excess heat, including hot showers and baths whenever you're bleeding. In addition, you should also avoid alcohol and aspirin, both of which inhibit blood clotting, preferably throughout the cycle. But the best thing you can do is to maintain a lifestyle of steady and vigorous exercise, which will indirectly lower the production of the excess estrogen that is causing your periods to be so heavy in the first place.

## Hot Flashes

> *Real women don't have hot flashes*
> *They have power surges.*
> —Anonymous

You may be one of the lucky minority who manage to coast through menopause with no discomfort whatsoever. Unfortunately, though, up to 85% of women experience hot flashes at one time or another during their menopausal years. They can start while your cycles are still regular and often continue through to about 2 years after your last menstrual period. In some women, they may persist several years longer. The unpleasant episodes may last anywhere from a few seconds to a few minutes. They may occur once a week or even once an hour! (Oh joy.)

You may experience hot flashes as nothing more than the feeling you get when you've just stuck your foot in your mouth at a dinner party—that familiar passing warmth on your face or upper body. But you may also experience them as a drenching sweat accompanied by chills. In rare cases of extreme intensity, they may even occur with heart palpitations and feelings of suffocation. Many women describe feeling an "aura" just before—a distinct sense that they are about to have a hot flash. Some even feel anxious, tense, dizzy, nauseous, or a tingling in the fingers a few seconds in advance.

Researchers believe hot flashes are caused by changes in the hypothalamus, the master gland in the brain that controls, among other things, the body temperature and cyclical fertility hormones. These changes are a result of declining levels of estrogen, which essentially trigger the body to turn on a misguided hormonal cooler. In essence then, hot flashes reflect an inappropriate lowering of the body's natural thermostat.

There are several practical things you can do that will make life easier while going through what may be a several-year transition. You should try to wear clothes made of cotton and other fibers that allow you to breathe, because the key is to literally stay cool. It's best to avoid hot weather, or at least have continual access to cold water. As with everything else, maintain a healthy well-balanced diet and get plenty of vigorous exercise. Finally, many women who chart may find a pattern to their hot flashes. Recording them can help you feel more in control, by allowing you to be psychologically prepared for when they return.

The most commonly prescribed medical treatment for hot flashes is hormone replacement therapy (HRT). By replacing the estrogen that has plummeted to such a low level, HRT is nearly 100% effective in eliminating the hot flashes. However, HRT is not without its side effects and potentially serious problems.

## *Vaginal Dryness*

One of the most commonly experienced and least discussed effects of menopause is the drying of vaginal tissue, again due to progressively dropping estrogen levels. Women are typically too embarrassed to talk about it, feeling that it must be their unique problem. But in fact most women find that their vaginas take longer to become sexually lubricated as menopause approaches. Some may even feel irritated by the type of stimulation that they previously found pleasurable.

While menopause can definitely lead to vaginal dryness, there are practical things you can try to keep your vagina lubricated, including taking more time for foreplay and using water-based lubricants such as K-Y Jelly. If you still find that you have vaginal dryness that makes intercourse uncomfortable or even painful, you may want to try estrogen therapy in cream form. This should relieve dryness or soreness in the vagina, usually within a week or two. Creams are often recommended over pills because they don't pose as many health risks.

## ৪৯ MENOPAUSE AND SEXUALITY

Menopause has a paradoxical effect on female sexuality. But just to set the record straight: It does not signal the end of a woman's sex life! While it's true that it tends to cause vaginal dryness, it finally frees women of the fear of pregnancy. The liberating feeling that results can be more than enough to compensate for the extra effort that it may take to become sexually lubricated. In fact, many women find their sex lives improve when they no longer have to worry about pregnancy or menstruation.

## ৪৯ HORMONE REPLACEMENT THERAPY

> *These days, it isn't raging hormonal imbalance that drives a postmenopausal woman berserk. It's raging medical debate. Some 30 to 40 million American women want a definitive answer on estrogen, and instead, they're getting the daily odds.*
>
> —Ellen Goodman

Probably no other phrase in medical terminology evokes more confusion and contradictory reactions than hormone replacement therapy. Should menopausal women take artificial hormones or not? The debate is often extremely heated, controversial, and ultimately inconclusive. The bottom line is that there is no ideal answer. Each woman's situation is unique, and will have to be thoughtfully discussed with her own physician.

Part of the controversy over HRT stems from the fact that when it was first prescribed in the 1930s, not much was known about the potential long-term effects of the therapy. It wasn't until years later that it was discovered that the type of estrogen therapy then being practiced would increase a woman's risk of uterine and breast cancer. In 1975, articles in the *New England Journal of Medicine* showed that women who took estrogen were several times more likely to develop cancer of the endometrial lining than those who did not.

Pharmaceutical companies and many doctors stress that things are different today. They cite several reasons for prescribing the new model of HRT:

- The new hormone therapies usually combine both estrogen and progestins (a form of progesterone). The progestins act to balance the estrogen, thus reducing the increased risk of cancer.
- The estrogen dosage today is typically lower than it was in the past.
- There is now strong evidence to show that estrogen is very effective in protecting older women from osteoporosis.

Today, one of the most commonly prescribed estrogens is Premarine. It's what is referred to as a conjugated estrogen, and is considered the most naturally occurring hormone. And where is it extracted from? The urine of pregnant horses, of course!*

## What Hormone Replacement Therapy Cannot Treat

It is often tempting for menopausal women to look to HRT as the magic pill that will resolve all sorts of problems. The fact is, there are a number of things that HRT will specifically not prevent, including wrinkled skin, weight gain (unfortunately, your metabolism slows down as you age), or depression—which is a common complaint during menopause. But it is true that HRT may make you feel better by treating the symptoms that cause your anxiety.

---

* In fact, that's how Premarine got its name:

| Pre | mar | ine |
|-----|-----|-----|
| (pregnant) | (mare's) | (urine) |

## What Hormone Replacement Therapy Can Treat

HRT can definitely treat certain menopausal complaints. There is no question that HRT can relieve hot flashes and vaginal dryness. It also helps maintain the acidity of the vagina, making it more resistant to infections. And far more significantly, most researchers agree that HRT can prevent osteoporosis.*

It should be made clear that HRT will only help these specific problems while you are taking the hormones. Once you discontinue, the problems will often return. This is particularly true with hot flashes. You should also remember that hormones will not restore bone density to their premenopausal level. It will simply prevent bone loss for as long as you remain on the therapy.

## Risks of Hormone Replacement Therapy

If HRT is so beneficial, why don't all menopausal women take it? There are several reasons, including some serious medical risks. Although the issue is still hotly disputed, there are many studies that suggest HRT increases the risk of breast cancer. Women with a family history of this disease are especially advised to avoid HRT. In addition, there are many experts who believe the increased risk of uterine cancer has not been eliminated, despite the addition of progestin to counter the adverse effects of estrogen. Thus women who may have a higher than normal risk of endometrial cancer, including those who are diabetic and substantially overweight, are advised against HRT.

## Side Effects

In addition to the increased medical risks, there can be annoying side effects. Among the more common are nausea (if taking high-dose estrogen), fluid retention, and fibroid enlargement. And of course you will continue to have cyclical vaginal bleeding, though it is usually shorter and lighter than typical menstruation.

## HRT: Balancing the Data

The reality of HRT is that potentially serious problems need to be weighed against some real and substantial benefits, with each individual woman judging

---

* There is also growing evidence that HRT may help prevent heart disease, but this is disputed.

how the pros and cons balance out when applied to her own situation. If you are considering HRT, you will definitely need to consult with an experienced clinician. This is clearly an important and complicated subject, and one in which I urge you to keep current. There are many factors to consider, but ultimately you can make an intelligent decision, so long as it is an informed one.

## ✿ FERTILITY AWARENESS DURING THE PREMENOPAUSAL YEARS

Some medical practitioners warn against using natural birth control when you begin to have menopausal signs because of the irregularity of cycles during this time, but this advice shows a misunderstanding of how the Fertility Awareness Method works. Yes, it is true that cycles tend to become more sporadic for women in their 40s. But the key to FAM is that each individual *day* is observed for possibly fertile conditions, and thus the cyclic consistency is almost irrelevant.

What *is* relevant is that many premenopausal women may have fertile cervical-fluid patterns for increasingly longer periods of time (such as preovulatory sticky day after day). This is both the potential frustration and irony of FAM in the years approaching menopause, for while the method's conservatism may tell a woman she is fertile more days than ever, the fact is that as she ages, her potential fertility is diminishing rapidly.

The truth is that using FAM during the menopausal years can be confusing, but depending on your own particular cycles, it may also be easier than ever before. Indeed, you may go for months at a time with nothing but dry, infertile days. Regardless, using FAM will provide you with an amazing window into the workings of your body as it travels through "yet another change."

### How to Determine Whether You Are Near Menopause

Using FAM during menopause may involve some modifications, but before using the special guidelines, you obviously need to determine how close to menopause you actually are. As discussed previously, you will generally have distinct symptoms to alert you, in addition to the fact that you will most likely be in your 40s as the transitional time arrives. As you know, the most distinct signs signaling the premenopausal transition period are menstrual cycle irregularities, hot flashes, and vaginal dryness.

## ℘ CHARTING YOUR FERTILITY AS
## MENOPAUSE APPROACHES

If you decide that you want to chart your cycles for birth control, brace yourself for quite a ride. You can still use the method effectively, but this phase may be quite a challenge. Whatever your choice, charting will reflect your hormonal changes, giving you a sense of control over your seemingly unpredictable body.

When charting premenopausally, anticipate significant changes in your typical fertility pattern. Each of your fertility signs will reflect your new hormonal fluctuations as your body prepares for the cessation of ovulatory cycles.

### Waking Temperatures

One of the most obvious reflections of your diminishing fertility will be your waking temperatures. Rather than seeing the usual thermal shifts every cycle, you will start seeing new variations. Initially, you may notice that your cycles become shorter and more frequent, and thus your thermal shifts occur sooner than usual. In addition, you may notice that the number of postovulatory temperatures decreases, reflecting shorter luteal phases than you normally have.

And finally, you'll notice more and more anovulatory cycles in which your temperature remains low throughout, indicating that you didn't release an egg that cycle. All of these variations in your temperature pattern are absolutely normal as you approach menopause, and should only serve to remind you of the benefits of charting to help you understand what is happening in your body.

### Cervical Fluid

As the number of follicles in your ovaries begins to decrease, you will stop ovulating as often. You will also produce progressively less estrogen, which in turn will decrease the amount of fertile-quality cervical fluid you produce. For example, if you used to observe about 3 days of eggwhite every cycle, you may now only have it one day, if at all. Yet without ovulation, progesterone won't be present to rapidly dry up what cervical fluid there is. All of this means that it may become harder to identify your Peak Day.

Your usual fertile pattern of cervical fluid will start to be replaced with more days of either dry, sticky, or even a watery secretion without any of the fertile characteristics such as slippery, stretchy, or lubricative. Your vaginal sensation may become a continuous, unchanging dry or sticky feeling. Or you may experience patches of cervical fluid, as your body makes noble attempts to ovulate in the face of impending menopause.

## Cervix

Being able to observe your cervix during phases of anovulation can be especially helpful, since such cycles can be fairly confusing. You will probably notice that as menopause approaches, your cervix is more often firm, closed, and low, confirming longer phases of infertility and clarifying confusing cervical fluid or temperature patterns.

## Secondary Fertility Signs

Along with the obvious changes you may notice in your three primary fertility signs, you will probably see changes in your secondary signs as well. You may even notice certain fertility signs for the first time as discussed below.

### Midcycle Spotting

If you're someone who never used to have midcycle spotting around ovulation, you may be surprised to start experiencing it now. This is because ovulatory spotting tends to be more common in long cycles, and one of the hallmarks of premenopausal cycles is their increasingly longer lengths.

### Mittelschmerz

If you are used to having midcycle pain around ovulation, you may notice that you don't experience it as often as you stop ovulating as frequently.

### Breast Tenderness

One of the nice benefits of anovulatory cycles is that you don't usually experience the postovulatory breast tenderness characteristic of normal cycles. This is because, when ovulation doesn't occur, there isn't any progesterone to cause the breast discomfort.

## ✣ THE CONTRACEPTIVE RULES AS MENOPAUSE APPROACHES

Once you have determined that you are indeed experiencing menopausal signs, the way you will use Fertility Awareness can be fairly straightforward: *You should follow all the standard rules of FAM discussed in Chapter 9, except that you should not rely on the First 5 Days Rule.*

What this means in practice is really quite simple. You should chart your cycles as you always have, but you should no longer assume that the first 5 days of the cycle are infertile. The reason for this is that your premenopausal cycles are subject to hormonal fluctuations which may cause a dramatically early ovulation.

Again, we are dealing with degrees of risk. Although there is little data to cite, it is likely that the first 3 days of a period are nearly as safe as the first 5 days were before you had that first hot flash. But to be most conservative, you should assume you're fertile until you can verify a *dry* day, which as you know, is essentially impossible as long as you're bleeding.

### *"Hard Cycles, Easy Cycles"*

As you approach menopause, you may find that you go for months without any dry days. Instead, you might have a continuous and extended preovulatory pattern of sticky days, perhaps interspersed with patches of wet cervical fluid. The occurrence of unchanging cervical fluid day after day is called a Basic Infertile Pattern (BIP) and is very common in premenopausal women. In such a case, you may want to use the BIP rules discussed in Appendix B. They allow women with a sticky BIP to count more days as infertile than would be possible under the standard FAM rules. However the BIP rules are admittedly more difficult to follow, and as you can read in Appendix B, they are somewhat riskier for premenopausal women.

Understandably, you might decide that using them is simply not worth the trouble. Yet before deciding anything definitively, I would encourage you to at least continue charting for several months. Aside from the fascinating record you'll have of your reproductive system going through the throes of biological angst, it is almost certain that your cycles will become both increasingly longer *and* dryer, making FAM easier than ever.

**Chart 19.1. A challenging premenopausal Basic Infertile Pattern.** Deborah has the misfortune of having a premenopausal BIP of sticky, day after day, interspersed with wet patches.

**Chart 19.2. An easy premenopausal Basic Infertile Pattern.** Later, Deborah develops a BIP of dry day after day. With charts like this one, FAM for birth control will be a breeze.

When all is said and done, each couple will have to decide what is best for themselves. You might decide that it's not worth waiting for easier cycles. If this is the case, you may want to consider more permanent forms of contraception. Personally, I feel that vasectomy is a better option than tubal ligation, because it is a cheaper and a less invasive procedure with fewer possible complications. But whatever you choose, remember that *menopausal women are considered potentially fertile for a full year after their last period.*

## ℘ MAINTAINING YOUR SANITY
## THROUGH THE MENOPAUSAL YEARS

In the end, how easily you glide through menopause will be determined in large part by your expectations before you get there. While the various menopausal signs can be a nuisance, they certainly don't have to be traumatizing. Reasonable solutions are available. So keep a sense of humor, and know that you're hardly alone.

Charting your cycles will offer you a unique opportunity to observe your body in a wondrous period of transformation. As your cycles veer from less than 3 weeks to 3 months or more, you'll always be on top of the hormonal turbulence within you. One day when you're about 50, after having gone all summer long without menstruating, you may have the opportunity to impress a friend. You'll be able to tell her that you know that you still have at least one more period to go, starting the following week. "How can you be sure?" she'll ask. "I know," you'll say, "because it says so on my chart."

CHAPTER ✍ 20

# Enriching Your Self-Esteem Through Knowledge About Your Body

*Once we are old enough to have had an education, the first step toward self-esteem for most of us is not to learn but to unlearn.*

—ANONYMOUS

> Luteal phase defect
> Hostile cervical mucus
> Incompetent cervix
> Inadequate pelvis
> Senile gravida
> Habitual aborter

*H*mm . . . let's see: defect, hostile, incompetent, inadequate, senile, aborter. Doesn't *that* paint a pretty picture? Regrettably, the list above merely describes women with fairly common conditions, such as those with a short luteal phase, nonfertile cervical fluid, a weak cervix, a narrow pelvis, a pregnancy after 35, and a tendency to miscarry. If you'd like to be further entertained, you can review the entire list of medical terminology still used in women's health today (see Appendix L).

You may think that this type of language doesn't affect self-esteem, because most women aren't even aware that these descriptions are recorded in their medical records. But many are matter-of-factly informed that they have the above conditions by well-meaning doctors who are oblivious to how insulting this terminology can be. These phrases reflect an antiquated medical system that is often insensitive to women and out of touch with their needs.

Instead of identifying with the above vocabulary, picture an altogether different scenario. Imagine growing up being told that your body is a marvel of biological beauty that will orchestrate amazing changes every cycle. Rather than thinking that you keep producing infectious discharges, you'd know to identify healthy cervical secretions as a reflection of the remarkable hormonal system working within. Imagine going to the doctor and feeling knowledgeable rather than vulnerable? And instead of succumbing to douche commercials that diminish self-confidence by implying that women are dirty, you could simply disregard them, knowing that just showering with soap and water will keep you clean and feminine.

What if teenagers acquired practical knowledge about their cycles and fertility even before the first day they menstruated? Not only would it increase their self-assurance, but it would enable them to identify both medical problems and normal biological occurrences, sparing them so much of the fear and confusion that comes with adolescence. And although FAM should not be promoted as a method of birth control among adolescents, the reality is that the practical knowledge it affords could reduce unplanned pregnancies in a population that, unfortunately, still believes among other things that you can't get pregnant the first time.

Imagine being able to utilize your body's own fertility signs to provide you with a completely natural, safe, and effective method of birth control that promotes shared responsibility and communication between you and your partner. Or envision what it would be like to know your own hormonal symphony so well that you could plan every aspect of your pregnancy, from the month you want to deliver your baby, to perhaps increasing the odds of conceiving the gender of your choice.

And if by chance you or your partner really do have a fertility problem, picture a dialogue of truly informed participants. Imagine you, your partner, and your doctor using your own charts to find the least invasive strategy first, before deciding that IVF or other high technologies are your last and only solution. Yes, it may be, but at least you would understand why.

On a more mundane note, wouldn't it be nice to experience PMS in a whole new light, finally understanding why you develop symptoms on a cyclical basis? Knowing there are steps you can take to alleviate the various pains and discomforts will always help, particularly if you take preemptive steps based on conveniently predictable patterns. In such a case, your fertility charts could serve as a biomedical data bank, perhaps helping you stave off that particularly unpleasant bloated feeling 3 days before your period.

And what if menopause was finally perceived for what it is—an inevitable, natural transition in a woman's life. If women were actually taught what to anticipate in the years leading up to their last period, they certainly wouldn't feel so confused and mystified by all the new changes. Indeed, women in their late 40s are hormonally like 13-year-old kids. Their bodies may create the biological equivalent of a Hollywood mystery, but like their adolescent daughters, these women can eliminate the confusion and take control as they enter the last phase of this long and curious journey.

There is a popular cliché that is as truthful as it is applicable: Knowledge is power. Unfortunately, so much of what people usually want to know is locked away in the secret papers of governmental, corporate, and academic bureaucracies. But there is also a treasure-trove of eminently practical information that in many ways serves to define your womanhood, and that knowledge is available to you whenever you want. Yes, it does take a couple of minutes a day to access, but it requires no particular job, connections, or even a computer. Fertility Awareness is certainly not high tech. But for all of you who are of reproductive age, the education it provides can reveal an entire world about which you may know so very little: yourself.

# APPENDICES

# Troubleshooting Your Cycle: Expecting the Unexpected

After you have started to chart, you may come across situations in which you need more clarification or guidance. What follows is a list of what I believe to be the most likely problem areas, based on my years of practice. They are categorized by symptom or fertility sign, with a cross-reference based on when the problem occurs in the cycle. While I know these pages can offer you a valuable resource, I hope your need for them will be minimal.*

## $\wp$ CATEGORIZED BY SYMPTOM OR FERTILITY SIGN

### Bleeding

### Waking Temperatures

* Many of the physical problems discussed in this appendix have potential solutions that you may wish to explore in Marilyn Shannon's *Fertility, Cycles, and Nutrition*.

## Cervical Fluid

## Cervix

## Intercourse

## CATEGORIZED BY WHEN IT OCCURS IN THE CYCLE

*Anytime in Cycle*

## SPOTTING BEFORE MENSTRUATION
## (AT THE END OF THE LUTEAL PHASE)

Spotting before menstruation can be considered normal if it follows at least 10 days of high temperatures *without* spotting. Otherwise, it can be an indication that the corpus luteum is starting to break down too early. Either way, Day 1 of the cycle is considered the first day of a true menstrual flow.

For pregnancy *avoiders,* this type of spotting is generally just a nuisance. But for pregnancy *achievers,* it may be a potential problem since it could indicate an insufficient luteal phase for implantation of the egg to occur. The two most common remedies are the use of progesterone vaginal suppositories and the ovulatory drug Clomid. The progesterone suppositories are prescribed to maintain the lining until implantation, and are considered less invasive. Clomid, on the other hand, acts to correct the preovulatory *and* postovulatory phases of the cycle. It is given orally and is thus considered a systemic drug, since it can affect the entire body.

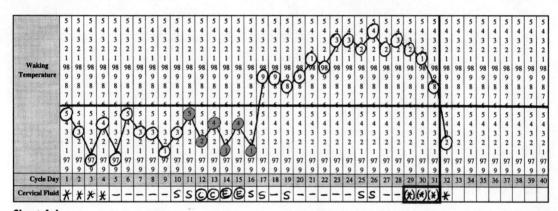

**Chart A.I.**

## VERY LIGHT OR HEAVY PERIODS

Exceptionally light or heavy periods can be the result of an anovulatory cycle —that is, a cycle in which an egg was not released. (This type of bleeding is especially common as women approach menopause.) You can determine if you ovulated by whether there was a thermal shift 12 to 16 days before this type of period. If there wasn't, you can be fairly certain that the bleeding you are experiencing is anovulatory. Technically, this is not a true menstrual period, since it did not follow the release of an egg. However, to maintain a point of reference, you would still consider it Day 1 of a new cycle.

It is critical that you differentiate between anovulatory bleeding and ovulatory spotting. Anovulatory bleeding occurs after an *absence* of a thermal shift (Chart A.2a). Ovulatory spotting occurs *within a couple of days of* a thermal shift, and is considered extremely fertile (Chart A.2b). It is usually due to the sudden drop in estrogen that precedes ovulation, and is actually considered a secondary fertility sign. If the bleeding appears to be unrelated to either, it might warrant a physical exam to rule out potential problems. (See pages 200– 203 for a discussion of possible causes of normal and abnormal bleeding.)

**Chart A.2a. Anovulatory bleeding.**

**Chart A.2b. Midcycle (ovulatory) spotting.**

## UNEXPLAINED BLEEDING

Once you know your cycle well, you won't need to be concerned if you occasionally spot in the day or so before your period or around ovulation. But, if you have red blood at inexplicable times, you should probably be checked by a doctor.

You should also be aware that if you become pregnant, you may have implantation spotting due to the fertilized egg burrowing into the lining. So if you have reason to think you might be pregnant, pay special attention to spotting that might occur from about a week or so after your thermal shift. Your temperature will verify whether you are indeed pregnant if they remain above the coverline for at least 18 days. Of course, anytime you suspect pregnancy, you should see a clinician to confirm it.

**Chart A.3.**

## MIDCYCLE SPOTTING

About 10% of women will notice that they occasionally have a day or two of spotting about midcycle, right around ovulation. In fact, they may even notice that the fertile cervical fluid (especially the eggwhite quality) is tinged with brown, red, or pink. This is a result of spotting mixed with cervical fluid. It is considered extremely fertile. It's usually due to the sudden drop in estrogen that precedes ovulation, and is nothing to be concerned about. If anything, it is a good secondary sign to record on your chart. It's typically more common in long cycles.

You can tell that it is ovulatory spotting because it occurs *within a couple of days of* a thermal shift (Chart A.4a). If, however, the spotting lasts more than a couple of days, is bright red, or you notice spotting at other times in the cycle that do *not* coincide with ovulation or the approach of your period, it could be an indication of a problem requiring medical attention (Chart A.4b), or possibly an early sign of pregnancy (see opposite page).

**Chart A.4a. Midcycle (ovulatory) spotting.**

**Chart A.4b. Spotting requiring medical attention.**

## SPOTTING ANYTIME FROM WEEK AFTER OVULATION TO EXPECTED PERIOD

If you experience spotting anytime from about a week after your temperature rises to the expected date of your period, it may be a sign of pregnancy. When the fertilized egg burrows into the uterine lining, it can cause implantation spotting. If you have reason to think you might be pregnant, pay special attention to your temperatures to see whether they remain above the coverline for at least 18 days (see page 142).

Please note that if you prefer to take a pregnancy test, even the most sensitive ones won't be valid until you've had at least 10 high temperatures. You should be aware that store-bought tests generally require a few more days because they are not as sensitive to the minute amounts of HCG that the embryo initially emits.

**Chart A.5.**

## WHEN TAKING ACCURATE TEMPERATURES IS NOT ALWAYS POSSIBLE

There are certain women who will be unable to take their waking temperatures at a consistent time. This may be because they have to work rotating shifts, or perhaps travel frequently across time zones. If you are ever in a situation where it is essentially impossible to obtain accurate waking temps, you can still use a modified form of the Natural Birth Control Method taught in this book. Unfortunately, it will require more days of abstinence or barriers.

This method relies exclusively on the Dry Day and Peak Day Rules as taught in Chapter 9. However, even after you have passed your Peak Day and counted to the 4th evening beyond, you should not assume that you are infertile unless you are dry. This is because without a thermal shift to verify the passing of ovulation, you risk being misled by the cervical fluid into thinking that you have ovulated when you actually have not. (This is often referred to as a "split peak," as discussed on page 120.)

To be most conservative, you should treat the presence of all cervical fluid and bleeding, including menses, as potentially fertile, no matter when it appears in the cycle. Unfortunately, this may mean using the "Peak + 4" rule more than once per cycle, although if the later patches of cervical fluid are only sticky and not wet you can get away with counting "Peak + 2" with little increase in risk. You should also know that if you are able to verify that your cervix remains in its most infertile state (low and closed with no wet cervical fluid at the cervical tip), your increased risk from intercourse during any sticky days should be quite small.

For pregnancy achievers, inability to observe a thermal shift will unfortunately prevent you from learning about numerous facets of your fertility. However, the basic goal of timing intercourse for your most fertile cervical fluid days remains the same.

## NO THERMAL SHIFT

Now and then, you may have an anovulatory cycle. If this occurs, you won't see a shift in temperatures from low to high because no progesterone will have been released to cause the temperatures to rise.

In addition, you could be one of the small percentage of women whose bodies don't respond to the effects of progesterone, and therefore don't show a thermal shift even if you have ovulated. As discussed in Chapter 14, one of the only ways to definitively determine if ovulation has occurred in this case is through ultrasound. Short of that, you could get a blood test in the second phase of the cycle to determine the presence of progesterone.

You also may be experiencing a temporary cause of anovulation such as illness, stress, or a medical problem such as a hormonal imbalance. Finally, you could be starting to approach menopause, in which case you will stop ovulating as often as you used to. Chapters 7 and 19 and Appendix B discuss these problems in more detail.

If you are using FAM for birth control and have established that you are indeed one of the few women whose temperatures simply do not reflect ovulation, you can use the Billings Method, which involves checking cervical fluid alone. While not as effective as the Fertility Awareness Method taught in this book, you can increase the effectiveness of the method by also charting cervical position, thus providing another sign to cross-check in cases of ambiguity.

If you do choose to use the Billings Method, you should be aware that you cannot use the First 5 Days Rule, because you can't prove that the bleeding you experience is menstruation and not ovulatory spotting. This is because you won't have the thermal shift to show that ovulation occurred 12 to 16 days before. And because you can't confirm that you've already ovulated, I strongly recommend that any wet cervical fluid or bleeding at *any* time during the cycle be considered fertile. Unfortunately, this may require you to apply the Peak Day Rule more than once per cycle.

**Chart A.6.**

## ERRATIC TEMPERATURES

Some women may find that their temperatures do not seem to follow the classic pattern of lows and highs. For these women, consider trying any of the following:

1. If using a digital thermometer, verify that the battery is not low.
2. Take your waking temperature vaginally rather than orally.
3. Consider using only a glass basal body thermometer since digitals may be less accurate for some women.
4. Be sure you take your temperature for the full 5 minutes with the glass thermometer.
5. Remember that certain factors can definitely increase waking temperatures, such as fever, drinking alcohol the night before, or not getting three consecutive hours of sleep.
6. Try to take your temperature about the same time everyday. You should know that for every half hour that you sleep *later* than normal, your temperature will tend to creep up about one-tenth of a degree. For every half hour that you wake up *earlier* than normal, it will tend to be about one-tenth of a degree lower. You should note the time you take it in the appropriate column. You should use the Rule of Thumb to discount aberrant temperatures that may result from sleeping late. (This will prevent you from attributing a high temperature to a thermal shift before it has actually occurred.)

**Chart A.7.**

## OUTLYING TEMPERATURES

If you have temperatures that are clearly out of line (for example, from fever, drinking alcohol the night before, or having slept in and taken your temperature late), just use the Rule of Thumb, covering any outlying temperatures with your thumb. Remember to draw a dotted line between the correct temperatures on either side of the outlying temperatures.

Remember that in calculating the coverline, you count the six low temperatures before the rise, *not* including the outlying temperature.

**Chart A.8.**

## HIGH TEMPERATURES DURING PERIOD

It is fairly common for women to experience several days of high temperatures during their period. This is usually the result of residual progesterone from the last cycle or fluctuating hormones that occur during menstruation. Draw a dotted line from the high temperatures during your period down to the normal-range temperatures. The high temperatures will probably be above the coverline, but you can simply disregard them by using the Rule of Thumb.

**Chart A.9.**

# HIGHER- OR LOWER-THAN-AVERAGE TEMPERATURES THROUGHOUT CYCLE

One of the most obvious symptoms of a possible thyroid problem is very high or low waking temperatures. (Most waking temperatures range between 97.0 to 97.5 degrees preovulatory and 97.6 to 98.6 degrees postovulatory.) If you find that you have any of the combination of symptoms below, you may want to see your doctor.

*Hyperthyroidism, or excessively high thyroid activity*
Symptoms of hyperthyroidism include high waking temperatures, scant menses, long cycles, and infertility.

*Hypothyroidism, or low thyroid function*
Symptoms of hypothyroidism include low waking temperatures, unusually long cycles, anovulatory cycles (with no thermal shift), prolonged phases of fertile-quality cervical fluid, heavy menses, or unexplained infertility.

**Chart A.10a. Possible hyperthyroid temperatures (high thyroid activity).**

**Chart A.10b. Possible hypothyroid temperatures (low thyroid function).**

## TEMPERATURE DIP BEFORE THE RISE

You may be one of the few women who consistently have a temperature pattern in which you see a conspicuous dip before your thermal shift. Or you may only occasionally notice this pattern. Either way, it is believed that it usually occurs on the day of ovulation and is the result of high levels of estrogen pushing your temperatures down.

For pregnancy avoiders, the dip does not affect your adherence to the preovulatory rules of contraception. For pregnancy achievers, this would be an excellent day to time intercourse (assuming, of course, your cervical fluid is fertile that day).

**Chart A.11.**

## TEMPERATURES RISE IN SPURTS (STAIR-STEP PATTERN)

One of the more common types of temperature patterns are those where the thermal shift occurs in an initial spurt of several days, followed by a type of bell curve. In other words, you will probably notice a cluster of 6 low temperatures followed by a shift of at least two-tenths higher for perhaps 3 or 4 days, followed by the final bell curve. The coverline is always drawn after the *first* shift of at least two-tenths higher than the cluster of six preceding low temperatures.

**Chart A.12.**

## TEMPERATURES RISE ONE-TENTH DEGREE AT A TIME (SLOW-RISE PATTERN)

Some women will notice that instead of their temperature shifting by at least two-tenths of a degree higher than the previous six lows, their temperatures rise by merely one-tenth of a degree at a time. While this type of shift can be fairly confusing to interpret, it can be done.

Wait for the first time your temperature rises at least one-tenth of a degree above the highest of the last six temperatures. On this chart, you would highlight Days 10 to 15 before the one-tenth-degree rise and draw the coverline straight through the elevated temperature on Day 16. Also note that in this particular case, Day 16 is in fact two-tenths of a degree above the previous day, but only one-tenth of a degree above the cluster of the previous six days. It is this latter fact that distinguishes the pattern as a slow-rise.

Once your temperature remained *above* the coverline for at least four days, you could be quite certain that you had ovulated. (Note that for pregnancy avoiders, to be conservative with this fairly rare temperature pattern, you should wait 4 rather than 3 days to consider yourself infertile. C'est la vie.) In addition, you should never consider yourself safe during such slow-rising temperatures unless you can corroborate your infertile phase with the Peak Day Rule.

If you are using FAM for *achieving* pregnancy, you should consider the postovulatory phase to be all the temperatures above the coverline, but realize that your ovulation probably occurred a day or more earlier. Remember that ovulation most likely occurs the day of, or the day after, the Peak Day, which is the last day of eggwhite-quality cervical fluid or lubricative vaginal sensation.

**Chart A.13.**

## DROP IN TEMPERATURE DAY 2 OF THERMAL SHIFT (FALL-BACK PATTERN)

Some women notice that they tend to have a pattern of a temperature drop on Day 2 of their thermal shift, followed by a sustained rise in temperature until their period. Unfortunately, to be conservative for birth control, you would want to start the count over again after the second sustained rise to be absolutely sure that the egg(s) are dead and gone.

If you don't want to wait the extra 2 days, you might rely on the Peak Day Rule to signal the start of the infertile phase. Admittedly, this could compromise contraceptive efficacy. However, if you verify that you are once again dry, *and* that your cervix has also returned to its infertile state, the increased risk of conception is quite small.

**Chart A.14.**

## TEMPERATURE BELOW COVERLINE WELL AFTER OVULATION

After ovulation (during the luteal phase), there is a second smaller surge of estrogen, which may cause a temporary drop in temperature and often coincides with a day or two of creamy cervical fluid. You need not be concerned, though, because it is not an indication of returning fertility. The egg is already dead and gone by then.

**Chart A.15.**

## DROP IN TEMPERATURE DAY BEFORE PERIOD BEGINS

Occasionally, you may notice an obvious drop in temperature the day before you get your period. While this is less common than when it occurs the day of menstruation itself, it is still considered part of the luteal phase (this sudden premenstrual drop is caused by the disintegration of the corpus luteum). Day 1 of the new cycle is not determined by the day of the drop, but by the first day of bleeding. This means that the luteal phase length is determined by the first day of the rise in temperature through to and including the last day before the red menstrual flow.

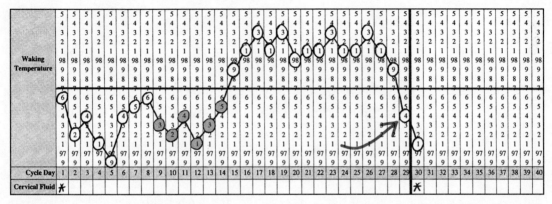

**Chart A.16.** Note that the luteal phase here is 15 days long because it goes from Day 15 through to and including Day 29, despite the fact there was a temperature drop on that day. Day 1 of the new cycle begins with the bleeding of the following day.

## FEVER

You will inevitably have a fever now and then while charting. Practically speaking, it is best handled by using the Rule of Thumb. Assuming the temperature is off the chart, you can simply circle and cross out the 99 temperature, noting the fever and other symptoms of illness in the miscellaneous column. Be sure to draw a dotted line between the normal temperatures on both sides of your fever. (Also remember that if you're using a BBT thermometer, you'll need to switch to a digital or glass for the days that you are sick.)

Depending on the intensity of the fever and when it occurs in the cycle, there are three possible impacts that it could have:

1. It could have no effect,
2. it could delay ovulation (causing a longer than usual cycle), or
3. it could suppress ovulation (causing an anovulatory cycle).

If the fever occurs *after* you've already ovulated, it will almost certainly have no effect. If it occurs before you've ovulated, any of the three listed above are possible.

Regardless, you can continue to use FAM as birth control using all the rules described in Chapter 9. However, if your illness is preovulatory, you obviously have to eliminate the temperatures discounted by the fever, and thus *you cannot begin the three day count for the Temperature Shift Rule until you are no longer sick. Never assume you've entered your postovulatory infertile phase until you can clearly verify a thermal shift of 3 consecutive high temperatures without the interference of any fever.* And before assuming that you're safe, verify that your other fertility signs also reflect continued infertility (Chart A.17a).

The one time in the cycle when this can be a bit tricky is if you get sick in the few days immediately leading up to ovulation (Chart A.17b). Still, you should be able to verify that ovulation has occurred, since once you're no longer sick, your temperatures will drop down to the higher range of temperatures that you would normally have after ovulating. If the fever delayed (or suppressed) ovulation, the temperatures would drop all the way to their lower preovulatory range.

**Chart A.17a.** On Day 8 of her cycle, Cindy awakens to a bad flu, which pushes her temperatures off the chart for three days. She uses the Rule of Thumb for Days 8–10, crossing out the highest temperature on the chart to reflect any ones that are 99 or above. After recovering, she is able to verify that she still has not ovulated, since her temperature returns to its lower preovulatory range on Day 11. As she continues to chart, her signs reflect a delayed ovulation, which in this case probably occurs about Day 20.

**Chart A.17b.** Eva awakens to a cold and low-grade fever, starting on Day 12. She uses the Rule of Thumb to discount Days 12–14. Completely well by Day 15, she carefully records her temperature and notices that it has only fallen to her relatively high postovulatory range. Thus she is able to start her temp count on Day 15, and by Day 17 she confirms through all her fertility signs that she has already ovulated. (Had her illness been intense enough to delay her ovulation, her temperature would have returned to its lower preovulatory range.)

## 10 OR FEWER DAYS OF HIGH TEMPERATURES ABOVE THE COVERLINE

If you have 10 or fewer days of postovulatory high temperatures above the coverline, it may indicate one of two things:

1. You have a short luteal phase (Chart A.18a).
   (For pregnancy achievers, this could be a problem. See page 138.)
2. Your temperatures may take a few days to reflect ovulation (Chart A.18b).

The way to determine what is occurring is to identify your Peak Day before the rise in temperature. Ovulation usually takes place within a day or so of that last day of wetness. If there is a large discrepancy between the Peak Day and the thermal shift, you can probably assume that your temperature takes several days to increase following ovulation. But the only way to definitively confirm that is through ultrasound, which would obviously be very impractical.

If you are using FAM for birth control and would like to take advantage of more safe days than your temperature would otherwise allow, you could choose to depend on the cervical fluid and cervical position to determine your safe postovulatory phase. But, of course, this is definitely not as conservative as also relying on the temperature.

And notice that if you only rely on cervical fluid and position, you can't assume that you've already ovulated. Thus any cervical fluid at any time in the cycle should be considered fertile, at least until a thermal shift verifies that ovulation has come and gone.

**Chart A.18a.** Note that her temperatures are probably an indication of a true short luteal phase (9 days in this case), because the shift coincides with her cervical fluid. She most likely ovulated about Day 16 on this chart, since ovulation usually occurs the day of, or the day after, the Peak Day.

**Chart A.18b.** By contrast, this chart shows that ovulation probably occurred earlier than the temperature reflected, because the Peak Day of cervical fluid was on Day 15, but the thermal shift wasn't until Day 21. Thus her body probably takes a few days to respond to the postovulatory progesterone, and she therefore does not really have a short luteal phase.

## 18 OR MORE HIGH TEMPERATURES AFTER OVULATION

If you have 18 or more consecutive high temperatures above the coverline with no sign of a period, it is almost always an indication of pregnancy. The sustained high temperatures are caused by the continual release of progesterone from the corpus luteum, which remains viable beyond the normal 12 to 16 days, once a pregnancy occurs. In fact, in many pregnant women, the pattern of high temperatures even increases into a third level caused by the additional progesterone in their body (see opposite page).

Remember that most women will have a very consistent luteal phase (the time from ovulation to menstruation). So, for example, if your own luteal phase is typically about 13 days, and your temperature remains high for 16 days, there is a good chance that you are pregnant. The point is to determine if the temperatures are staying high longer than what is normal for you.

Another possible reason for 18 high temperatures is that occasionally a woman may develop a *corpus luteum cyst,* a rare condition in which the corpus luteum continues to live beyond the normal 12 to 16 days—even when she isn't pregnant. If this should happen, the temperature may continue to remain high due to the progesterone that is still being emitted from the persistent corpus luteum. Of course, if the progesterone doesn't drop, the uterine lining is not shed during menstruation. It would therefore *appear* that you were pregnant.

You may also notice light spotting and mild pain about the time your period is due. A pregnancy test combined with a manual exam of the uterus may be warranted to rule out such an occurrence. If it turns out that you do have a corpus luteum cyst, the good news is that they usually dissipate on their own.

**Chart A.19.**

## TWO LEVELS OF HIGH TEMPERATURES AFTER OVULATION (TRIPHASIC PATTERN)

As mentioned in the previous section, a triphasic pattern of temperatures is virtually always caused by pregnancy. It is the result of additional progesterone circulating in the woman's body, and increases about the time of implantation of the egg. While there is apparently no discussion of this phenomenon in the medical literature, my professional experience is that this triphasic pattern seems to occur in most pregnant women who chart. (See page 6 of color insert.)

**Chart A.20.**

## CONTINUAL STICKY CERVICAL FLUID DAY AFTER DAY (BASIC INFERTILE PATTERN)

Some women notice that they have a continuous, nonchanging cervical fluid, even during their infertile phase. You may want to get it checked to rule out any type of infection or cervical problem. If there is none, you should then consider such cervical fluid part of your Basic Infertile Pattern (BIP).

With a BIP, you will usually experience day after day of sticky cervical fluid. In order to establish a Basic Infertile Pattern, you must observe your cervical fluid very carefully for 2 weeks without the interference of semen, spermicides, douches, or anything else that may make your observations difficult.

Once you have established your BIP, any days with this pattern are treated as if they were dry, whether you are trying to avoid or achieve pregnancy. The trick is to learn to detect the *change* to a wetter fertile-quality cervical fluid. For complete instructions on how to use FAM for birth control while you have a BIP with normal ovulatory cycles, see page 116.

| Cycle Day | 1 | 2 | 3 | 4 | 5 | 6 | 7 | 8 | 9 | 10 | 11 | 12 | 13 | 14 | 15 | 16 | 17 | 18 | 19 | 20 | 21 | 22 | 23 | 24 | 25 | 26 | 27 | 28 | 29 | 30 | 31 | 32 | 33 | 34 | 35 | 36 | 37 | 38 | 39 | 40 |
|---|---|---|---|---|---|---|---|---|---|---|---|---|---|---|---|---|---|---|---|---|---|---|---|---|---|---|---|---|---|---|---|---|---|---|---|---|---|---|---|---|
| Cervical Fluid | ✱ | ✱ | ✱ | ✱ | S | S | S | S | S | S | S | © | © | © | S | S | S | S | S | S | S | S | S | S | S | S | S | S | ✱ | | | | | | | | | | | |
| Peak Day | | | | | | | | | | | | | | | | | | | | | | | | | | | | | | | | | | | | | | | | |
| Vaginal Sensation | | | | | dry | = | = | sticky | = | = | wet | wet | lube | dry | = | = | = | = | = | = | = | = | = | = | = | = | = | = | | | | | | | | | | | | |
| Cervix | | | | | | | | | | | | | | | | | | | | | | | | | | | | | | | | | | | | | | | | |
| Cervical Fluid Description | | | | | scant, crumbly | crumbly | dryish, sticky | sticky | more, but still sticky | crumbly | sticky | white lotion | more lotion | 2" clear stretch | sticky | | | | | | | | | | | | | | | | | | | | | | | | | |

**Chart A.21.**

## CONTINUAL WET CERVICAL FLUID DAY AFTER DAY

If you notice continuous creamy or eggwhite-quality cervical fluid that extends for weeks at a time, it could be an indication of excessively high levels of estrogen or low thyroid function (hypothyroidism). Some of the other symptoms of the latter condition include unusually long cycles with low waking temperatures. If you suspect you have either of these problems, you should see a doctor.

| Cycle Day | 1 | 2 | 3 | 4 | 5 | 6 | 7 | 8 | 9 | 10 | 11 | 12 | 13 | 14 | 15 | 16 | 17 | 18 | 19 | 20 | 21 | 22 | 23 | 24 | 25 | 26 | 27 | 28 | 29 | 30 | 31 | 32 | 33 | 34 | 35 | 36 | 37 | 38 | 39 | 40 |
|---|---|---|---|---|---|---|---|---|---|---|---|---|---|---|---|---|---|---|---|---|---|---|---|---|---|---|---|---|---|---|---|---|---|---|---|---|---|---|---|---|
| Cervical Fluid | ✶ | ✶ | ✶ | ✶ | – | – | S | Ⓔ | Ⓔ | Ⓔ | Ⓔ | Ⓔ | Ⓔ | Ⓔ | Ⓔ | Ⓔ | Ⓔ | Ⓔ | Ⓔ | Ⓔ | Ⓔ | Ⓔ | Ⓒ | Ⓒ | S | S | – | – | – | – | S | S | – | S | – | – | S | – | ✶ | | |

**Chart A.22.**

## WATERY CERVICAL FLUID RATHER THAN CREAMY

Occasionally, you may only have a watery cervical fluid that is either completely clear or the consistency and look of nonfat milk. In either case, you may wish to use your own symbol, such as Ⓦ for watery, or wet. Regardless, you should treat it as fertile, just as you would creamy or eggwhite-quality cervical fluid.

| Cycle Day | 1 | 2 | 3 | 4 | 5 | 6 | 7 | 8 | 9 | 10 | 11 | 12 | 13 | 14 | 15 | 16 | 17 | 18 | 19 | 20 | 21 | 22 | 23 | 24 | 25 | 26 | 27 | 28 | 29 | 30 | 31 | 32 | 33 | 34 | 35 | 36 | 37 | 38 | 39 | 40 |
|---|---|---|---|---|---|---|---|---|---|---|---|---|---|---|---|---|---|---|---|---|---|---|---|---|---|---|---|---|---|---|---|---|---|---|---|---|---|---|---|---|
| Cervical Fluid | ✳ | ✳ | ✳ | ✳ | ⊛ | – | – | S | S | S | Ⓦ | Ⓦ | Ⓔ | – | – | – | – | – | – | – | – | – | – | – | – | – | ✳ | | | | | | | | | | | | | |
| Peak Day | | | | | | | | | | | | | | | | | | | | | | | | | | | | | | | | | | | | | | | | |
| Vaginal Sensation | | | | | | | | | | | dry | dry | dry | wet | wet | wet! | | | | | | | | | | | | | | | | | | | | | | | | |
| Cervix | | | | | | | | | | | | | | | | | | | | | | | | | | | | | | | | | | | | | | | | |
| Cervical Fluid Description | | | | | | | | | | | milky, watery | " | 4" clear stretch | | | | | | | | | | | | | | | | | | | | | | | | | | | |

**Chart A.23.**

## ABSENCE OF ANY EGGWHITE-QUALITY CERVICAL FLUID

You may find that you never notice eggwhite-quality cervical fluid, or rarely see it. Or you observe stretchy cervical fluid, but it is opaque rather than clear. Remember that fertile-quality cervical fluid is on a continuum, from dry to extremely wet, with the most fertile quality being the wettest. The wettest you produce may be just creamy. Either way, your Peak Day of fertility is always your last day of the wettest cervical fluid or vaginal sensation that you produce as described on page 83.

Note that it is still very possible to get pregnant when eggwhite is absent, assuming you produce *some* wetness capable of sustaining sperm. However, cycles that do not produce eggwhite are not as fertile as those that do.

| Cycle Day | 1 | 2 | 3 | 4 | 5 | 6 | 7 | 8 | 9 | 10 | 11 | 12 | 13 | 14 | 15 | 16 | 17 | 18 | 19 | 20 | 21 | 22 | 23 | 24 | 25 | 26 | 27 | 28 | 29 | 30 | 31 | 32 | 33 | 34 | 35 | 36 | 37 | 38 | 39 | 40 |
|---|---|---|---|---|---|---|---|---|---|---|---|---|---|---|---|---|---|---|---|---|---|---|---|---|---|---|---|---|---|---|---|---|---|---|---|---|---|---|---|---|
| Cervical Fluid | ✳ | ✳ | ✳ | ✳ | — | — | s | s | ⓒ | ⓒ | ⓒ | ⓒ | — | — | — | — | — | — | — | — | — | — | — | — | — | — | — | ✳ | | | | | | | | | | | | |
| Peak Day | | | | | | | | | | | | | | | | | | | | | | | | | | | | | | | | | | | | | | | | |
| Vaginal Sensation | | | | | | | | | wet | cold | cold | wet | | | | | | | | | | | | | | | | | | | | | | | | | | | | |
| Cervix | | | | | | | | | | | | | | | | | | | | | | | | | | | | | | | | | | | | | | | | |
| | | | | | | | | | | | | | | | | | | | | | | | | | | | | | | | | | | | | | | | | |
| Cervical Fluid Description | | | | | | | | | creamy, watery = | creamy, thick, a lot " = more | | | | | | | | | | | | | | | | | | | | | | | | | | | | | | |

**Chart A.24.**

## PATCHES OF WET CERVICAL FLUID INTERSPERSED OVER LONG CYCLES

Occasionally, during the various phases in your life in which ovulation occurs less frequently, your body may go through episodes of trying to ovulate before it actually does. Eventually, after weeks or months of experiencing "false starts" in the form of patches of cervical fluid, you should be able to verify ovulation took place by the arrival of a thermal shift. Until you can do this, however, all cervical fluid must be seen as preovulatory and potentially fertile.

For contraceptors, this transitional pattern can be frustrating in that the sympto-thermal rules require you to abstain or use barriers every day from the first day that you get your first patch of cervical fluid. Technically, this would even include the dry days that follow (as long as there is no thermal shift to show that ovulation has passed).

However, if you have this pattern, you can apply the Billings Method with only a slightly increased risk. This method allows you to discard the Temperature Shift Rule and simply apply the Peak Day Rule (meaning you are safe the evening of the 4th day after your Peak Day, as described on page 119). If you do this though, remember you must continue to carefully check your cervical fluid everyday, at least until you can observe a thermal shift which verifies that you have ovulated. And with every *new* patch of cervical fluid, you must apply the Peak Day Rule again.

If you are *trying* to get pregnant, remember that you are still considered fertile during wet days as long as you have not seen your temperature rise.

**Chart A.25.** When Courtney traveled to France for the summer, her cycle was thrown off kilter, and thus she actually didn't ovulate until about Day 76 (note that this chart starts with cycle Day 40). Several times over the summer her body "prepared" to ovulate, but then stopped short, as seen by the sporadic patches of cervical fluid in the weeks leading up to her thermal shift. With this extended cycle, she chose to use the Billings Method, which does not use the Temperature Shift Rule. Thus, she considers herself infertile the evening of the 4th day after *each* one of her Peak Days, through to the following patch of cervical fluid. (Infertile evenings are boxed in red.)

## WET, CREAMY CERVICAL FLUID WELL AFTER OVULATION

After ovulation, there is a second smaller surge of estrogen well into the luteal phase, which occasionally causes a day or two of creamy cervical fluid. This often coincides with a temporary drop in temperatures. Pregnancy avoiders need not be concerned, assuming the Temperature Shift and Peak Day rules have clearly shown ovulation has already occurred. If you're not sure, don't take risks.

**Chart A.26.**

## WET SENSATION OR EGGWHITE BEFORE MENSTRUATION

Having a very wet, watery sensation, or even an eggwhite-quality substance about a day or two before your period is absolutely normal. It is merely an indication that the corpus luteum has disintegrated, as it does before menstruation. The first part of the lining that typically flows out when progesterone drops is the water that comprised part of the endometrial lining. This watery substance is not to be confused with fertile-quality cervical fluid. It has no bearing on your fertility. By definition, if it comes out just before your period and after you have established that you are in your infertile phase, then you are indeed infertile at that time.

**Chart A.27.**

## INFECTION MASKING CERVICAL FLUID

Vaginal infections produce many aggravations, including their ability to mask cervical fluid. What typically differentiates most infections from healthy cervical fluid is that infections usually have at least one of the following symptoms:

1. True discharge, which is perhaps gray, green, foamy, or even like cottage cheese
2. Itching or irritation such as stinging
3. An unpleasant or unusual odor
4. Discoloration of the vagina, such as redness
5. Potential swelling of the vagina and vaginal opening

If you suspect that you have an infection, you should record a question mark in the box for Cervical Fluid. It is imperative that you abstain from intercourse during this time in order to allow your body a chance to heal, and to prevent passing it back and forth between you and your partner. If nothing else, it can be extremely painful to have sex when you have an infection!

| Cycle Day | 1 | 2 | 3 | 4 | 5 | 6 | 7 | 8 | 9 | 10 | 11 | 12 | 13 | 14 | 15 | 16 | 17 | 18 | 19 | 20 | 21 | 22 | 23 | 24 | 25 | 26 | 27 | 28 | 29 | 30 | 31 | 32 | 33 | 34 | 35 | 36 | 37 | 38 | 39 | 40 |
|---|---|---|---|---|---|---|---|---|---|---|---|---|---|---|---|---|---|---|---|---|---|---|---|---|---|---|---|---|---|---|---|---|---|---|---|---|---|---|---|---|
| Cervical Fluid | * | * | * | * | – | – | ? | ? | ? | ? | ? | ? | ? | ? | © | © | s | – | – | – | – | – | – | – | – | – | – | – | – | – | – | * | | | | | | | | |

**Chart A.28.**

## WET CERVICAL FLUID FOUND AT THE CERVIX BUT NOT AT THE VAGINAL OPENING

Women who check their cervical fluid at the cervical tip may notice that it seems wetter or more abundant than what they simultaneously observe at the vaginal opening. This is logical, since it can take a few hours for the cervical fluid to trickle down.

Remember to keep in mind that if you check internally, you will always have at least a slight moisture on your finger that should not be confused with cervical fluid. Simply wave your finger in the air for a few seconds. If the dampness dissipates, then you know it was only the moisture from the vagina itself.

If you find a slight white filmy substance on your finger but your vaginal sensation is *dry,* you may then consider that day a dry day. This is because women will usually have such a substance internally even when it appears as if they are dry externally. This would still be considered infertile.

| Cycle Day | 1 | 2 | 3 | 4 | 5 | 6 | 7 | 8 | 9 | 10 | 11 | 12 | 13 | 14 | 15 | 16 | 17 | 18 | 19 | 20 | 21 | 22 | 23 | 24 | 25 | 26 | 27 | 28 | 29 | 30 | 31 | 32 | 33 | 34 | 35 | 36 | 37 | 38 | 39 | 40 |
|---|---|---|---|---|---|---|---|---|---|---|---|---|---|---|---|---|---|---|---|---|---|---|---|---|---|---|---|---|---|---|---|---|---|---|---|---|---|---|---|---|
| Cervical Fluid | ✳ | ✳ | ✳ | ✳ | – | – | – | – | S | S | S | Ⓒ | Ⓒ | Ⓔ | – | – | – | – | – | – | – | – | – | – | – | – | ✳ | | | | | | | | | | | | | |
| Peak Day | | | | | | | | | | | | | | | | | | | | | | | | | | | | | | | | | | | | | | | | |
| Vaginal Sensation | | | | | | | | | dry | dry | dry | cold | wet | WET | | | | | | | | | | | | | | | | | | | | | | | | | | |
| Cervix | | | | | | | | | | | | | | | | | | | | | | | | | | | | | | | | | | | | | | | | |
| Cervical Fluid Description | | | | | | | | | scant sticky | sticky (film at cervix) | sticky (scant cream-cervix) | creamy | thick white cream | 2" clear slippery | | | | | | | | | | | | | | | | | | | | | | | | | | |

**Chart A.29.** Note that cervical fluid that is wetter at the cervical tip than externally, as well as any filmlike substance, can be recorded in the Cervical Fluid Description column. But the symbols you record in the Cervical Fluid column should reflect what you observe at the external vaginal opening. You may prefer to use Chart 3 in Appendix K. It is specifically designed for recording both internal and external cervical fluid observations.

## CERVIX THAT CAN'T BE FOUND

Although at times you may think your cervix has migrated up your body and out your ear, believe me, it's still there. When a woman is approaching ovulation, her cervix rises, often becoming so high it feels inaccessible. If this is the case, trust your body. If you have been able to feel it before, it probably means that you are just very fertile at that time. In such a case, simply record a question mark in the cervix column on the days that you can't actually feel it.

| Cycle Day | 1 | 2 | 3 | 4 | 5 | 6 | 7 | 8 | 9 | 10 | 11 | 12 | 13 | 14 | 15 | 16 | 17 | 18 | 19 | 20 | 21 | 22 | 23 | 24 | 25 | 26 | 27 | 28 | 29 | 30 | 31 | 32 | 33 | 34 | 35 | 36 | 37 | 38 | 39 | 40 |
|---|---|---|---|---|---|---|---|---|---|---|---|---|---|---|---|---|---|---|---|---|---|---|---|---|---|---|---|---|---|---|---|---|---|---|---|---|---|---|---|---|
| Cervical Fluid | | | | | | | | | | | | | | | | | | | | | | | | | | | | | | | | | | | | | | | | |
| Peak Day | | | | | | | | | | | | | | | | | | | | | | | | | | | | | | | | | | | | | | | | |
| Vaginal Sensation | | | | | | | | | | | | | | | | | | | | | | | | | | | | | | | | | | | | | | | | |
| Cervix | | | | | | • | • | • | o | o | o | o | ? | ? | ? | • | • | • | • | • | • | • | • | • | • | • | • | • | • | • | | | | | | | | | | |

Chart A.30.

## CERVIX THAT NEVER FULLY CLOSES

Women who have delivered a child vaginally usually have a cervix that never completely closes during the infertile phase. On infertile days, rather than feeling a tiny dimple, it feels more like a horizontal, slight opening. The trick is to learn how to differentiate between the subtle changes in the oval-shaped opening as ovulation approaches.

| Cycle Day | 1 | 2 | 3 | 4 | 5 | 6 | 7 | 8 | 9 | 10 | 11 | 12 | 13 | 14 | 15 | 16 | 17 | 18 | 19 | 20 | 21 | 22 | 23 | 24 | 25 | 26 | 27 | 28 | 29 | 30 | 31 | 32 | 33 | 34 | 35 | 36 | 37 | 38 | 39 | 40 |
|---|---|---|---|---|---|---|---|---|---|---|---|---|---|---|---|---|---|---|---|---|---|---|---|---|---|---|---|---|---|---|---|---|---|---|---|---|---|---|---|---|
| Cervical Fluid | | | | | | | | | | | | | | | | | | | | | | | | | | | | | | | | | | | | | | | | |
| Peak Day | | | | | | | | | | | | | | | | | | | | | | | | | | | | | | | | | | | | | | | | |
| Vaginal Sensation | | | | | | | | | | | | | | | | | | | | | | | | | | | | | | | | | | | | | | | | |
| Cervix | | | | o | o | o | o | O | O | O | o | | | | | | | | | | | | | | | | | | | | | | | | | | | | | |

Chart A.31.

## BUMPS ON THE SURFACE OF THE CERVIX

Many women notice bumps that feel like large, hard granules of sand just under the skin of the cervix. They are called nabothian cysts and are usually considered harmless and tend to disappear on their own. Still, you may want to have a clinician confirm your suspicion the first time you feel one. Some women notice that they come and go with the cycle. Of course, a woman would probably never realize she had them unless she checked her cervix.

## PELVIC PAIN DURING INTERCOURSE

You may occasionally feel a deep pain during intercourse, depending on where you are in your cycle and the position you use. One of the causes of such pain may be the height of the cervix at the time. When a woman is not in her fertile phase, the cervix is at its lowest point and can actually be hit by her partner's penis during intercourse, especially if she straddles atop him. This is because this position tends to push the cervix down to its lowest point. To remedy the problem, simply be aware of how high your cervix is on any given day and avoid the position that causes pain.

Another cause could be from even the slightest jarring of the already tender ovary about to release an egg. Even a full bladder could cause pain during intercourse. Of course, if you experience severe pain, you should seek medical attention to rule out anything more serious.

**Chart A.32.**

## SPOTTING AFTER INTERCOURSE

Some women will notice occasional spotting after making love. It is usually caused by the cervix being tapped with the penis. This is especially likely when the cervix is lowest and most vulnerable to being hit. There may be no problem at all. However, if the bleeding is heavy or occurs often, you should consult a doctor to make sure it isn't anything more serious such as an infection or even cervical cancer.

**Chart A.33.**

# Using FAM During Special Circumstances (Stress, Breastfeeding, Premenopause, etc.)

> Please note: Before reading this appendix, you should have internalized the basic principles of Chapters 6 and 9. However, there is no reason to read it if your charting has revealed that you are ovulating normally. Breastfeeding women should read this appendix as well as the following one specifically devoted to using FAM while nursing.

The typical woman will experience about 400 periods in her lifetime. (OK, OK, kvetch and moan, if you must.) But remember, not every bleeding episode is preceded by ovulation, and therefore, technically, such anovulatory bleeding is not menstruation. Teenagers and breastfeeding or premenopausal women may go months without ovulating but may still experience menstrual-like bleeding.

Even excluding these groups, it is possible that the average woman may have an anovulatory cycle about once every year or two. And, occasionally, women may go for months without any bleeding at all. What all of this means is that if you bleed it may or may not imply that you ovulated, but if you ovulate you will bleed (unless, of course, you get pregnant).

When a woman isn't ovulating, it would seem obvious that she isn't fertile, right? Well, yes and no. When women don't ovulate, of course they aren't fertile. But ironically, anovulatory cycles can be a little more challenging to interpret, because the obvious patterns of fertility don't occur. In essence, then, the woman must act as if she is continually in a preovulatory phase, since ovulation *could* still occur. This situation is very different from a typical cycle in which the fertility signs reflect the obvious approach and passing of ovulation.

Anovulation can be a temporary phase lasting no more than a month or two, or it could last up to several years. As described above, long periods of time without menstruation often occur during phases such as adolescence, breastfeeding, and premenopause. In addition, women coming off the Pill or other hormones, or those who exercise strenuously and whose body fat is extremely low, may also go for a long time without ovulating. There may be physiological conditions that affect the hormone system. And finally, other factors which could delay ovulation for short or long phases are situations such as stress, illness, or travel.

## YOUR BASIC INFERTILE PATTERN (BIP) WHEN NOT OVULATING

During anovulatory cycles, you will usually experience a *Basic Infertile Pattern* (BIP) unlike what you are normally used to. Many women who experience a long phase of anovulation are continually dry, day after day. Other women may notice that instead of experiencing dry days when not ovulating, they have the same type of sticky cervical fluid day after day.

Regardless, if you also have a dry vaginal sensation, these days are treated as *if* they were dry days, but only after you have clearly established your BIP. While this modification is considered safe, there may be a small increase in risk, and therefore, I strongly suggest that if you have a sticky BIP, it is best to check your cervical tip before intercourse to verify that there is no *wet* cervical fluid present. If there is, do not consider yourself safe.

## ESTABLISHING YOUR BASIC INFERTILE PATTERN

In order to establish a BIP, you must observe your cervical fluid very carefully for 2 weeks without the interference of semen, spermicides, douches, or anything else that may mask its observation. Ideally you should abstain during this time.

Once you have charted your cervical fluid for 2 consecutive weeks, and have established that you are continually dry, or have the same sticky-type cervical fluid, you have established your Basic Infertile Pattern. *Only then may you apply the two anovulatory rules described in this chapter.*

| Cycle Day | 1 | 2 | 3 | 4 | 5 | 6 | 7 | 8 | 9 | 10 | 11 | 12 | 13 | 14 | 15 | 16 | 17 | 18 | 19 | 20 | 21 | 22 | 23 | 24 | 25 | 26 | 27 | 28 | 29 | 30 | 31 | 32 | 33 | 34 | 35 | 36 | 37 | 38 | 39 | 40 |
|---|---|---|---|---|---|---|---|---|---|---|---|---|---|---|---|---|---|---|---|---|---|---|---|---|---|---|---|---|---|---|---|---|---|---|---|---|---|---|---|---|
| Cervical Fluid | S | S | S | S | S | S | S | S | S | S | S | S | S | S | S | S | S | S | S | S | S | S | S | S | S | S | S | S | S | S | S | S | S | S | S | S | S | S | S | S |
| Peak Day | | | | | | | | | | | | | | | | | | | | | | | | | | | | | | | | | | | | | | | | |
| Vaginal Sensation | | | *2-week BIP of sticky is established* | | | | | | | | | | | | | | | | | | | | | | | | | | | | | | | | | | | | | |

**Chart B.1. Basic Infertile Pattern of sticky days.** (Infertile evenings are boxed in red.)

### UNCHANGING DAY RULE

If your 2-week Basic Infertile Pattern (BIP) is dry or the same-quality sticky cervical fluid day after day, you are safe for unprotected intercourse the evening of every dry or unchanging sticky day. (Women with a BIP of wet cervical fluid must unfortunately consider themselves fertile.)

## The Unchanging Day Rule Applied

Thus, if your 2-week BIP is *sticky* day after day, you are safe to have intercourse the evenings of sticky days (as if they were dry), as shown in Chart B.1.

## A Basic Infertile Pattern of Both Dry and Sticky Cervical Fluid

You may observe a pattern of dry *and* sticky over the 2-week observation time in which you determine your BIP. If you are a new user of FAM, I would encourage you to only consider the evening of a dry day as safe. For experienced users of FAM, you may choose to use such a combination pattern as your BIP, paying special attention to any *change* to a wet-type cervical fluid. But you should be aware that you are taking a slightly greater risk when you consider a combination of dry and sticky as a Basic Infertile Pattern. If you have this type of BIP, I would particularly urge you to verify that you have no wet cervical fluid at your cervical tip before having intercourse.

### A Word About Semen Masking Cervical Fluid

If there is semen or spermicide present the day after intercourse, you should note it with a question mark since it could mask cervical fluid. The day of semen is then considered potentially fertile.

As mentioned in the bottom of the box on page 85, a trick to eliminate the semen from your body following intercourse is to do SETs, or Semen Emitting Technique. If the day after intercourse you experience the same unchanged cervical fluid, you are safe for unprotected sex again that evening.

## 🙠 SIGNS OF IMPENDING OVULATION

Occasionally, during the various phases in your life in which ovulation doesn't occur, your body may go through episodes of trying to ovulate before it actually does. During this time, after weeks or months of experiencing the same BIP, you may notice *patches* of more fertile cervical fluid interspersed with the dry or sticky days. It is critical to be attentive to such changes because it is your body's way of reflecting hormonal activity that may lead to ovulation again. So, if you notice patches of more fertile cervical fluid interspersed among the dry or sticky phases, you must follow the rule below.

> **PATCH RULE**
>
> You are safe the evening of every day that your 2-week Basic Infertile Pattern remains the same. But as soon as you see a *change* in your BIP, you must consider yourself fertile until the fourth consecutive evening after the Peak Day. The Peak Day is the last day of the more fertile patch of cervical fluid or lubricative vaginal sensation in your BIP. Obviously, any type of *wet* cervical fluid or bleeding must be considered a fertile patch.

### The Patch Rule Applied

So, for example, if your 2-week BIP is dry day after day, you are considered safe the evening of any dry day. But if you get a patch of any type of cervical fluid following the 2-week observation time, you must consider those days potentially fertile through to the fourth consecutive evening after your Peak Day (Chart B.2).

**Chart B.2. Patch Rule with Basic Infertile Pattern of dry days.** When she developed patches of spotting, sticky, or wet cervical fluid interspersed throughout her dry days, she considered herself fertile until she could identify the Peak Day plus 1,2,3,4. So in this chart the first patch she considered fertile started on Day 57 and continued through until Peak plus 4, or the evening of Day 62. She then considered herself safe all the evenings of dry days until her next patch on Day 66. Also note that if cycles extend beyond 40 days, you can renumber Day 1 of the chart as 41, as seen above. (Infertile evenings are boxed in red.)

| Cycle Day | 1 | 2 | 3 | 4 | 5 | 6 | 7 | 8 | 9 | 10 | 11 | 12 | 13 | 14 | 15 | 16 | 17 | 18 | 19 | 20 | 21 | 22 | 23 | 24 | 25 | 26 | 27 | 28 | 29 | 30 | 31 | 32 | 33 | 34 | 35 | 36 | 37 | 38 | 39 | 40 |
|---|---|---|---|---|---|---|---|---|---|---|---|---|---|---|---|---|---|---|---|---|---|---|---|---|---|---|---|---|---|---|---|---|---|---|---|---|---|---|---|---|
| Cervical Fluid | S | S | S | S | S | S | S | S | S | S | S | S | S | S | S | S | S | C | C | E | S | S | S | S | S | S | S | S | S | S | S | C | S | S | S | S | S | S | S | S |
| Peak Day |  |  |  |  |  |  |  |  |  |  |  |  |  |  |  |  |  |  | PK | 1 | 2 | 3 | 4 |  |  |  |  |  |  |  | PK | 1 | 2 | 3 | 4 |  |  |  |  |  |
| Vaginal Sensation | 2-week BIP of sticky |
| Cervix | already established |

**Chart B.3. Patch Rule with Basic Infertile Pattern of sticky days.** When she developed patches of spotting or wet cervical fluid interspersed throughout her sticky days, she considered herself fertile until she could identify the Peak Day plus 1,2,3,4. So in this chart the first patch she considered fertile started on Day 57 and continued through until Peak plus 4, or the evening of Day 63. She then considered herself safe all the evenings of sticky days until her next patch on Day 72. (Infertile evenings are boxed in red.)

If your 2-week BIP is sticky day after day, you are considered safe the evening of any sticky day. But if you get a patch of any type of wet cervical fluid following the 2-week observation time, you must consider those days potentially fertile through to the fourth consecutive evening after your Peak Day (Chart B.3, above).

## A Less Conservative Approach

Some clinicians believe if the patch is of a *sticky*- rather than wet-quality cervical fluid, you need only wait until the second night (rather than the fourth) beyond your Peak Day (Chart B.4, below).

This less conservative approach is still considered very safe, but if you absolutely can't risk a pregnancy, you should either wait until the fourth night beyond, or verify that there is no cervical fluid at the cervical tip before having intercourse.

| Cycle Day | 1 | 2 | 3 | 4 | 5 | 6 | 7 | 8 | 9 | 10 | 11 | 12 | 13 | 14 | 15 | 16 | 17 | 18 | 19 | 20 | 21 | 22 | 23 | 24 | 25 | 26 | 27 | 28 | 29 | 30 | 31 | 32 | 33 | 34 | 35 | 36 | 37 | 38 | 39 | 40 |
|---|---|---|---|---|---|---|---|---|---|---|---|---|---|---|---|---|---|---|---|---|---|---|---|---|---|---|---|---|---|---|---|---|---|---|---|---|---|---|---|---|
| Cervical Fluid | – | – | – | – | – | – | – | – | – | – | – | – | – | – | – | – | – | – | – | C | C | – | – | – | – | – | – | – | – | – | S | S | S | – | – | – | – | – | – | – |
| Peak Day |  |  |  |  |  |  |  |  |  |  |  |  |  |  |  |  |  |  | PK | 1 | 2 | 3 | 4 |  |  |  |  |  |  |  | PK | 1 | 2 |  |  |  |  |  |  |  |
| Vaginal Sensation | 2-week BIP of dry |
| Cervix | already established |

**Chart B.4. Less conservative Patch Rule with Basic Infertile Pattern of dry days.** She still counts 4 days after any patch of wet cervical fluid (or spotting), and thus with the cervical patch of Days 59 and 60, she does not consider herself safe until the evening of Day 64. However, she chose to be a little less conservative with patches that were only *sticky,* and thus with the patch ending Day 73, she considers herself infertile on the evening of Day 75, just 2 days after it ended. (Infertile evenings are boxed in red.)

**Bleeding During Anovulatory Phases**

When women experience episodes of bleeding during phases of anovulation, it is imperative that they treat those particular days as *potentially fertile*. The bleeding could be an indication of either ovulatory spotting or the start of hormonal activity preparing for ovulation. The key to determining *true* menstruation is the observation of a thermal shift 12 to 16 days prior.

Deciding what to call Day 1 of the cycle can be somewhat confusing when the bleeding is not true menstrual bleeding. You can either choose to start a new chart each time you have an episode of bleeding, or continue as if you are experiencing one continuous, potentially months-long cycle with intermittent phases of bleeding. The critical point is to be able to identify when the bleeding is true menstruation.

Of course, this is where the basal temperatures will indicate once you've really ovulated. Remember that you normally have a thermal shift about 12 to 16 days prior to true menstruation. But when you are starting to resume cycling for the first time in months, your luteal phase may be initially shorter until your cycles get back to normal.

**Changes in your BIP**

If a new cervical fluid pattern continues to be the same day after day for at least 2 weeks, that patch now becomes your *new* Basic Infertile Pattern, from which you must be on the lookout for yet another change. So, for example, if you had been dry day after day, then had a patch of sticky cervical fluid that lasted more than 2 weeks, that sticky quality would become your new BIP. You would then be considered safe all of those subsequent evenings until you observe a more fertile-quality patch (such as creamy) or experience spotting or bleeding. You must treat those patches as possibly fertile until you can apply the Patch Rule described on page 297.

**A Word of Caution for Premenopausal Women**

Unfortunately, premenopausal women who follow the BIP rules could be at somewhat greater risk of pregnancy than their younger peers. While it is true that women are less fertile in their 40s, fertility signs shift more quickly than usual premenopausally. Thus, a woman who has a BIP pattern of sticky days may find herself becoming creamy or eggwhite faster than before, when a gradual transition occurred over a few days. As a result, the body may progress faster toward ovulation than in earlier years. Therefore, some FAM experts feel that a premenopausal woman should limit preovulatory intercourse to the evening of *dry* days only, since sperm will die in just a few hours in that environment.

I agree that premenopausal women may be taking a slightly greater risk in following the BIP rules. However, I believe that the increased risk can be kept to a minimum *if you check your cervical fluid internally at the cervical tip to verify that there is no wet fluid present before having intercourse.* By taking this precaution, you are minimizing the possibility of a quick transition to the fertile wet cervical fluid needed for sperm survival.

## ✍ CONCLUDING REMARKS ON FAM AND ANOVULATORY PHASES

The most important point to remember when experiencing anovulation is to constantly be on the lookout for a *change* in cervical fluid that could indicate approaching ovulation. Ideally, you should continue to take your temperature to confirm that you are not ovulating. However, if you find this tedious during long months of not seeing a thermal shift, you could choose to wait to take your temperature until you see your cervical fluid change. Either way, remember that you always have the benefit of checking your cervix during times of uncertainty.

These rules are admittedly more complex than the standard FAM rules. Until you internalize them, you can always use the rules discussed in Chapter 9, but this means that in doing so, you may have to consider yourself fertile more days than you would probably care to.

Finally, you should know that you will usually have ample warning of cycles resuming by the buildup of patches of cervical fluid as your body tries to ovulate. Just keep in mind that phases of anovulation can be confusing, so you need to be on the lookout for changes. And while it may be frustrating at times, remember that anovulatory phases will probably be a very small part of your reproductive life.

## ✌ SUMMARY OF NATURAL BIRTH CONTROL RULES WHILE EXPERIENCING ANOVULATION

### UNCHANGING DAY RULE

If your 2-week Basic Infertile Pattern (BIP) is dry or the same-quality sticky cervical fluid day after day, you are safe for unprotected intercourse the evening of every dry or unchanging sticky day. (Women with a BIP of wet cervical fluid must consider themselves fertile.)

### PATCH RULE

You are safe the evening of every day that your 2-week Basic Infertile Pattern remains the same. But as soon as you see a *change* in your BIP, you must consider yourself fertile until the fourth consecutive evening after the Peak Day. The Peak Day is the last day of the more fertile patch of cervical fluid or lubricative vaginal sensation in your BIP. Any type of *wet* cervical fluid or bleeding must be considered a fertile patch.

# Using FAM While Nursing Your Baby

> Please note: This chapter will be confusing if you haven't first internalized the basic principles and rules discussed in the preceding appendix.

For those optimists who think you'll actually have *time* for lovemaking after having a baby, this appendix is for you. While breastfeeding is a wonderful and gratifying experience for most women, it can be difficult to identify when fertility will return, especially for those who haven't charted before. So let's set the record straight right from the beginning: Women *can* get pregnant while breastfeeding!

So why all the confusion over whether or not women are fertile while breastfeeding? Everybody has a neighbor, friend, or relative who swears they did or didn't get pregnant while nursing. These nursing women then become the standard by which people judge the effectiveness of breastfeeding for birth control.

Actually, the answer to the question of fertility during breastfeeding lies in how we define breastfeeding. It's true that the majority of women who breastfeed "on request," meaning throughout the day and night and every time the baby is hungry, may not see their periods resume for as long as a year or more. However, most women's fertility will only be suppressed by such intense breastfeeding if they also limit pacifiers and supplements, including water. It's simple biology.

This is because every time a baby suckles at the breast, it indirectly suppresses the hormones that trigger ovulation. But in order for breastfeeding to efficiently prevent the release of eggs, the baby must suckle at least every 4 hours during the day and every 6 hours at night. Thus, the key to determining when your cycles will return is to remember that *the longer and more often your baby is away from your breast, the sooner you will start ovulating again.*

## ∮ LEVEL OF BREASTFEEDING THAT AFFECTS FERTILITY

The chart on page 306 is a simple synopsis of the factors that will determine what rules of natural birth control to use until your cycles resume after childbirth. As a new mother, you will choose to do one of the following:

- Fully or nearly fully breastfeed on request
- Partially breastfeed
- Not breastfeed at all

### *Full or Nearly Full Breastfeeding*

One of the best gifts you can give your baby is the life-long health benefit provided by breastfeeding. Not only is it excellent nourishment, but it offers important immunological protection against disease and allergies. Yet in order to fully attain such advantages, you should breastfeed around the clock, whenever your baby is hungry. Ideally, no supplements should be given during the first 6 months.

While such a disciplined regimen may be difficult to maintain, nature will reward you with one of the simplest and most effective forms of natural contraception available. You will be able to use the Lactational Amenorrhea Method (LAM)* if you meet the following three criteria:

> **LACTATIONAL AMENORRHEA METHOD (LAM)**
>
> - Your menses have not returned.
> - You are fully or nearly fully breastfeeding.
> - Your baby is less than 6 months old.

The first criterion of LAM is that you have not resumed menstruating. What this means in practice is that any vaginal bleeding before the 56th day is almost always anovulatory (and therefore can be ignored), assuming you are

---

* "Lactational" means pertaining to the production of milk and "amenorrhea" means lack of menstruation.

fully or nearly fully breastfeeding. However, any bleeding after the 56th day should be considered a sign of resumed ovulation.

*Full* breastfeeding means that you are not giving your baby *any* supplements or pacifiers. However, the Institute of Reproductive Health at Georgetown University has shown through extensive studies that the contraceptive effectiveness of LAM is maintained even if your breastfeeding is *nearly* full, meaning that you supplement no more than 15% of all feedings. Of course the risk of resumed ovulation is on a continuum, and thus you should try to breastfeed as close to fully as possible. In addition, full or nearly full breastfeeding means that intervals between feedings should not exceed 4 hours during the day or 6 hours at night.

With LAM, you don't need to chart at all if you meet the boxed criteria, since it is considered to be at least 98% effective. This is a tremendous advantage because charting while breastfeeding can be somewhat challenging. However, if you do not meet the LAM criteria, you will need to follow the FAM rules for breastfeeding discussed below.

### Partially Breastfeeding

Partially breastfeeding means that supplements such as juices and solids are regularly given. It also means that you are nursing less frequently than every 4 hours during the day, and less than every 6 hours at night. Charting while partially breastfeeding is particularly challenging because it's harder to know when you will resume ovulating. Basically, you should follow the two anovulatory rules discussed in the preceding appendix (Unchanging-Day Rule and Patch Rule). But keep in mind that ovulation may return soon, since any supplements or long periods between nursing can lead to the early resumption of cycling. Of course, once true menstruation resumes, you should revert back to the four standard FAM rules covered in Chapter 9.

When you are establishing your Basic Infertile Pattern discussed on page 295, chart your cervical fluid for 2 weeks following the stopping of lochia, the postchildbirth spotting. Ideally, you should abstain during this time in order to get an accurate reflection of what type of cervical fluid you produce while breastfeeding. (Chances are, if you've just had a baby, intercourse isn't top on your list of favorite activities, anyway.)*

---

* In fact, one of the most common complaints of breastfeeding mothers is that their vaginas tend to be dry, often making intercourse uncomfortable. This is due to the low levels of estrogen indirectly caused from circulating prolactin. But as your body gets closer to finally resuming cycling again after childbirth, this condition should dissipate on its own.

Once you start introducing supplements to your baby's diet, especially at about 6 months of age, you should breastfeed your baby *before* giving the supplement. The benefit of this approach is that your breast milk provides your baby with protection against disease, while nursing helps to suppress the return of your ovulation.

## Not Breastfeeding at All (Strictly Bottle-Feeding)

Women who don't breastfeed find that their cycles resume very quickly—as early as 4 to 10 weeks after childbirth. If you aren't breastfeeding following the birth of your baby, you should start charting shortly after birth, since you can be fairly sure that your cycles will soon return. Note that in following the standard FAM rules, you must assume that you are in a preovulatory state until a temperature shift confirms that you have ovulated that first time after childbirth.

## ❧ THE TRANSITION TO RESUMED FERTILITY FOR ALL BREASTFEEDING WOMEN

Breastfeeding women will almost always have a warning of returning fertility through their cervical fluid. In fact, the episodes of cervical fluid may tend to be somewhat longer than normal as the body attempts to finally ovulate after months of anovulation. You will probably notice quite a few "false starts" in which you see longer and longer patches of fertile-quality cervical fluid as your body tries to finally pass over the estrogen threshold necessary to release an egg.

One of the most important points to understand regarding the transition to fertility relates to what is considered fertile-quality cervical fluid. Once your cycles resume (as reflected by a thermal shift), *any* preovulatory cervical fluid is considered fertile. In other words, the type of sticky cervical fluid that may have previously reflected infertility (your Basic Infertile Pattern) must now be considered fertile *once you start cycling again*. The bottom line is that you must go back to the four standard rules used for normal cycles discussed in Chapter 9.

# NATURAL BIRTH CONTROL RULES WHILE BREASTFEEDING

| Degree of Breastfeeding | Natural Birth Control Method | Natural Birth Control Rules | When to Resume Taking Waking Temperatures | Comments |
|---|---|---|---|---|
| **Not Breast-feeding at All** | FAM with: *Standard* rules | First 5 Days Rule<br>Dry Day Rule<br>Temperature Shift Rule<br>Peak Day Rule | By Day 14 after baby's birth | Cycles may resume within 4 weeks of child-birth.<br><br>You must consider your-self preovulatory until you can confirm that ovulation has resumed by temperature shift prior to a menstruation. |
| **Partial Breastfeeding**<br><br>Partial breastfeeding means that supplements such as bottle-feeding, juices, and solids are frequently given.<br><br>It also means nursing less frequently than every 4 hours during the day or every 6 hours at night. | FAM with: *Anovulatory* rules | Unchanging Day Rule<br>Patch Rule | • when you notice a change in your Basic Infertile Pattern of cervical fluid<br>or<br>• when you have a bleeding episode<br>or<br>• when your baby suddenly decreases suckling<br>or<br>• when you introduce solid foods<br>(whichever comes first) | Partially breastfeeding is the most challenging to chart because it is harder to predict when you will resume ovulating.<br><br>You must consider your-self preovulatory until you can confirm that ovulation has resumed by temperature shift prior to a menstruation. |
| **Full or Nearly Full Breast-feeding**<br><br>Full breastfeeding means not giving supplements at all, whereas *nearly* full means that supplements are given, but for no more than 15% of feedings.<br><br>It also means nursing at intervals of at least every 4 hours during the day and at least every 6 hours at night.<br><br>(A critical point: for contraceptive purposes, the first two criteria listed to the far right must also apply.) | Lactational Amenorrhea Method (LAM) | None, so long as the LAM criteria in the right column are met. | • when you have your first bleeding episode which is over 56 days since childbirth<br>or<br>• when the baby is 5–6 months old<br>or<br>• when you increase the use of solids or supplements to more than 15% of feedings, or no longer nurse your baby at least every 4 hours during the day and every 6 hours at night<br>(whichever comes first) | LAM provides over 98% protection against pregnancy so long as you meet the following three criteria:<br><br>1. Menses has not yet resumed (you can ignore bleeding before 56 days postpartum)<br><br>2. The baby is under 6 months old<br><br>3. You are fully or nearly fully breastfeeding, as defined by the first column.<br><br>If any of these three criteria are no longer met, you'll need to use the appropriate FAM rules listed in the above rows. |

## ஐ CONCLUDING REMARKS ON NATURAL BIRTH CONTROL WHILE BREASTFEEDING

The most important point to remember when experiencing the transition from childbirth to resumed cycling is to constantly be on the lookout for a *change* in cervical fluid that could indicate approaching ovulation. You may prefer to not take your temperature until you see that change. And, of course, you can always have the benefit of checking your cervical position during times of uncertainty.

You should also not be surprised if you go through weeks or even months of wet cervical fluid before you return to normal cycles. (In such a case, you'll need to decide whether you want to abstain or use a barrier method.)

Remember that your body has not ovulated in a long time, and it may take a while for it to get back into its usual pattern of fertility. This can be frustrating, but try to keep it all in perspective. Before you know it, your baby will be dating and you'll be dealing with bigger issues than your *own* contraceptive concerns!

# The Contraceptive Effectiveness of Natural Birth Control

*Why do mice have such small balls? Because only 10% can dance!*
—A JOKE TOLD AMONG BIOSTATISTICIANS,
WHO NO DOUBT GOT IT QUICKER THAN THE REST OF US

Before any couple decides to use a method of contraception, they should know its rate of effectiveness. The only "guaranteed birth control" is abstinence, and thus, for any sexually active woman of reproductive age, there is always some risk of pregnancy. A critical question in selecting a contraceptive is ascertaining the *degree of risk* you personally find acceptable.

The Fertility Awareness Method as taught in this book, *if understood thoroughly and always used correctly,* is extremely effective in preventing pregnancies. Indeed, it is so effective that the weakest link will be the barrier method you use, if you choose to have intercourse during your fertile phase. If used perfectly *and* you abstain during your fertile phase (as is done with Natural Family Planning), the chance of becoming pregnant would be approximately 2% over the course of a typical year. According to the 1994 edition of *Contraceptive Technology,* this is a lower failure rate than that of any barrier method. If you correctly use a barrier throughout the fertile phase, then your chance of becoming pregnant would be close to the method failure rate of the barrier you use. The table on page 313 will help to put this data in context.

Indeed, putting contraceptive data into proper social and biostatistical perspective is an important undertaking that is worth the few minutes it takes to read this appendix. You should know that when scientists discuss the efficacy of a contraceptive, there are in fact two different types of effectiveness ratings. One is called *method failure* rate, and refers specifically to the ability of a given form of birth control to prevent pregnancies when that method is *used* *correctly for every act of intercourse.* What is considered correct usage is usually defined by set guidelines, often spelled out by contraceptive manufacturers. For the Fertility Awareness Method, correct usage is detailed in Chapter 9 of this book.*

In many ways, what is more important than the method failure rate of any contraceptive is the *user* failure rate, for that is where you can see what occurs in the real world. User failure is generally defined as the rate of unwanted pregnancies for the population as a whole, taking into account both correct and incorrect usage. For example, the method failure of the condom is estimated by *Contraceptive Technology* at 3%, but user failure is closer to 12%, in part because men sometimes fail to put it on in a way that avoids leakage. This means that over the course of the first year of use, 12% of regular condom users will become pregnant. Fortunately, user failure rates for almost all contraceptives tend to drop after the first 12 months.

As you can imagine, there are some birth control methods in which the method and user failure rates are nearly identical, for the method chosen does not rely on the behavior of the user. Male and female surgical sterilization is the best example of this, with both method and user failure at or below .4%. Their disadvantages aside, it's true that long-term hormonal treatments such as Norplant and Depo-Provera are also exceptionally effective, with both method and user failure rates even lower than sterilization!

Standard birth control pills have a method failure rate of 1% or lower, but typical user failure rises to 3% or higher, depending on the study. This is primarily because women may forget to take the Pill for a few days. As the chart shows, the condom has a lower method failure rate than the other barrier methods, with all barriers showing user failure rates substantially higher than their corresponding method rates. This is because some people are not sure how to use the particular contraceptive, or more likely, because people are somewhat careless in their employment of the various devices.

* "Method effectiveness rates," as opposed to "failure rates," are expressed as a positive number showing how many sexually active women would *not* become pregnant over the course of a year were the method in question used perfectly (correctly, every time). Thus if a diaphragm manufacturer claims a method effective-ness of 94%, it is another way of saying that over the course of that year, 6% of women using that method are likely to get pregnant, assuming they use it perfectly.

It should be noted that while manufacturers certainly prefer to express the positive (94% effective), rather than the negative (6% failure), it is more accurate to discuss contraceptive statistics in terms of *failure* rates than *efficacy* rates. This is because in the real world, a 6% failure rate does not actually translate into a 94% success rate. Why? Because only about 85% of sexually active women of reproductive age would get pregnant over the course of a year even if they used *no* method. Also, given that women are fertile only a few days per cycle, it is clear that barrier method effectiveness rates will always be overstated. In this discussion, I will use the more statistically accurate failure rates.

Where does this leave NFP among the major contraceptive methods? (For the rest of this appendix, I will usually refer to NFP and not FAM, unless dealing specifically with barrier method issues. This is because research on the effectiveness rates of natural methods should be uncompromised by barrier method failures.) As I have already stated, the method failure rate of the rules as taught in this book is estimated at 2%. However, the user failure rates are much harder to pinpoint, because quite frankly, the medical literature is filled with studies showing such rates ranging widely, from 1% to certain studies claiming user failure as high as 20%.*

With such a wide discrepancy in data, is it possible to use the rules with the confidence you need? In fact, yes, very much so, but first you need to know where the data arise and why the discrepancy in reported rates is really not such a mystery. Finally, you need to really think about what the data *do* imply in terms of the type of people who should, and should not, use NFP or FAM as their contraceptive choice.

## ❧ NATURAL FAMILY PLANNING: HIGHLY EFFECTIVE, HIGHLY UNFORGIVING

NFP is highly effective when used correctly, but more than any other method, it is extremely unforgiving of improper use, or more specifically, "cheating." The reason for this is quite logical. If, for example, you misuse a diaphragm or condom or even forget to take a pill, the chances are that for any individual act of intercourse it probably wouldn't matter anyway since you most likely wouldn't be in the fertile phase of your cycle. NFP, of course, is the exact opposite, in that if you disregard the rules, you are by definition having unprotected intercourse precisely when you *are* potentially fertile. To use NFP effectively, you need to understand this, and most important, you need the necessary motivation to avoid pregnancy. As the major studies make clear, if you lack the latter, you will indeed be taking substantial and foolish risks.

As mentioned, various studies show that in the real world, NFP user failure rates vary greatly. Still, 10 to 12% per year seems close to the average reported in the medical literature for the sympto-thermal rules taught in Chapter 9. But

---

* These data refer specifically to the sympto-thermal method, the technical name given for the natural birth control rules detailed in Chapter 9. It involves observing *both* waking temperature and cervical fluid as well as the option of observing cervical position. Generally, other methods of natural birth control only observe waking temperature or cervical fluid. And the Rhythm Method (often referred to as the Calendar Method) doesn't involve observing any fertility signs.

what is equally important is that all these studies clearly suggest that in a large percentage of pregnancies that occur while "using" NFP, the cause of conception was due to *intentional violation of the method rules*. Simply put, many couples without sufficient motivation did cheat, and many of those paid the price.*

Ultimately it is a question of semantics as to whether those couples are reflective of user failure or simply should be considered nonusers, but you can see why NFP and FAM instructors get frustrated when they hear that the method is "not really considered effective." Indeed, a man using a condom who gets his wife pregnant because he remains inside her too long after ejaculation can certainly be included in the user failure rate. But if just one day he gets lazy and leaves the condom in the drawer, is this seriously a user failure if a pregnancy results? I would suggest that for any contraceptive, intentional and complete abandonment of the method in question reflects a category of nonusage that simply cannot be seen within the user failure paradigm.

More than any method, motivation to avoid pregnancy dramatically affects the user failure results. Some of the studies have in fact separated the test groups into motivational categories, such that for example, couples who used NFP to avoid pregnancy were put in one group whereas those who used NFP merely to better space their children were put in another. Not surprisingly, the "spacers" would invariably take greater chances, resulting in user failure rates substantially higher than the "avoiders," who showed user failure rates as low as 2%. (In fact, user failure rates well below 1% have been documented, but usually when intercourse is limited to the postovulatory infertile phase.)

## 🙰 NFP, MOTIVATION, AND RESPONSIBILITY

I write all of this not to simply tell you that the medical literature (and mainstream media) is inherently biased against NFP in its effectiveness reporting.

* One major study in the *American Journal of Obstetrics and Gynecology* (October 15, 1981, p. 368) reported without irony that "Couples who stated that they had used the fertile phase of the cycle in an attempt to achieve pregnancy accounted for 9.8% . . . of pregnancies. Since these couples did not give advance notification of their desires to attempt pregnancy, these . . . were attributed to the respective method."(!) It's also clear that a significant percent of the other failures, while not *trying* to get pregnant, were quite happy to take chances during the fertile phase. In fact, this particular article is actually a good and quite representative example of the numerous studies cited in the medical and scientific journals. In this report, over 100 women representing more than 1,600 total months of sexual exposure were monitored for contraceptive failure rates in use of the sympto-thermal method used in this book. Perhaps the most interesting result reported was that the authors concluded after intensive follow-up interviews that there were *no method failures whatsoever.*

The fact is that the numbers do tell us something quite valuable, that each one of you should contemplate before deciding whether NFP is the right method for you. Simply stated, the wide variance in user and method failure rates shows that the very "device-free" nature of the method means that it is extremely easy to slip into a "taking chances" mentality. Indeed, NFP is not a difficult method to learn, and learn well, but it is unfortunately an easy method to practice poorly, which by its very nature really means to not practice at all.

The bottom line on NFP as a contraceptive choice is this: *No one truly wishing to avoid pregnancy should be using it if they do not thoroughly understand the rules of the method, and most important, have the necessary discipline to follow those rules correctly and consistently.* If you do not completely understand the method as presented in this book, I urge you to get training through one of the institutions listed in Appendix M before relying on NFP as a contraceptive choice. Ultimately, natural methods of contraception are only appropriate for those couples with the maturity and self-respect necessary to not take foolish risks.

## &#8450; FERTILITY AWARENESS, BARRIERS, AND THE FERTILE PHASE: ASSESSING THE ODDS

There are a number of tangential issues related to Fertility Awareness efficacy rates that should be briefly addressed so that all couples can make the most appropriate contraceptive decisions. As I have mentioned, studies have shown that the method failure of NFP is estimated at 2%. However, you should realize that there is a higher risk of pregnancy for those couples who use barrier methods rather than abstain when the woman is fertile.

The statistical reality is actually quite intuitive. For those couples who choose to use a barrier method over abstinence *throughout* the fertile phase, the method and user failure rates of FAM will always be at least as high as the failure rates of the barrier they choose to use. It is for this reason that I suggest that couples who do not abstain use a condom as their method of choice. At approximately 3% method failure and 12% estimated user failure, it is a better barrier than any of the others, as seen in the table on page 313. (Of course the very fact that you'll know that you *are* fertile should encourage the type of diligent behavior necessary for keeping your own user failure rate at a minimum.)

For those couples who are determined to absolutely minimize their risk yet do not want to practice abstinence for the *full* fertile period, there are

## CONTRACEPTIVE METHOD EFFECTIVENESS TABLE*

| Method | Typical User Failure | Method Failure |
|---|---|---|
| Chance | 85 | 85 |
| Sponge[a] | 18 | 9 |
| Cervical cap[b] (w/jelly/foam) | 18 | 9 |
| Diaphragm (w/jelly/foam) | 18 | 6 |
| Spermicides (vaginal suppositories) | 21 | 6 |
| Female condom ("Reality") | 21 | 5 |
| Withdrawal | 19 | 4 |
| Male condom (without jelly/foam) | 12 | 3 |
| IUD[c] | ≥ 2 | ≥ 1.5 |
| The Pill[d] | 3 | ≥ .5 |
| Sterilization (male and female) | ≥ .4 | ≥ .4 |
| Norplant/Depo-Provera | ≥ .3 | ≥ .3 |
| NFP[e] (FAM w/sympto-thermal rules, and abstinence during fertile phase) | (See footnote e.) | 2 |

* All data in this table are adapted from *Contraceptive Technology, Sixteenth Revised Edition,* 1994.

a. For women who have given birth, the failure rates are substantially worse, at 36% and 20%, respectively.

b. For women who have given birth, the failure rates are substantially worse, at 36% and 26%, respectively.

c. Failure rates vary with type of IUD chosen.

d. Method failure rate varies with type of Pill chosen.

e. *Contraceptive Technology* puts NFP *method* failure of the sympto-thermal rules taught in this book at 2%. The sympto-thermal *user* failure rate is not listed. Based on the various studies throughout the medical literature, the traditionally calculated user failure rate appears to be about 10 to 12%. However, when *intentional violation of the method rules* is factored out, this number falls substantially.

reasonable compromises. In reality, the vast majority of conceptions will occur from intercourse that takes place when the woman has creamy or eggwhite cervical fluid. This is the time not only closest to ovulation, but also the time that sperm have the best odds of survival. If a barrier failure is going to result in pregnancy, it is very likely to happen at this point in the cycle. Fortunately, for most women this phase lasts 5 days or less. Thus for those determined to avoid pregnancy, I suggest you consider alternatives to intercourse for that short period of time.

## 🙙 FAM/NFP AND THE RISK CONTINUUM

In discussing the contraceptive rules and the temptation to stray from them, it should be clear that there is in fact a range of possible acts that make up the entire pregnancy-risk continuum. Given this, I would like to address the increased risks associated with what I know to be the specific times most couples are tempted to "cheat."

### Unprotected Intercourse When the Two Postovulatory Rules Don't Coincide

Some women may notice that the Temperature Shift and Peak Day rules do not always reflect infertility on the same day. The safest approach is to consider yourself fertile until both rules say that you are not (the line "farthest to the right" as described on page 121). However, it is also true that you run only a slightly increased risk in using the following modified guideline: If your temperatures clearly reveal that you're safe on one day, but your cervical fluid reveals you're not safe until a day or so later, you may shave off the last day that the cervical fluid says you are still fertile. It should be stressed that the reverse does not apply. This is because three high temperatures are stronger evidence than "Peak plus 4" that the egg(s) are already dead and gone. If you would like to use this modified guideline but are still a bit hesitant, you can always check your cervix. If it is at its lowest, most closed position, your increased risk of pregnancy is virtually nill.

### Unprotected Intercourse on Preovulatory Dry Days Before 6 P.M.

One of the most common questions I am asked is what is the risk associated with unprotected intercourse on preovulatory dry days *before* 6 P.M. As you know, the 6 P.M. rule is there in order to give the cervical fluid a chance to descend to the vaginal opening, lest unprotected intercourse that morning be greeted by unseen cervical fluid wet enough to nurture the sperm that noon. Unfortunately, I have not found any studies on this particular issue (you could imagine the logistical problems in organizing such a survey).

However, my years of teaching this method have convinced me that the increased risk is very small *if you can verify before intercourse that there is no cervical fluid at your cervical tip and your cervix remains in the lowest infertile position.* The physiological possibility that sperm can survive in such a dry vaginal environment long enough for the cervical and hormonal changes that are necessary for their survival must be remote, and thus I personally would not consider this to be an unreasonable risk. But until studies verify my personal beliefs, unprotected intercourse at such times in the cycle must still be considered abandonment of the rules taught in this book.

## Unprotected Intercourse on Preovulatory Sticky Days

A directly related question is how risky unprotected intercourse is during the preovulatory sticky cervical-fluid phase. In reality, the only women who can have unprotected sex during this time with only a small rise in risk are those who have clearly established that they have a Basic Infertile Pattern of sticky days, as discussed in Appendix B.

For all other women, you should not take the risk. The truth is that you are not extremely fertile at this time, because sperm need wet cervical fluid to survive beyond a few hours, and anyone with stickiness is probably still a few days from ovulation. However, it is also a fact that if you're just a little unlucky, sticky fluid can turn to wet in the few hours before sperm will die, thus preparing the way for a conception in the days to follow.

Unprotected sex at this point is therefore the type of cheating that significantly increases the "user failure" rates in all Fertility Awareness studies. I would argue that such acts are nonuse of the method. But if you still decide to take the increased risk, I strongly urge you to verify that there is no *wet* cervical fluid at the cervical tip before having sex. If there is, intercourse without a barrier would be downright foolish.

## &#x266C; A FINAL WORD ON CERVICAL POSITION AND CONTRACEPTIVE EFFICACY

By now, it should be obvious that your cervical position can play an important role in confirming your fertility status. Indeed, for those of you determined to take the absolute lowest risk of pregnancy while still using natural birth control, I suggest that you continue to use the standard rules but limit intercourse to when your cervix is in its lowest, most infertile position (with no wet cervical fluid at the cervical tip). Although no studies have been done, I believe that if women did this, NFP method failure would fall from 2% to well below 1% per year. Admittedly, you may find that such a guideline results in an extra day or so of abstinence, but this may be a trade-off that you're happy to accept.

## &#x266C; A NOTE ABOUT THE BILLINGS METHOD

Finally, I should mention here that many people around the world practice a simplified form of Fertility Awareness called the Billings Method. The primary way that it differs from the Fertility Awareness Method used in this book is that it relies exclusively on observing cervical fluid to determine the fertile phase. Because it does not use basal body temperature to verify the occurrence of ovulation, failure rates are somewhat higher, though method failure is still listed at only 3% by *Contraceptive Technology*. The problem is with *user* failure, which is generally quite a bit higher than the corresponding sympto-thermal rates. For this reason, I personally urge you to use a basal body thermometer in order to maximize both contraceptive efficacy as well as the number of days considered safe from pregnancy.

# The Menstrual Cycle:
# A Summary of Events Through
# the Use of a 28-Day Model

Note: You should refer to page 5 of the color insert while reading this appendix.

The main text of this book provided a brief overview of how the female reproductive system works. Still, I believe it is worth taking a few pages here to give a somewhat more detailed description of the typical menstrual cycle. For those of you who have often wondered how and why your body does what it does, this summary can offer a more complete introduction to the topic. Should you find it interesting, I would encourage you to explore a more thorough discussion of the subject in biology and medical texts, especially if you experience gynecological conditions that stray considerably from the norm.

Like so much in nature, your body is a highly complex system of continuous feedback loops. If they are functioning smoothly, the menstrual cycle's hormonal influences will ultimately create an intricate self-correcting thermostat. Of course the principle goal of the system is a much more ambitious project than keeping a room at 72 degrees. Every cycle, your body works to produce an egg capable of being fertilized, and the conditions necessary to nurture it for the duration of a pregnancy.

In order to explore how this happens, I'll take the prototype 28-day cycle and analyze the hormonal developments that occur in chronological progression. I will also overlay the major fertility signs so that you can review how the pieces all fit together. *Please remember that what will follow is a description of a perfectly functioning 28-day cycle, but as you certainly know by now, what is 28 days for Jane Doe may be a completely normal 24 to 36 days for you.* \*

## ❧ THE KEY HORMONES

Before beginning, it's advisable to review the primary function and sources of the five most important female sex hormones. While your reproductive system has more than a dozen hormones, these are the five key ones that I think women should know. They are:

**1. Estrogen:** Although there are many types of estrogen, we are most concerned with B-estradiol, the type produced by the follicles that develop within your ovaries as you progress from menstruation to ovulation. Other forms of estrogen are responsible for promoting the maturation of female sex organs as well as secondary sexual characteristics. There is very little estrogen in your system as a new cycle begins.

**2. Progesterone:** The heat-producing hormone primarily manufactured by the corpus luteum, beginning immediately following ovulation. It is the hormone most responsible for nurturing and maintaining the endometrium in the postovulatory phase. As you have learned, the corpus luteum is the follicular body on the interior of the ovarian wall that is left behind by the ovulated egg. The immediate cause of menstruation is the cessation of progesterone production, triggered by the disintegration of the corpus luteum a couple of days earlier.

**3. Follicle Stimulating Hormone (FSH):** The hormone most responsible for the initial development of a select few follicles each cycle. Under the influence of FSH, a dozen or so follicles evolve from tiny and immature (primordial), to relatively large and partially matured (vesicular). As this occurs, the eggs within each follicle gradually approach the capacity to be ovulated. FSH is produced in the anterior part of the pituitary, but absorbed by FSH receptor cells on the follicular wall. The pituitary is a gland at the base of the brain located between the brain stem and the hypothalamus. There is little FSH in the system as menstruation begins.

---

\* In fact, even the *mean* average cycle length among fertile women is believed to be 29.5 days, and not 28. This is based on what is thought to be the most extensive study ever done on this topic, by Dr. Rudi F. Vollman, a Swiss gynecologist whose name is synonymous with research in this field.

**4. Luteinizing Hormone (LH):** The other major hormone produced in the anterior pituitary, LH is responsible for both stimulating and completing follicular growth (with FSH), as well as the luteinization of the ruptured follicle in order to transform it into a corpus luteum following ovulation. LH is best known for the "LH surge," that dramatic increase in LH production that serves as the immediate trigger to ovulation, which follows a day or so later. Together, FSH and LH are called the pituitary or gonadotropin hormones. There is little LH in the system as menstruation begins.

**5. Gonadotropin Releasing Hormone (GnRH):** That hormone produced in the hypothalamus, which when secreted, causes the anterior pituitary to increase production of the gonadotropin hormones, specifically FSH and LH. The hypothalamus is located just above the pituitary, and essentially forms the floor and lower walls of the brain. It is for this reason that some speculate stress and other environmental factors can play such havoc with the length of menstrual cycles. It is believed that stress directly affects the hypothalamus and its manufacture of GnRH, which in turn affects output of FSH, LH, and so on down the cyclical line.

It should be pointed out that knowledge of GnRH is somewhat more speculative than that of the other hormones. This is because it is harder to monitor since it operates between the hypothalamus and pituitary within the brain. It is known that it is released in pulses that last about an hour or so, and that various experiments have shown that it is indeed these GnRH pulses that stimulate FSH and LH production within the anterior pituitary. However, there is still some uncertainty as to the intensity and timing of GnRH production within the hormonal system. (It is for these reasons that GnRH is not charted on the graph in the color insert.)

## ❧ THE ROAD TO OVULATION

Day 1 of any cycle is the first day of menstruation. As you've learned by now, it is hardly the most important day, for that distinction belongs to the day of ovulation. Yet for women the world over, it certainly is the most noticeable event. The majority simply accept their menstrual fate, and some (though I suspect not most) have even learned to celebrate it. In any case, why the bleeding, and why now?

Like any recurring cycle, you can't simply pick a given day, call it the first, and then explain what is going on without at least acknowledging that what happens on Day 1 is a direct result of what happened on the last days of the previous cycle. In this case, it was the sudden plunge in progesterone, the hormone that had kept the endometrial wall nourished and in place, which now causes the dramatic menstrual events that mark the first phase of the reproductive cycle. It is also worth noting that as menstruation begins, none of the key hormones are present in significant quantity.

In the days before you begin to menstruate, the endometrium on the uterine wall has reached its full maturity, approximately 5 to 6 millimeters thick. Cellular proliferation in the endometrium has been accompanied by swelling and secretory development, as well as an increased supply of nutrients and blood vessels that have built up over the previous cycle. In brief, the endometrium has reached the goal necessary for its only purpose: to provide the appropriate conditions to nurture a fertilized ovum.

Now, on Day 1, with neither progesterone nor the HCG (human chorionic gonadotropin) that an implanted embryo would supply, the endometrial wall begins to disintegrate. Over a period of approximately 5 days, the uterine lining is gradually washed away as the blood vessels that supply it with nutrients and oxygen begin to constrict. Menstrual blood begins to flow from the uterus through the cervix and out the vagina. The secretion that results also contains matter from the collapsing endometrium. Over the course of your period, you will generally lose anywhere from 1 to 8 ounces of blood and other fluids, though 2.5 ounces appears to be more typical.

As soon as you have begun to menstruate, your body's endocrine system has started to take action. Even before the first day of the new cycle, the pituitary gland has already begun to secrete small but ever-increasing amounts of FSH, the hormone that begins to develop the dozen or so follicles in the ovary that will later compete for the prize of ovulation a couple of weeks later. It is generally believed that the plunging levels of progesterone and estrogen in the last few days of the previous cycle is what allows for the increased production of FSH. In other words, it was the high levels of progesterone (and to a lesser extent estrogen) that had been blocking FSH production.

By about Day 5, or just as menstruation is ending, the pituitary also begins to release small but increasing amounts of LH. It is believed that LH production within this stage of the cycle is about 3 days behind production of FSH. In fact, the gradual release of LH is a direct result of a positive feedback system triggered by the previous production of FSH. As the FSH begins to act on the handful of ovarian follicles that move toward ovulatory potential, they begin to develop a new coating of granulosa cells, cells which in turn begin to secrete the first amounts of estrogen for the new cycle.

It is this new estrogen that apparently signals the hypothalamus to release GnRH, which in turn triggers the gradually increasing secretion of LH. This newly released LH, working in biochemical unison with FSH, continues to develop those follicles whose growth now extends this positive feedback system of follicular development for the next several days. As your period ends, the hormonal game plan is now well on its way to creating the conditions necessary for ovulation. Indeed, follicular growth during menstruation has already doubled the size of the several primordial follicles that have started to mature for that cycle.

By Day 7 or 8, and for reasons not completely understood, one of the follicles begins to emerge as dominant, while the others begin to disintegrate in a process called atresia. Many endocrinologists believe that the dominant follicle has begun to secrete so much estrogen in the week or so following menstruation (Days 6 to 12), that LH and FSH production is somewhat decreased. It is believed that the increased estrogen begins to signal the hypothalamus to reduce production of GnRH, thus slowing the manufacture of LH and FSH. And it is this slowdown that leads to the atresia of most of the other primary follicles, though the dominant follicle continues to mature. (In cases of multiple ovulation, two or more follicles progress to complete maturation.)

While creation of FSH and LH is therefore reduced in Days 6 to 12, estrogen production from the emerging dominant follicle begins to rise dramatically. This rising level of estrogen begins to act on your uterus, in both noticeable and subtle ways. As the estrogen rises, the endometrial cycle also begins anew, with the beginning creation of stromal and epithelial cells within the uterus. By about Day 12, this building process has resulted in an endometrial wall approaching 3 to 4 millimeters thick, whereas when menstruation had ended a week earlier, there was virtually no such structure in existence.

As this process moves forward, the rising levels of estrogen are also beginning to produce the fertility signs that form the foundation of this book. Usually by about Day 8 or 9, its effect on the cervical glands have triggered the first flow of cervical fluid, although this early in the process it is generally a sticky quality. But as estrogen production from the developing follicles within the ovaries rises to its highest levels on Days 10 through 13, the cervical fluid gradually changes to creamy, and then to eggwhite. Typically by Day 13, estrogenic levels have reached their peak, with the resulting cervical fluid having reached its most lubricative consistency. By now, the cervix itself is soft, high, and open.

On Day 12 or 13, something dramatic happens in the hormonal feedback system. As already stated, increasing levels of estrogen are believed to be the reason FSH and LH production are kept relatively low in Days 6 to 13. But at a certain point, for reasons we don't truly understand, estrogen production reaches a threshold level in which its hormonal effect on the pituitary abruptly reverses. LH secretion by the anterior pituitary gland suddenly surges six to ten times its normal rate, peaking at about 12 to 16 hours before ovulation. Within hours of this LH surge, a less dramatic FSH surge follows. In combination, the two cause a negative feedback effect which suddenly shuts down the production of estrogen in the remaining dominant follicle. The follicle has now fully matured, reaching a size of 1 to 1.5 centimeters. For this 28-day journey, you have now reached the halfway point, and thus ovulation is imminent.

On Day 14, under direct stimulation from the soaring levels of the gonadotropin hormones, the dominant follicle begins to ooze liquid from a protrusion that has formed on its surface. Simultaneously, it begins to swell, severely weakening the follicular wall. Sometime during the next few hours, the follicle ruptures, with the interior ovum being propelled through the ovarian wall into the abdominal cavity. Ovulation has now taken place.

Most likely, your cervical fluid has reached its last day of eggwhite (and in fact has already begun to rapidly dry up), your cervical position has reached its most fertile (i.e., soft, high, and open), and that morning, you had your last low basal temperature before the thermal shift. For many of you, Day 14 will also produce *mittelschmerz,* that secondary fertility sign in which an occasionally sharp pain around your abdomen verifies indeed that ovulation is about to, or has already occurred.

## ℘ COMPLETING THE CYCLE

The newly released ovum now begins its long journey through the fimbria and down the fallopian tube. Assuming there are no sperm to fertilize it, it will disintegrate within the next 6 to 24 hours. Meanwhile, the body's own hormonal progression continues unabated into the next phase. Back in the ovary from which ovulation took place, the left-over granulosa cells of the dominant follicle are quickly being transformed into luteinizing cells by the high amount of LH. Within hours, these cells have formed the corpus luteum on the interior of the ovarian wall, and it in turn has already begun to secrete heavy doses of progesterone into the body. Waking up on Day 15, you can usually see the result, as this heat-producing hormone triggers your thermal shift.

From Day 15 until about Day 26, the corpus luteum continues to secrete large amounts of progesterone, as well as a modest amount of estrogen. There are several things that immediately result from this combination of hormonal stimulants. With the dramatic fall of estrogen production caused by the hormonal events immediately preceding ovulation, the fertile cervical signs quickly reverse. By Day 16, there is generally no more cervical fluid, and the cervical position has returned to firm, low, and closed. (In fact, cervical fluid dries up so quickly you are frequently already dry on the very day you are actually ovulating!)

Still, the corpus luteum continues to release enough estrogen to continue building up the endometrial wall. In addition, progesterone both holds the wall in place as well as contributes to additional endometrial swelling and development, so that by Day 26 the endometrium has reached a thickness of 5 to 6 millimeters. Were a fertilized egg able to reach the endometrium any time from Day 21 onward (which is likely the first day it could have if ovulation was a week earlier), this uterine shelter would now be ready to house the new embryo.

In the days following ovulation, the combination of high progesterone and low estrogen creates other hormonal effects. Most important, the anterior pituitary and hypothalamus are now alerted by the progesterone to sharply curtail production of GnRH, LH, and FSH. Thus production of these hormones will stay very low from ovulation until near the end of the cycle, or about Day 27. Meanwhile, the corpus luteum itself continues to grow under the initial influence of the LH surge, but peaks in size about a week after ovulation. By Day 21, it can be up to 1.5 centimeters, and has generally reached full maturity.

Without the continued presence of LH to sustain it, the corpus luteum now begins to deteriorate. It continues to secrete large but decreasing amounts of progesterone (thus sustaining the endometrium), but by about Day 26, its secretory function is extinguished and cellular degeneration occurs rapidly. Had there been a pregnancy, release of HCG from the developing fetus would have signaled the corpus luteum to remain viable for several more months.

Thus by Day 27, the body's release of progesterone (as well as estrogen) has plummeted, setting the stage for the hormonal transition to the next menstruation, and the beginning of another cycle. As soon as the corpus luteum dies, the absence of ovarian hormones allows for the initial buildup of FSH. And most dramatically and as previously discussed, the plunge in progesterone production quickly triggers the disintegration of the endometrial wall, and the beginning of your next period. We are now once again where this voyage began.

## ✌ KEEPING TRACK OF THE MENSTRUAL JOURNEY

I would like to conclude by repeating what I hope this book has already made clear: While the prototypical 28-day cycle is a useful tool for charting chronological order and biological cause and effect, it is in fact not the cyclical experience of most women most of the time! As you have already learned, typical cycle lengths vary between women from 24 to 36 days, and of course, within individual women, there are great variations over time due to stress, diet, and other influences. You already know that given these factors, it's not possible to predict the length of the preovulatory phase, and thus the preceding description was accurate as to order of events, but not as to the actual day of occurrence. I hope that if nothing else, this book has taught you that in matters of fertility, you simply need to chart if you want to know where you are within your cycle.

# Most Commonly Asked Questions

As a FAM instructor, I have been asked just about every possible question regarding fertility. I have chosen to address the most frequently asked among them in this appendix. They are categorized by subject, but are more thoroughly discussed in relevant sections of the book. These pages simply serve as a review, or perhaps as an introduction for your friends, who may want to know more about such a fundamental aspect of their lives.

## ℱ THE FERTILITY AWARENESS METHOD (FAM)

### HOW EFFECTIVE IS FAM FOR BIRTH CONTROL?

If *used correctly every cycle,* and you abstain during the fertile phase, the FAM rules taught in this book have a failure rate of approximately 2% per year for the typical couple. This is considered lower than any barrier method, including the condom. (Sterilization and chemical methods such as Norplant and the Pill have an even lower equivalent failure rate of 1% or less.) However, for those couples who choose to have sex throughout the fertile phase while using a barrier method, the overall failure rate will naturally be no lower than the rate of the barrier the couple chooses to use. For most women, the fertile phrase is usually about 8 to 10 days per cycle.

In actual use, studies show that failure rates vary greatly, from about 1% to 20% per year, with most of the variance being a direct function of the *motivation* of the couples involved. For a more thorough discussion of Fertility Awareness and contraceptive effectiveness, see Appendix D.

## WHAT IS THE DIFFERENCE BETWEEN THE FERTILITY AWARENESS METHOD AND THE RHYTHM METHOD?

Probably a more appropriate question is what do they have in common? The only thing they have in common is that both are natural methods of birth control. The Rhythm Method is an obsolete, ineffective method of identifying the fertile phase using statistical prediction based on *past* cycles. The Fertility Awareness Method, however, is a scientifically validated method involving the observation of the three primary fertility signs: waking temperature, cervical fluid, and cervical position. FAM is considered very effective because the woman's fertility is determined on a day-to-day basis.

## HOW MUCH TIME IS REQUIRED TO LEARN AND USE THE METHOD?

How long it takes to learn the method will vary with each woman. I hope that many of you will be able to assimilate all you need to know by thoroughly reading the relevant chapters of this book. Others may need to take a class from a qualified instructor, which typically involves two 3-hour sessions and an individual 1- or 2-hour follow-up consultation (see Appendix M for class resources). It usually takes one or two cycles of observation to feel confident enough to rely on FAM for birth control.

Charting usually requires under 2 minutes per day: About 1 minute to take your temperature with a digital thermometer on awakening, and about a minute or so to check and record the other fertility signs. If you eventually use the short-cut method as described in Chapter 10, you will need to chart about 10 days per cycle, for a total time commitment of about 20 minutes a month.

I should reiterate here that while it is true that the short-cut method does not compromise contraceptive efficacy, I personally recommend charting every day of your cycle (outside menstruation), especially for the first few cycles that you chart. I should also point out that some women may not be able to use the digital thermometers if they do not reflect an obvious temperature pattern reflecting ovulation. In that case, those women would have to use a glass basal body thermometer, which requires 5 minutes upon awakening.

## IS FAM A GOOD METHOD FOR EVERYBODY?

No, not as a method of birth control. It is only appropriate for those women who have the discipline to learn the method well, and then to follow the rules once they have internalized them. In addition, it is only recommended for monogamous couples, given the danger of AIDS and other STDs.

However, as a method of pregnancy achievement, FAM is highly advised as the first step every couple should take to maximize their chances of conception, and to determine if there may be anything impeding their ability to get pregnant. In addition, Fertility Awareness can be very effective in helping couples plan the timing of their baby's birth.

FAM is also highly beneficial for all women who simply want to educate themselves about their bodies. So even if you have no interest in using the method for avoiding or achieving pregnancy, it is an empowering means of taking control of your gynecological health.

## HOW MANY DAYS DO YOU HAVE TO ABSTAIN WHEN USING THE FERTILITY AWARENESS METHOD FOR BIRTH CONTROL?

You never have to abstain when using the Fertility Awareness Method. This is different than *Natural Family Planning,* which does require abstinence during the fertile phase. However, if you do have intercourse when you are potentially fertile, you must use a barrior method of contraception to avoid pregnancy. The fertile phase will vary, but in practice this means that the average couple would have to use barriers about 8 to 10 days per cycle. The average cycle is 27 to 31 days, and thus for the typical couple, barriers (or abstinence) would be required for about 30% of the cycle.

## DO WOMEN EVER HAVE TRULY "DRY" DAYS?

When a woman charts, she identifies her cervical fluid by various degrees of wetness, and records a dash (–) if no cervical fluid is present at the vaginal opening. This symbol for dry refers to a lack of cervical fluid, and not to internal vaginal moisture, which is present to some degree all of the time. It's easy to distinguish between cervical fluid and vaginal moisture. Cervical fluid on your finger will stay moist for minutes or longer, whereas vaginal moisture —like that inside your mouth—will dissipate from your finger within seconds.

## DO I HAVE TO WAKE UP EVERY DAY AT THE SAME TIME IN ORDER TO TAKE MY TEMPERATURE?

No, although you should try to be as consistent as possible. In general, waking temperatures tend to creep up about two-tenths of a degree for every extra hour you sleep in. Thus, if you take it substantially later than usual, it may result in a reading that is outside the range of your usual pattern. If you wake up *earlier* than usual, you should take your temperature upon awakening, so long as you have had 3 hours of consecutive sleep.

Regardless, an occasional aberrant temperature can easily be dealt with by following the Rule of Thumb (see page 75). You should also be aware that if taking your temperature feels like a burden, you can in fact take it for only about a third of the cycle without sacrificing contraceptive efficacy as described in Chapter 10.

### HOW CAN TEMPERATURES BE RELIED ON IF I SOMETIMES GET A FEVER?

There may be several influences, from fever to alcohol to lack of sleep that could affect your waking temperature. But this doesn't compromise your ability to rely on it while charting. This is because you ultimately want to identify a *pattern* of low and high temperatures, rather than focusing on individual ones. Outlying temperatures can be effectively dealt with by using the Rule of Thumb, which basically allows you to ignore them in interpreting your chart (see page 75). In addition, you will generally be able to use your other two signs to cross-check your fertility in situations such as these.

### IS THERE REALLY A RISK OF PREGNANCY IF I ONLY HAVE STICKY (NONWET) CERVICAL FLUID?

Yes. While sticky cervical fluid is certainly less fertile than creamy or eggwhite, it is still possible to conceive from preovulatory intercourse on a sticky day. See page 315 for a more complete discussion of this question.

### IS IT WORTH CHECKING MY CERVICAL POSITION?

Although it is not necessary to check your cervix in order to practice FAM effectively, I urge you to learn how to do so. At a minimum, I think you should practice checking in the days leading up to and just past ovulation, for the first few cycles that you're learning the method. Once you recognize how your cervical position reflects your fertility, you will always be able to use it as a cross-check whenever you find the slightest ambiguity in your other two fertility signs. The bottom line is that complete familiarity with the changes in your cervix will greatly increase the confidence with which you observe your fertility and overall gynecological health. Since it only takes *seconds* a day to check, my attitude is that for those relevant several days per cycle, you should just do it!

A distinct but closely related question is whether you should ever check your cervical *fluid* at the cervical tip. The short answer is that it isn't necessary, although if you want to be even more conservative than the FAM rules require, or if you simply want to know your cervical fluid status ahead of time, it certainly couldn't hurt. (Remember that the cervical fluid you normally check at the vaginal opening might have taken several hours to trickle down from the cervical tip.) Finally, checking this way may provide some couples with more time for unprotected sex (see pages 314–315).

## ✆ OVULATION

### DO WOMEN ALWAYS OVULATE ON DAY 14 OF THEIR CYCLE?

No! The day of ovulation can vary among women as well as within each individual woman. However, once a woman ovulates, the time between ovulation and her menstruation is very consistent, almost always between 12 and 16 days. Within most *individual* women, this length of time generally doesn't change by more than a day or two. In other words, if there is going to be variation in the cycle, it is the first preovulatory phase that may vary. The second (postovulatory) phase remains fairly constant.

### CAN A WOMAN OVULATE MORE THAN ONCE PER CYCLE?

No. Have you ever heard of a woman getting pregnant on Monday, and then again that following Friday, and then two weeks later on Thursday? Certainly not, because once a woman ovulates, her body cannot release any more eggs that cycle. Ovulation is an event that may take place over approximately 24 hours, but just once per cycle. During those 24 hours, one or more eggs may be released (as in the case of fraternal twins). But once ovulation has occurred, it is virtually impossible for a woman to release another egg until the next cycle.

### WHAT IS MULTIPLE OVULATION?

Multiple ovulation is the release of two or more eggs in a single cycle. It occurs within 24 hours or less, after which no more eggs will be released until the following cycle. It is responsible for the birth of *fraternal* twins, as opposed to identical twins, which are the result of a single egg that divides after fertilization.

Multiple ovulation appears to be more common than once thought. While it is true that less than 1 in 100 American deliveries are fraternal twins, researchers now realize that there are many more fraternal *conceptions*. Most of these second fetuses miscarry in what is called the "vanishing twin phenomenon." Taking this into account, one could speculate that multiple ovulation may actually occur as frequently as 5 to 10% of all cycles.

## DO WOMEN FEEL MORE SEXUAL AROUND OVULATION?

Many women do. Because estrogen peaks around ovulation, women typically experience a wet, slippery sensation due to the fertile cervical fluid produced. This cervical fluid feels similar to sexual lubrication, and can therefore be experienced as a sexual feeling. A woman who practices FAM needn't worry about confusing the two, because cervical fluid is checked periodically throughout the day, and *not* when she is sexually aroused.

## CAN ORGASM CAUSE OVULATION?

No. Orgasms and ovulations are unrelated. In order to ovulate, estrogen must build up in the woman's system gradually, usually over a period of days. Orgasms, however, can occur at *any* time in the cycle!

##   FERTILITY AND CYCLES

## WHAT PERCENT OF A WOMAN'S CYCLE IS FERTILE?

The answer to this question is somewhat tricky. The general answer is that most women are fertile for only a few days of their cycle. However, there are several factors to consider:

1. The woman's egg can only live up to 24 hours. Two or more eggs may be released over a maximum of 24 hours. So, in a vacuum, a woman is only fertile for about a day or two. But the man's sperm can live up to 5 days, so the combined fertility of the two individuals is about a week.
2. For a couple trying to get pregnant, the woman's fertile phase is as long as she has fertile-quality cervical fluid, up through ovulation. That might be several days, or as few as one.
3. For a couple trying to prevent pregnancy, FAM adds a buffer zone

of a few days to assure that an unplanned pregnancy does not occur.

## IS IT TRUE THAT A WOMAN CAN GET PREGNANT ANYTIME DURING HER CYCLE?

No, it is not. It is true that ovulation can vary greatly from cycle to cycle, but once a woman ovulates, she cannot ovulate again for the remainder of that cycle.

## CAN A WOMAN GET PREGNANT DURING HER PERIOD?

The answer lies in the wording of the question. More precisely, it is essentially impossible for a woman to get pregnant *during* her period, but on rare occasions it is possible for a woman to get pregnant from *intercourse* during her period. Since sperm can live for 5 days, a couple could have sex near the end of the woman's period, and the sperm could then live long enough to fertilize an egg several days later, if the woman had a very early ovulation. (Conception is more likely in these cases if intercourse occurs at the end of a 6- or 7-day menstruation.) It's also possible that women who think they got pregnant from intercourse during their period were actually having sex during ovulatory spotting.

## CAN A WOMAN GET PREGNANT IF SHE HASN'T BEEN MENSTRUATING?

Yes. Since a woman releases an egg 12 to 16 days *before* menstruation, it is possible to get pregnant without actually having periods. So women who are not menstruating due to any reason such as excessively low body fat, breastfeeding, or being premenopausal, are always at risk of ovulating at any point. This is because the underlying condition causing the lack of menstruation could change, thus unexpectedly triggering the release of an egg.

The bottom line is that women who don't menstruate cannot count on their condition as reliable contraception. Thus, the only practical way to know if ovulation is approaching is through charting your cycles, and more specifically, observing the change in your cervical fluid.

Of course, for those couples desiring to get pregnant, the reality is that you will definitely want to resolve the underlying problem preventing menstruation. Until you do so, your chances of conception will be very low.

## CAN STRESS AFFECT YOUR FERTILITY?

The role stress plays on one's fertility is often exaggerated. It may prevent ovulation altogether, but more likely, it will delay it by temporarily suppressing the hormones necessary for ovulation to occur.

If a couple adheres to the myth of ovulation always occurring on Day 14, they may inadvertently prevent pregnancy by timing intercourse at the wrong time, thus triggering a vicious circle of misperceived infertility causing more stress. Charting the cycle would allow the couple to regain the control necessary to identify the woman's fertile phase.

## HOW MANY DAYS CAN SPERM SURVIVE?

Sperm can generally survive a maximum of 5 days in the fertile-quality cervical fluid that the woman produces around the time of ovulation. There is some suggestion in the medical literature that on extremely rare occasions, sperm can survive from 6 to 8 days. It is much more likely sperm will survive a maximum of 3 days, and only a few hours in drier, less fertile types of cervical fluid. If there is *no* cervical fluid present, the sperm will probably die within a couple of hours.

## HOW LONG CAN A HUMAN EGG SURVIVE?

Most ova probably survive about 6 to 12 hours after ovulation, but for the purpose of contraception, you must count on a 24-hour survival period.

## HOW DOES THE PILL WORK?

In essence, the Pill works by tricking the body into thinking it's already pregnant. It does this by manipulating the normal hormonal feedback system. The end result is that the body doesn't release the hormones necessary to stimulate the ovary to release an egg.

As a back-up, every other facet of the woman's reproductive system is also altered. Most important, the uterine lining is obstructed from producing a rich site for egg implantation, and the cervical fluid is prevented from forming a wet fertile quality necessary for sperm survival.

# The Difference Between Natural Methods of Birth Control

|  | Rhythm Method | Billings (Ovulation) Method | BBT (Basal Body Temperature) Method | FAM/NFP* (Sympto-Thermal Method) |
|---|---|---|---|---|
| Fertility Signs That Are Observed | None<br><br>A mathematical formula based on past cycle lengths is used to predict future fertile phase. | Cervical fluid | Waking temperature | Waking temperature and cervical fluid<br><br>Cervical position is optional, as are any number of secondary signs such as ovulatory pain or midcycle spotting. |

* The difference between the Fertility Awareness Method (FAM) and Natural Family Planning (NFP) is that those who practice NFP choose to abstain during the fertile phase, whereas those who practice FAM allow themselves to use a barrier during this time.

# Optional Coverline

There is an optional way of drawing the coverline that is easier than that taught on page 73. In this option, you simply *draw the coverline one-tenth degree above the highest temperature during the first 10 days of your cycle.* For a lot of women, this system works well, but I personally don't use it because the only temperatures that are hormonally significant are the six or so that precede the rise confirming ovulation. In addition, many women have elevated temperatures during the first week or more of the cycle that precludes its effective use.

**Chart H.1. The type of temperature pattern that allows for the simpler coverline rule.** Because all of the temperatures in the first part of the cycle are conspicuously below those in the second part, you can easily draw the coverline one-tenth degree above the highest of the first 10 days.

**Chart H.2. The type of temperature pattern that would not allow for the simpler coverline rule.** Note that many of the early temperatures are too high, preventing the drawing of an effective coverline one tenth of a degree above the highest of the first 10 days. Thus, this pattern requires the standard coverline drawn one-tenth degree above the highest of the previous 6 days.

# Optional Cervical Fluid Symbols

You may find that you prefer to use your own symbols to describe your cervical fluid. There are advantages and disadvantages to using various symbols. After a lot of consideration, I chose the ones in this book because I think they are the most intuitive and best describe the type most women experience. However, if you find that those symbols are not as reflective of your own cervical fluid, you should develop your own, or use others such as those listed below:

| | | |
|---|---|---|
| **D** | Dry | No cervical fluid present. |
| **N** | Nonwet | Sticky, flaky, crumbly, or pasty cervical fluid. |
| Ⓦ | Wet | Watery, creamy, slippery, or stretchy cervical fluid. |

Previous books have also used the combination of the three symbols below:

| | | |
|---|---|---|
| **D** | Dry | No cervical fluid present. |
| **M** | Mucus, *not* wet | Sticky, flaky, crumbly, or pasty cervical fluid. |
| Ⓜ | Mucus, wet | Watery, creamy, slippery, or stretchy cervical fluid. |

# Drugs That Can Affect
# the Cervical Fluid (CF)

*by Hanna Klaus, M.D.*

*Current Medical Research*                                    *Natural Family Planning*

| Drug | Usually Prescribed For | Site of Effect | Type of Effect |
|---|---|---|---|
| **Acetylcystene** (mucomist) | Asthma, Cystic fibrosis | Local | If sufficiently absorbed, could increase or thin cervical fluid (CF). |
| **Alpha Antitrypsin** | Cystic fibrosis | Local | Could increase or thin cervical fluid. |
| **Ampicillin** | Infections | Local | Could increase or thin cervical fluid. |
| **Antidepressants/ Antipsychotics:** e.g., Thorazine, Mellaril, Triavil, Parnate, Valium, Prozac, MAO (Monoamino Oxidase) Inhibitors | Depression | Local and systemic | A variety of menstrual disturbances ranging from menorrhagia to menopause have at times been reported with Prozac (*Physicians' Desk Reference* 1991). |
| **Antiestrogens**   (*see Tamoxifen or Clomiphene*) | | | |
| **Antigonadotropins**   (*see Danazol, Buserelin, Leuprolide*) | | | |
| **Antihistamines** | Cough, Colds | Local | Can decrease amount of CF, can cause thickening or dryness. |
| **Antitumor drugs:** e.g., Busulfan, Cyclophosphamide, Cytotoxic agents, Mercaptopurine, Chlorambucil, Actinomycin | Used to treat tumors. (*Actinomycin is also used for systemic fungus infection.*) | Systemic | Suppresses ovulation, induces menopausal (high) levels of FSH, LH. |
| **Atropine** | Antispasmodic | Local | Can decrease amount of CF, can cause thickening or dryness. |
| **Belladonna** | Antispasmodic | Local | Can decrease amount of CF, can cause thickening or dryness. |
| **Buserelin** | Antigonadotropin used to treat endometriosis, etc. | Hypothalamus | A variety of menstrual disturbances ranging from menorrhagia to menopause could occur. |

| | | | |
|---|---|---|---|
| **Cimetidine** (*Tagamet*) | Used to treat peptic ulcers | Local and systemic at level of hypothalamus or above | A variety of menstrual disturbances ranging from menorrhagia to menopause. Inhibits histamine, also pituitary gonadotropins. |
| **Clomiphene** (*Clomid*) | Ovulation Induction Antiestrogen drug | Systemic | Reduces or suppresses cervical fluid. A variety of menstrual disturbances ranging from menorrhagia to menopause could occur. |
| **Cough mixtures** with Antihistamines, e.g., Phenylephrine | Cough | Local | Can decrease amount of CF, can cause thickening or dryness. |
| **Danazol** | Antigonadotropin, used to treat endometriosis, etc. | Systemic | A variety of menstrual disturbances ranging from menorrhagia to menopause could occur. |
| **Dicyclomine** | Antispasmodic | Local | Can decrease amount of cervical fluid, can cause thickening or dryness. |
| **Estrogens** | | Local and systemic | Produces CF with fertile signs; may also produce strong cholinergic action, i.e., *may* cause dryness whether local or systemic. |
| **Expectorants** (*see Potassium iodide, Guafenesin*) | | | |
| **Guafenesin (such as Robitussin)** | Expectorant found in cough syrups | Local | Could increase or thin cervical fluid. |
| **Leuprolide** | Antigonadotropin, used in treatment of endometriosis, etc. | Systemic | A variety of menstrual disturbances ranging from menorrhagia to menopause could occur. |
| **Oral contraceptives** | Contraception | Local and systemic | Produce sticky, yellow, or white opaque CF (*Progestine effect*). |
| **Potassium iodide** | Expectorant found in cough syrups | Local | Could increase or thin cervical fluid. |
| **Progesterones** | | Local and pituitary | Produce sticky, yellow, or white, opaque CF. |
| **Propantheline** | Antispasmodic | Local | Can decrease amount of CF, can cause thickening or dryness. |
| **Tamoxifen** | Used to treat breast cancer | Systemic | Antiestrogen, reduces or suppresses CF. A variety of menstrual disturbances ranging from menorrhagia to menopause could occur. |
| **Urecholine** (*Bethanechol*) | Cholinergic agent—urinary retention | Local and systemic | Theoretically could thin secretions. |

**Miscellaneous Notes**
• **Vitamin B6** may suppress Prolactin, a caution to nursing mothers. Some think that B complex increases cervical fluid.
• **Any increase in exercise,** any rapid change in weight may suppress ovulation.
• **Perfumed toilet paper, fabric softener,** and **tampons** are said to increase or distort recognition of cervical fluid.
• **Smoking**—*active and passive*—has been associated with high-nicotine and -cotinine levels in cervical fluid, which in turn are associated with dysplasia. No observable physical change has been reported.

*This fact sheet has been prepared for the DDP for NFP, NCCB, by Hanna Klaus, M.D. NFP Center of Washington, D.C., Inc., 1991 with the kind assistance of Sr. Paulette Elking, D. Ph.*

# Optional Master Charts (for Recording Exercise, PMS, or Internal/External Cervical Fluid)

*One of the most entertaining charts I've seen was that of Leah and David, who recorded not only his and her exercise and weight, but also "latte consumption." But it was not enough that they charted if and when they drank lattes. They also recorded whether the lattes were nonfat or 2 percent, short or tall, and single or double! Only in Seattle.*

After observing your fertility signs for a few cycles, you may find that you would prefer a chart that meets your needs better than the master chart on the last page of the book. Once you've internalized the various symbols in the key at the bottom of the chart, you will probably prefer to use that space for more notes. So I've included three other charts, two of which have omitted the key to allow extra blank space. All three have a column labeled "Ovulatory Pain." When you copy any of the charts, you'll need to enlarge them by about 125%.

Chart 1: Same type as the master chart on the last page, but with four columns for color-coding PMS signs, such as those shown on page 7 of the color insert.

Chart 2: Chart with a column for recording exercise as well as six columns for color-coding PMS signs.

Chart 3: Chart with separate columns to record both internal and external cervical fluid checking as well as six columns for color-coding PMS signs.

If you would prefer to develop your own chart, you may want to use the same program I chose—Microsoft Excel.

# Fertility Cycle # _____

| Last 12 Cycles | Shortest _____ | Longest _____ | Month _____ | Year _____ | This cycle length: _____ |

| Cycle Day | 1 | 2 | 3 | 4 | 5 | 6 | 7 | 8 | 9 | 10 | 11 | 12 | 13 | 14 | 15 | 16 | 17 | 18 | 19 | 20 | 21 | 22 | 23 | 24 | 25 | 26 | 27 | 28 | 29 | 30 | 31 | 32 | 33 | 34 | 35 | 36 | 37 | 38 | 39 | 40 |
|---|---|---|---|---|---|---|---|---|---|---|---|---|---|---|---|---|---|---|---|---|---|---|---|---|---|---|---|---|---|---|---|---|---|---|---|---|---|---|---|---|
| Date | | | | | | | | | | | | | | | | | | | | | | | | | | | | | | | | | | | | | | | | |
| Day of Week | | | | | | | | | | | | | | | | | | | | | | | | | | | | | | | | | | | | | | | | |
| Intercourse | | | | | | | | | | | | | | | | | | | | | | | | | | | | | | | | | | | | | | | | |
| Birth Control Method Used | | | | | | | | | | | | | | | | | | | | | | | | | | | | | | | | | | | | | | | | |
| Time Temp Taken | | | | | | | | | | | | | | | | | | | | | | | | | | | | | | | | | | | | | | | | |
| Temp Count | | | | | | | | | | | | | | | | | | | | | | | | | | | | | | | | | | | | | | | | |

Waking Temperature grid (each cell contains the temperature scale):
99 9 8 7 6 5 4 3 2 1 98 9 8 7 6 5 4 3 2 1 97 9 (repeated across all 40 cycle days)

| Cycle Day | 1 | 2 | 3 | 4 | 5 | 6 | 7 | 8 | 9 | 10 | 11 | 12 | 13 | 14 | 15 | 16 | 17 | 18 | 19 | 20 | 21 | 22 | 23 | 24 | 25 | 26 | 27 | 28 | 29 | 30 | 31 | 32 | 33 | 34 | 35 | 36 | 37 | 38 | 39 | 40 |
|---|---|---|---|---|---|---|---|---|---|---|---|---|---|---|---|---|---|---|---|---|---|---|---|---|---|---|---|---|---|---|---|---|---|---|---|---|---|---|---|---|
| Cervical Fluid | | | | | | | | | | | | | | | | | | | | | | | | | | | | | | | | | | | | | | | | |
| Peak Day | | | | | | | | | | | | | | | | | | | | | | | | | | | | | | | | | | | | | | | | |
| Vaginal Sensation | | | | | | | | | | | | | | | | | | | | | | | | | | | | | | | | | | | | | | | | |
| Cervix | | | | | | | | | | | | | | | | | | | | | | | | | | | | | | | | | | | | | | | | |
| Cervical Fluid Description | | | | | | | | | | | | | | | | | | | | | | | | | | | | | | | | | | | | | | | | |
| Ovulatory Pain | | | | | | | | | | | | | | | | | | | | | | | | | | | | | | | | | | | | | | | | |
| Miscellaneous | | | | | | | BSE | | | | | | | | | | | | | | | | | | | | | | | | | | | | | | | | | |

| Cervical Fluid Symbols | ✳ Menses | (✳) Spotting | — No Cervical Fluid | S Sticky | ⓒ Creamy | Ⓔ Eggwhite |
|---|---|---|---|---|---|---|
| | Bright Red | Pink or Brown | Nothing | Sticky, Crumbly, Gummy, or Rubbery Yellow or White | Creamy, Lotiony, Milky, or Smooth Yellow or White | Slippery and Usually Stretchy Clear, Streaked or Opaque |
| Vaginal Sensation | | Moist or Dry | Dry | Dry or Sticky | Wet and/or Cold | Lubricative and Very Wet, May Feel Humid |
| Cervix Symbols | • o O | | | | | |
| | F M S | F = Firm  M = Medium  S = Soft | | • = Closed  o = Partly Open  O = Open | | |

**Chart I**

# Fertility Cycle # _____

| Cycle Day | 1 | 2 | 3 | 4 | 5 | 6 | 7 | 8 | 9 | 10 | 11 | 12 | 13 | 14 | 15 | 16 | 17 | 18 | 19 | 20 | 21 | 22 | 23 | 24 | 25 | 26 | 27 | 28 | 29 | 30 | 31 | 32 | 33 | 34 | 35 | 36 | 37 | 38 | 39 | 40 |
|---|---|---|---|---|---|---|---|---|---|---|---|---|---|---|---|---|---|---|---|---|---|---|---|---|---|---|---|---|---|---|---|---|---|---|---|---|---|---|---|---|
| Date | | | | | | | | | | | | | | | | | | | | | | | | | | | | | | | | | | | | | | | | |
| Day of Week | | | | | | | | | | | | | | | | | | | | | | | | | | | | | | | | | | | | | | | | |
| Intercourse | | | | | | | | | | | | | | | | | | | | | | | | | | | | | | | | | | | | | | | | |
| Birth Control Method Used | | | | | | | | | | | | | | | | | | | | | | | | | | | | | | | | | | | | | | | | |
| Time Temp Taken | | | | | | | | | | | | | | | | | | | | | | | | | | | | | | | | | | | | | | | | |
| Temp Count | | | | | | | | | | | | | | | | | | | | | | | | | | | | | | | | | | | | | | | | |

**Waking Temperature**

Each cell column reads top to bottom: 99 9 8 7 6 5 4 3 2 1 / 98 9 8 7 6 5 4 3 2 1 / 97 9 (repeated across all 40 day columns)

| Cycle Day | 1 | 2 | 3 | 4 | 5 | 6 | 7 | 8 | 9 | 10 | 11 | 12 | 13 | 14 | 15 | 16 | 17 | 18 | 19 | 20 | 21 | 22 | 23 | 24 | 25 | 26 | 27 | 28 | 29 | 30 | 31 | 32 | 33 | 34 | 35 | 36 | 37 | 38 | 39 | 40 |
|---|---|---|---|---|---|---|---|---|---|---|---|---|---|---|---|---|---|---|---|---|---|---|---|---|---|---|---|---|---|---|---|---|---|---|---|---|---|---|---|---|
| Cervical Fluid | | | | | | | | | | | | | | | | | | | | | | | | | | | | | | | | | | | | | | | | |
| Peak Day | | | | | | | | | | | | | | | | | | | | | | | | | | | | | | | | | | | | | | | | |
| Vaginal Sensation | | | | | | | | | | | | | | | | | | | | | | | | | | | | | | | | | | | | | | | | |
| Cervix | | | | | | | | | | | | | | | | | | | | | | | | | | | | | | | | | | | | | | | | |
| Cervical Fluid Description | | | | | | | | | | | | | | | | | | | | | | | | | | | | | | | | | | | | | | | | |
| Ovulatory Pain | | | | | | | | | | | | | | | | | | | | | | | | | | | | | | | | | | | | | | | | |
| Miscellaneous | | | | | | BSE | | | | | | | | | | | | | | | | | | | | | | | | | | | | | | | | | | |
| Exercise | | | | | | | | | | | | | | | | | | | | | | | | | | | | | | | | | | | | | | | | |

Chart 2

# Fertility Cycle # _____

| Cycle Day | 1 | 2 | 3 | 4 | 5 | 6 | 7 | 8 | 9 | 10 | 11 | 12 | 13 | 14 | 15 | 16 | 17 | 18 | 19 | 20 | 21 | 22 | 23 | 24 | 25 | 26 | 27 | 28 | 29 | 30 | 31 | 32 | 33 | 34 | 35 | 36 | 37 | 38 | 39 | 40 |
|---|---|---|---|---|---|---|---|---|---|---|---|---|---|---|---|---|---|---|---|---|---|---|---|---|---|---|---|---|---|---|---|---|---|---|---|---|---|---|---|---|
| Date | | | | | | | | | | | | | | | | | | | | | | | | | | | | | | | | | | | | | | | | |
| Day of Week | | | | | | | | | | | | | | | | | | | | | | | | | | | | | | | | | | | | | | | | |
| Intercourse | | | | | | | | | | | | | | | | | | | | | | | | | | | | | | | | | | | | | | | | |
| Birth Control Method Used | | | | | | | | | | | | | | | | | | | | | | | | | | | | | | | | | | | | | | | | |
| Time Temp Taken | | | | | | | | | | | | | | | | | | | | | | | | | | | | | | | | | | | | | | | | |
| Temp Count | | | | | | | | | | | | | | | | | | | | | | | | | | | | | | | | | | | | | | | | |

### Waking Temperature

Temperature grid with values 99, 9, 8, 7, 6, 5, 4, 3, 2, 1, 98, 9, 8, 7, 6, 5, 4, 3, 2, 1, 97, 9 repeated across all 40 cycle days.

| Cycle Day | 1 | 2 | 3 | 4 | 5 | 6 | 7 | 8 | 9 | 10 | 11 | 12 | 13 | 14 | 15 | 16 | 17 | 18 | 19 | 20 | 21 | 22 | 23 | 24 | 25 | 26 | 27 | 28 | 29 | 30 | 31 | 32 | 33 | 34 | 35 | 36 | 37 | 38 | 39 | 40 |
|---|---|---|---|---|---|---|---|---|---|---|---|---|---|---|---|---|---|---|---|---|---|---|---|---|---|---|---|---|---|---|---|---|---|---|---|---|---|---|---|---|
| CF at Vulva | | | | | | | | | | | | | | | | | | | | | | | | | | | | | | | | | | | | | | | | |
| CF at Cervix | | | | | | | | | | | | | | | | | | | | | | | | | | | | | | | | | | | | | | | | |
| Peak Day | | | | | | | | | | | | | | | | | | | | | | | | | | | | | | | | | | | | | | | | |
| Vaginal Sensation | | | | | | | | | | | | | | | | | | | | | | | | | | | | | | | | | | | | | | | | |
| Cervix | | | | | | | | | | | | | | | | | | | | | | | | | | | | | | | | | | | | | | | | |
| Cervical Fluid at Vulva | | | | | | | | | | | | | | | | | | | | | | | | | | | | | | | | | | | | | | | | |
| Cervical Fluid at Cervix | | | | | | | | | | | | | | | | | | | | | | | | | | | | | | | | | | | | | | | | |
| Ovulatory Pain | | | | | | | | | | | | | | | | | | | | | | | | | | | | | | | | | | | | | | | | |
| Miscellaneous | | | | | | BSE | | | | | | | | | | | | | | | | | | | | | | | | | | | | | | | | | | |

Chart 3

# Offensive Terminology in Women's Health

If you think women's health terminology is harmless, the following should make you think again. It's a list of medical terms used to describe female conditions and functions. Glance down the left side of the list first, then review what those terms really mean.

| | |
|---|---|
| Luteal phase defect | Short luteal phase (less than 10 days) |
| Dysfunctional uterine bleeding | Irregular or anovulatory bleeding (the bleeding that occurs in a cycle in which the woman didn't ovulate) |
| Discharge | Used to describe healthy, cyclical cervical fluid, as well as a true infection with symptoms of unhealthy secretions |
| Hostile cervical mucus | Infertile-quality cervical fluid that doesn't support sperm survival |
| Incompetent cervix | Cervix that tends to dilate prematurely during pregnancy |
| Inadequate pelvis | Pelvis considered too narrow to allow a vaginal birth |
| Senile gravida | A pregnant woman, 35 or over |
| Elderly prima gravida | First-time pregnant woman 35 and over |
| Advanced geriatric status | Women over 35 |

| | |
|---|---|
| Premature ovarian failure | Early menopause |
| Expected date of confinement (EDC) | The due date for childbirth |
| Habitual aborter | A woman who tends to have recurring, spontaneous miscarriages |
| Spontaneous abortion | Miscarriage |
| Threatened abortion | Bleeding while pregnant |
| Products of conception | Fetus that is delivered dead |
| Pregnancy wastage | Same as above |
| Fibrocystic breast disease | Fibrocystic breasts or breasts that tend to have benign lumpiness |
| Senile vaginitis | Dry vagina of (postmenopausal) woman after her estrogen levels have subsided |
| Vaginal atrophy | Same as above |
| Hysterectomy | In ancient Greek, literally means "removal of hysteria" (the Greek word for "womb" came from the belief that disturbances in the uterus caused female insanity) |
| Pudendum | Literally means "that of which we are ashamed." Actually means the soft padding that covers the pubic bone |
| Vagina clean | Terminology recorded in a woman's medical records to indicate no infections. (Is the implication that others are dirty?) |

Some of the terms are included here simply because their etymologies are of particular interest. Obviously, I am not suggesting that words as embedded in the lay vocabulary as "hysterectomy" should be changed at this point. However, I don't think it's unreasonable to suggest that the English language is capable of producing more gender-sensitive terms than "senile vaginitis" or "incompetent cervix." I suspect that no man is ever told he has a medically incompetent anything, but if a female doctor ever did, he might start to understand why I compiled this list.

# Fertility Awareness Resources

The organizations listed below should be able to help you locate a Fertility Awareness instructor in your area. The majority specifically teach Natural Family Planning, which, as you know, requires abstinence during the fertile phase. Ultimately, of course, the information taught is virtually the same as the Fertility Awareness Method, but you should be aware that NFP instruction often comes with a religious orientation that you may or may not appreciate. If you would prefer to use barriers during the fertile phase, try to find a FAM instructor first. Both the NFP organizations themselves and some of the Community Resources listed afterward may be able to refer you to one.

## ℘ NFP ORGANIZATIONS

No matter which one you choose, you may want to verify that they teach the Sympto-Thermal Method, which involves the observation of both waking temperatures and cervical fluid. Many NFP organizations only teach the Billings Method, which relies exclusively on the observation of cervical fluid.

**American Academy of National Family Planning**
615 South Ballas Road
St. Louis, Missouri 63141-7018
Phone: (314) 569-6495 (no fax number at time of publication)

**Billings Ovulation Method Association-USA**
316 North 7th Avenue
St. Cloud, Minnesota 56303-3633
Phone: (888) NFP-NFP-1 (637-6371)   Fax: (612) 252-2877

**Couple to Couple League**
PO Box 111184
Cincinnati, Ohio 45211-1184
Phone: (513) 661-7612    Fax: (513) 389-3885

**Diocesan Development Program for NFP**
3211 4th Street NE
Washington, DC 20017-1194
Phone: (202) 541-3240    Fax: (202) 541-3054

**Family of the Americas Foundation**
PO Box 1170
Dunkirk, Maryland 20754-1170
Phone: (800) 443-3395    Fax: (301) 627-0847

**Natural Family Planning of Corpus Christi**
4639 Corona Drive, Suite 13B
Corpus Christi, Texas 78411-4315
Phone: (512) 852-0222    Fax: (512) 851-2067

**NFP Center of Washington, D.C.**
8514 Bradmoor Drive
Bethesda, Maryland 20817-3810
Mailing Address: PO Box 30239, Bethesda, Maryland 20824-0239
Phone: (301) 897-9323    Fax: (301) 897-9323 (then hit *)

**Northwest Family Services**
4805 NE Glisan
Portland, Oregon 97213-2957
Phone: (503) 215-6377    Fax: (503) 731-6940

**Pope Paul VI Institute**
6901 Mercy Road
Omaha, Nebraska 68106-2604
Phone: (402) 390-6600    Fax: (402) 390-9851

**Serena Canada**
151 Holland Avenue
Ottawa, Ontario K1Y 0Y2
Canada
Phone: (613) 728-6536 (No fax number at time of publication)

**St. Francis Regional Medical Center**
Natural Family Planning
929 North St. Francis
Wichita, Kansas 67214-3882
Phone: (316) 268-5993   Fax: (316) 291-7945

## ℘ COMMUNITY RESOURCES

You might also try contacting any of the following, which may be able to point you in the right direction:

Catholic churches and dioceses
Family planning clinics
Health food stores and co-ops
Hospital education departments
Planned Parenthood
Public health departments
University health clinics
Women's clinics

## ℘ INFERTILITY SUPPORT

If you are facing fertility problems and would like to be a part of an organized community dealing with similar issues, I particularly recommend contacting RESOLVE, the wonderful organization listed below. It has local chapters throughout the United States and provides support groups, education, and monthly meetings, among other services. The Ferre Institute provides informative materials, including a newsletter.

**RESOLVE, Inc.**
1310 Broadway
Somerville, Massachusetts 02144-1731
Phone: Business—(617) 623-1156   Help Line—(617) 623-0744
Fax: (617) 623-0252

**Ferre Institute, Inc.**
258 Genesee Street, Suite 302
Utica, New York 13502-4629
Phone (315) 724-4348   Fax: (315) 724-1360

**Infertility Awareness Association of Canada, Inc.**
774 Echo Drive, Suite 523
Ottawa, Ontario K1S 5N8
Canada
Phone: (613) 730-1322
(800) 263-2929 (from Canada only)
Fax: (613) 730-1323

# Recommended Books

The following list of books is not comprehensive. There are numerous excellent women's health books continually being written. I have simply chosen several that I've had the opportunity to read and found particularly useful.

## FERTILITY AWARENESS

Billings, Evelyn, M.D., and Westmore, Ann. *The Billings Method: Controlling Fertility Without Drugs or Devices*. New York: Ballantine, 1986.

Kass-Annese, Barbara, R.N., CNP, and Danzer, Hal, M.D. *The Fertility Awareness Handbook*. Alameda, CA: Hunter House, 1992.

Pfeiffer, Regina Asaph, and Whitlock, Katherine. *Fertility Awareness: How to Become Pregnant When You Want to, and Avoid Pregnancy When You Don't*. Englewood Cliffs, NJ: Prentice-Hall, 1984.

## PREGNANCY ACHIEVEMENT

Berger, Gary, M.D., and Goldstein, Marc, M.D. *The Couple's Guide to Fertility*. New York: Doubleday, 1989.

Scher, Jonathan, M.D. *Preventing Miscarriage*. New York: HarperPerennial, 1990.

Silber, Sherman, M.D. *How to Get Pregnant with the New Technology*. New York: Warner, 1991.

## WOMEN'S HEALTH

Ammer, Christine. *The New A to Z of Women's Health: A Concise Encyclopedia*. New York: Everest House, 1989.

Boston Women's Health Book Collective. *The New Our Bodies, Ourselves*. New York: Simon & Schuster, 1992.

Madaras, Lynda, and Patterson, Jane, M.D. *Womancare*. New York: Avon, 1984.

Stewart, Felicia, M.D., et al. *Understanding Your Body*. New York: Bantam, 1987.

## PMS

Lark, Susan, M.D. *PMS Self-Help Book*. Berkeley, CA: Celestial Arts, 1984.

Martorano, Joseph, M.D., and Morgan, Maureen, C.S.W., R.N. *Unmasking PMS*. New York: M. Evans, 1993.

## MENOPAUSE

Lark, Susan, M.D. *Menopause Self-Help Book*. Berkeley, CA: Celestial Arts, 1990.

Perry, Susan, and O'Hanlan, Katherine A., M.D. *Natural Menopause*. Reading, MA: Addison-Wesley, 1992.

Sheehy, Gail. *The Silent Passage*. New York: Pocket Books, 1993.

## MISCELLANEOUS

The Burton Goldberg Group. *Alternative Medicine: The Definitive Guide*. Puyallup, WA: Future Medicine Publishing, 1993.

Castleman, Michael. *Sexual Solutions*. New York: Touchstone, 1989.

Cutler, Winnifred, Ph.D. *Love Cycles*. New York: Villard, 1991.

Kippley, Sheila. *Breastfeeding and Natural Child Spacing*. Cincinnati, OH: The Couple to Couple League International, 1989.

Murray, Michael, N.D., and Pizzorno, Joseph, N.D. *Encyclopedia of Natural Medicine*. Rocklin, CA: Prima Publishing, 1990.

Shannon, Marilyn. *Fertility, Cycles, and Nutrition*. Cincinnati, OH: The Couple to Couple League International, 1992.

Shettles, Landrum, M.D., Ph.D., and Rorvik, David. *How to Choose the Sex of Your Baby*. New York: Doubleday, 1989.

Sloane, Ethel. *The Biology of Women*. Albany, NY: Delmar Publishers, 1993.

# Glossary

**Adhesion:** Fibrous tissue that abnormally binds organs or other body parts. It is usually the result of inflammation or abnormal healing of a surgical wound.

**AI:** See **Artificial Insemination.**

**AIDS:** Acquired immune deficiency syndrome. A fatal disease that is most often transmitted sexually. It is caused by a virus that damages the body's immune system, resulting in infections and cancers.

**Amenorrhea:** Prolonged absence of menstruation. Causes include stress, fatigue, psychological disturbances, obesity, weight loss, anorexia nervosa, hormonal contraceptives, and medical disorders.

**Amniocentesis:** Puncture of the fluid sac surrounding the fetus through the abdominal wall and uterus to obtain a sample of the amniotic fluid for testing. The procedure, performed around the sixteenth week of pregnancy, can be used to identify various birth defects.

**Androgens:** Male sex hormones, responsible for the development of male secondary sex characteristics, including facial hair and a deep voice. Most androgens, including the principal one, testosterone, are produced in the testes. Small amounts of androgens are also produced in a woman's ovaries and adrenal glands.

**Anovulation:** The absence of ovulation.

**Anovulatory (anovular) cycle:** A cycle in which ovulation does not occur.

**Arousal fluid:** The colorless, lubricative fluid secreted around the vaginal opening in response to sexual stimulation, in preparation for intercourse. Arousal fluid should not be confused with fertile cervical fluid, which is secreted in a cyclical pattern around ovulation.

**Artificial Insemination:** A procedure in which sperm is deposited just outside the cervix, or inside the uterus. (See **IUI.**)

**Bartholins glands:** Small glands that produce a colorless lubricative fluid around the vaginal opening in response to sexual stimulation. This fluid is often termed **arousal fluid.**

**Basal body temperature (BBT):** See **Waking temperature.**

**Basic Infertile Pattern (BIP):** An extended, unchanging pattern of cervical fluid or dryness that women occasionally experience instead of the normal pattern of progressively wetter (and more fertile) cervical fluid. Such a pattern generally indicates relative inactivity of the ovaries and low estrogen levels.

**BBT method:** Basal body temperature method. A type of natural birth control in which the postovulatory infertile phase of the menstrual cycle is identified exclusively by a sustained rise in basal body temperature. Because those who use this method do not chart cervical fluid, they must either abstain or use barriers during the entire preovulatory phase of the cycle.

**Billings method:** A natural birth control method in which days of fertility are identified exclusively by observations of cervical fluid at the vaginal opening. Developed by Drs. John and Evelyn Billings.

**BIP:** See **Basic Infertile Pattern.**

**Biphasic temperature pattern:** A temperature chart that shows a pattern of relatively low temperatures in the preovulatory phase of the cycle, followed by a postovulatory higher level for about 12 to 16 days, until the next menstruation.

**Blastocyst:** The newly created fertilized ovum, before implantation occurs.

**Blighted ovum:** A pregnancy in which no fetus ever developed in the pregnancy sac.

**Breakthrough bleeding:** Bleeding due to excessive estrogen production, which causes the endometrium to grow beyond the point that it can sustain itself. It usually occurs during anovulatory cycles.

**Breastfeeding:** The act of suckling on the part of the infant, and the act of giving milk from the breast directly to the infant on the part of the mother. *Full* breastfeeding means that you are not giving your baby *any* supplements or pacifiers; *nearly full* breastfeeding means that you supplement no more than 15% of all feedings. Both mean that intervals between feedings should not exceed 4 hours during the day or 6 hours at night. *Partially* breastfeeding means that supplements such as juices and solids are regularly given. It also means that you are nursing less frequently than every 4 hours during the day, and less than every 6 hours at night.

**Cervical crypts:** Pockets in the lining of the cervix that secrete cervical fluid.

**Cervical erosion:** The condition of the cervix when the cells lining the cervical canal grow over the lip of the cervix.

**Cervical fluid:** The secretion produced within the cervix that acts as a medium in which sperm can travel. Its presence and quality are directly related to the production of estrogen and progesterone. Analogous to a man's seminal fluid, it is one of the three primary fertility signs, along with cervical position and waking temperature. Cervical fluid typically gets progressively wetter as ovulation approaches. See **Sticky, Creamy,** and **Eggwhite-quality cervical fluid.**

**Cervical mucus:** See **cervical fluid.**

**Cervical os:** The opening of the cervix.

**Cervical palpation:** Feeling the cervix with your middle finger to determine its height, softness, and opening.

**Cervical polyp:** A soft, noncancerous tumor that develops high up in the cervical canal, often protruding through the cervix. It may cause no symptoms at all, or it may cause bleeding or cramping.

**Cervical position:** The term used to describe one of the three primary fertility signs. In this book, cervical position refers to three facets of the cervix: its height, softness, and opening.

**Cervical tip:** The opening of the cervix, often referred to as the **cervical os.**

**Cervix:** The lower portion of the uterus that projects into the vagina.

**Chlamydia:** A highly prevalent sexually transmitted disease. It can lead to infertility through scarring of the fallopian tubes.

**Chromosome:** One of the 46 microscopic units within each cell that carries the genetic material responsible for inherited characteristics.

**Clomid (clomiphene citrate):** A commonly prescribed drug primarily used to induce ovulation.

**Colposcopy:** A procedure used to examine the vagina and cervix under magnification through an instrument known as a colposcope. It is of particular value in the early detection of cancer of the cervix.

**Corpus luteum:** The yellow gland formed by the ruptured follicle after ovulation. If the egg is fertilized, the corpus luteum continues to produce progesterone to support the early pregnancy until the palcenta is formed. If fertilization does not occur, the corpus luteum degenerates within 12 to 16 days.

**Corpus luteum cyst:** A rare and temporary condition in which the corpus luteum doesn't disintegrate after its typical 12-to-16-day life span. It may lead women to mistakenly believe they are pregnant by delaying their periods and maintaining their high postovulatory temperatures beyond 16 days.

**Coverline:** A line used to help delineate pre- and postovulatory temperatures on a fertility chart.

**Cowper's gland:** One of a pair of small glands that secretes the lubricative preejaculatory fluid in the male, changing the urethra from acidic to alkaline.

**Creamy cervical fluid:** The quality of cervical fluid that is generally wet and often similar to the consistency of hand lotion. It is considered fertile, although not as fertile as the eggwhite cervical fluid that usually follows it.

**Creighton model/ovulation method:** A cervical fluid method developed by Dr. Thomas Hilgers.

**D and C:** See **Dilation and curettage.**

**Danazol:** A synthetic hormone used to treat endometriosis.

**Dilation and curettage ("D and C"):** A surgical procedure used to scrape the surface of the endometrium with an instrument called a curette. Prior to the curettage, the cervix is gradually opened with instruments called dilators.

**Discharge:** An emission from the vagina. In this book, it refers to an unhealthy symptom of an infection.

**Double ovulation:** The release of two separate eggs in one menstrual cycle. Both eggs are released within a 24-hour period.

**Dry Day Rule:** One of the four natural birth control rules. It states that before ovulation, you are safe for unprotected intercourse the evening of every dry day (after 6 P.M.).

**Dry days:** Days when you observe no cervical fluid or bleeding and have a dry vaginal sensation.

**Dysmenorrhea:** Painful menstruation. Painful spasmodic contractions of the uterus, which usually arise just prior to or for the first few hours of menstruation, and then gradually subside.

**Dyspareunia:** Painful or difficult intercourse.

**Ectopic pregnancy:** The implantation and development of a fertilized ovum outside the uterus, usually in the fallopian tube.

**Eggwhite-quality cervical fluid:** The most fertile type of cervical fluid a woman produces. It typically resembles raw eggwhite and tends to be clear, slippery, and stretchy. It usually appears in the 2 or 3 days preceding ovulation.

**Embryo:** The initial stages of development from the fertilized egg to around six weeks after conception.

**Endocrinologist:** A physician who specializes in the function of hormones.

**Endometrial biopsy:** The removal of a small part of the uterine lining (endometrium) for examination under the microscope. Used to determine whether the woman's lining is developing appropriately.

**Endometriosis:** The growth of endometrial tissue in areas other than the uterus, for example, in the fallopian tubes or the ovaries. A woman may be asymptomatic, or she may have lower abdominal pain which worsens during menstruation, pain during intercourse, and unusually long menstrual periods. Hormone therapy, surgery, and pregnancy may improve the condition. Endometriosis may cause infertility.

**Endometrium:** The lining of the uterus which is shed during menstruation. If conception occurs, the fertilized egg implants within it.

**Epididymis:** The beginning of the sperm duct, where sperm are stored, matured, and transported. It is attached to the testicles.

**Estrogen:** The hormone produced mainly in the ovaries, responsible for the development of female secondary sex characteristics, as well as one of the primary hormones that control the menstrual cycle. Increasing estrogen levels in the first part of the menstrual cycle produce significant changes in the cervical fluid and cervix, indicating fertility.

**Fallback temperature shift pattern:** A type of thermal shift in which the temperature drops on or below the coverline on the second day after having already risen above it.

**Fallopian tube:** One of a pair of tubes through which the ripened ovum is transported from the ovary towards the uterus. Sperm swim from the uterus toward the outer end of the fallopian tube where fertilization may take place.

**False temperature rise:** A temperature rise due to causes other than ovulation, such as fever, restless sleep, or drinking alcohol the night before. It can also be caused by taking your temperature substantially later than usual.

**Ferning:** The characteristic pattern produced by fertile cervical fluid when dried on a glass slide. So named because it resembles a fern.

**Fertile phase:** The days of the menstrual cycle during which sexual intercourse or insemination may result in pregnancy. It includes several days leading up to and immediately following ovulation.

**Fertile-quality cervical fluid:** Cervical fluid that is wet, slippery, stretchy, or resembles raw eggwhite. This type of cervical fluid appears around the time of ovulation, allowing sperm to live and travel in it for about 3 to 5 days.

**Fertility Awareness Method:** A means of determining one's fertility through observing the three primary fertility signs: waking temperature, cervical fluid, and cervical position.

**Fertility drugs:** Drugs used to stimulate ovulation. The two most common are Clomid and Pergonal.

**Fetus:** A name for a developing embryo from 6 weeks after fertilization until the time of birth.

**Fibrocystic breast disease:** A misleading term for nothing more than a common benign disorder characterized by the formulation of fluid-filled sacs in one or both breasts.

**Fibroid:** A fibrous and muscular growth of tissue in or on the wall of the uterus.

**Fimbria:** The end of the fallopian tube near the ovary. The fimbriae pick up the egg immediately after ovulation.

**First 5 Days Rule:** One of the four natural birth control rules. It states that you are safe the first five days of the menstrual cycle *if* you had an obvious temperature shift 12 to 16 days before. This rule is considered less effective if you have had cycles of 25 days or less or have premenopausal symptoms.

**Follicle:** A small fluid-filled structure in the ovary that contains the egg (ovum). The follicle ruptures the surface of the ovary, releasing the ovum at ovulation.

**Follicle-stimulating hormone (FSH):** The hormone produced by the pituitary gland that stimulates the ovaries to produce mature ova and the hormone estrogen.

**Gamete:** The mature reproductive cells of the sperm and ovum.

**Gamete Intra-fallopian Transfer:** See **GIFT.**

**Gestation:** The period of development from conception to the end of pregnancy and birth.

**GIFT:** Gamete Intra-fallopian Transfer. A procedure in which the woman's eggs are removed from her ovaries and then placed in her fallopian tube with her partner's sperm. Unlike IVF, fertilization takes place in the fallopian tube, not a petri dish.

**Gonadotropin Releasing Hormone (GnRH):** A chemical substance produced by the hypothalamus in the brain. It stimulates the pituitary gland to produce and release both FSH and LH, hormones which in turn lead to follicular development and ovulation.

**Gonadotropins:** The hormones produced by the pituitary gland of males and females that regulate maturation of the sperm and egg. The most important gonadotropins are FSH and LH.

**Gonads:** The primary sex glands of the ovaries and testes.

**HCG:** Human chorionic gonadotropin, typically referred to as the "pregnancy hormone." It is produced by the developing embryo when it implants into the uterine lining. Its main action is to maintain the corpus luteum and hence the secretion of estrogen and progesterone until the placenta has developed sufficiently to take over hormonal production. See **Pregnancy test.**

**Hormone:** A chemical substance produced in one organ and carried by the blood to another organ where it exerts its effect. An example is FSH, which is produced in the pituitary gland and travels via the blood to the ovary, where it stimulates the growth and maturation of follicles.

**Hormone replacement therapy:** The use of manufactured hormones, particularly estrogen, to replace the perimenopausal woman's diminished natural supply of hormones. Prescribed to alleviate menopausal symptoms such as vaginal dryness and hot flashes, as well as to prevent osteoporosis.

**HSG:** Hysterosalpingogram. An X ray taken after a special dye is injected through the cervix to produce an image of the inside of the uterus and fallopian tubes. Used to determine whether the tubes are blocked or have scarring.

**Hypothalamus:** A part of the brain located just above the pituitary gland that controls several functions of the body. It produces hormones that influence the pituitary gland and regulate the development and activity of the ovaries and testes.

**Hysteroscopy:** Exploratory surgery to view the inside of the uterus.

**Idiopathic infertility:** Infertility of unknown cause.

**Implantation:** The process by which the fertilized egg imbeds in the uterine lining, or endometrium.

**Infertile phases:** The phases of the cycle when pregnancy cannot occur. Women have a preovulatory and postovulatory infertile phase.

**Infertile-quality cervical fluid:** A thick, sticky, or opaque-quality cervical fluid that produces a vaginal sensation of dryness or stickiness. It is very difficult for sperm to survive within it.

**Intermenstrual pain:** See *Mittelschmerz.*

**Intra-Uterine Insemination:** See **IUI.**

**In Vitro Fertilization:** See **IVF.**

**IUI:** Intra-Uterine Insemination. A procedure in which a catheter is used to insert the man's sperm through the cervix directly into the uterus.

**IVF:** In Vitro Fertilization. A procedure in which several eggs from the woman's ovaries are fertilized with her partner's sperm in a petri dish outside her body, then placed in the uterus 2 days later.

**Kegel exercise:** An exercise to contract and relax the vaginal muscles, in order to help strengthen them. It is also used to help push cervical fluid and semen out of the vaginal opening.

**Lactational Amenorrhea Method (LAM):** A natural method of family planning used by breastfeeding women whose periods have not yet returned. It is considered highly effective if they are fully or nearly fully breastfeeding and are less than 6 months postpartum.

**Laparoscopy:** A procedure in which a laparoscope, a thin telescope instrument, is inserted through a small incision in the navel to examine the inside of the abdomen, particularly the ovaries.

**Laparotomy:** A surgical operation involving opening the abdomen.

**Lochia:** Bloody secretions from the uterus and vagina the first few weeks after childbirth.

**Lubricative sensation:** The slippery and wet vaginal sensation you feel, usually when fertile-quality cervical fluid is present. If you feel it when no cervical fluid is present, you are still fertile.

**LUFS:** Luteinized unruptured follicle syndrome, a condition in which the ovum remains stuck within the luteinized follicle, unable to pass through the ovarian wall to a possible conception. It is now believed to be a major cause of unexplained infertility.

**Luteal phase:** The phase of the menstrual cycle from ovulation to the onset of the next menstruation. It typically lasts from 12 to 16 days, but rarely varies by more than a day or 2 within individual women.

**Luteinizing hormone (LH):** A pituitary hormone that is released in a surge, causing ovulation and development of the corpus luteum.

**Menarche:** The first menstrual period in a girl's life.

**Menorrhagia:** Exceptionally heavy bleeding during regular menstrual periods.

**Menses:** See **Menstruation.**

**Menstrual cycle:** The cyclical changes in the ovaries, cervix, and endometrium under the influence of the sex hormones. The length of the menstrual cycle is calculated from the first day of menstruation to the day before the following menstruation.

**Menstrual cycle, phases of:** There are three specific phases in the menstrual cycle:

1. The preovulatory infertile phase, which starts at the onset of menstruation and ends at the onset of the fertile phase.
2. The fertile phase, which includes the days before and immediately after ovulation when intercourse may result in pregnancy.
3. The postovulatory infertile phase, which starts at the completion of the fertile phase and ends at the onset of the next menstruation.

**Menstruation:** The cyclical bleeding from the uterus as the endometrium is shed. True menstruation is preceded by ovulation usually 12 to 16 days earlier.

**Method failure rate:** This refers to the effectiveness of a contraceptive method under ideal conditions, when always used correctly.

**Micromanipulation:** A procedure in which a single sperm is inserted directly into the ovum through the assistance of high-tech instruments. The newly created embryo is then transferred from the petri dish to the woman's uterus.

**Midcycle spotting:** Light bleeding between two menstrual periods. Usually occurs around the time of ovulation, and is often considered a secondary fertility sign.

*Mittelschmerz:* Lower abdominal pain occurring around the time of ovulation.

**Monophasic temperature pattern:** A chart that does not show the biphasic pattern of low and high temperatures, usually indicating an absence of ovulation that cycle.

**Mucus plug:** The accumulation of sticky, infertile-quality cervical fluid in the cervical opening. It generally impedes the passage of sperm through the cervix.

**Multiple ovulation:** The release of at least two separate eggs in one menstrual cycle. Each of the eggs is released within the same 24-hour period of time.

**Nabothian cyst:** A harmless cyst on the surface of the cervix.

**Natural Family Planning (NFP):** Methods for planning or preventing pregnancy by observation of the naturally occurring signs of the fertile and infertile phases of the menstrual cycle. Unlike the Fertility Awareness Method, users of NFP abstain rather than use contraceptive barriers during the fertile phase.

**Ova:** Plural of **ovum.**

**Ovary:** One of a pair of female sex organs that produce mature **ova,** which in turn produce estrogen.

**Ovulation:** The release of a mature egg **(ovum)** from the ovarian follicle.

**Ovulation predictor kits (OPK):** Kits that detect the impending release of an egg, usually by testing urine for the presence of LH.

**Ovulatory cycle:** A cycle in which **ovulation** occurs.

**Ovulatory pain:** Often called *Mittelschmerz.* Lower abdominal pain occurring around the time of ovulation. It may be caused by the irritation of the pelvic lining due to a slight amount of blood loss or from the actual breakthrough of the egg through the ovarian wall. Considered a **secondary fertility sign.**

**Ovulatory spotting:** See **Midcycle spotting.**

**Ovum:** The mature female sex cell, or egg. The plural is **ova.** Analogous to the male sperm.

**Ovum transfer:** A procedure in which a man's sperm is used to fertilize the egg of a donor woman. The resulting embryo is then placed in the uterus of his partner, who may even be postmenopausal.

**Patch Rule:** One of the two natural birth control rules used during phases of anovulation. It states that you are safe the evening of every day that your 2-week Basic Infertile Pattern remains the same. But as soon as you see a *change* in your BIP, you must consider yourself fertile until the fourth evening after the Peak Day.

**PC muscles:** Popular term for the pubococcygeous muscles of the pelvic floor. Their function is to support the bladder, rectum, and uterus.

**Peak Day:** The last day that you produce your most fertile cervical fluid, have spotting, or have a lubricative vaginal sensation for any given cycle. It usually occurs either a day before you ovulate or on the day of ovulation itself.

**Peak Day Rule:** One of the four natural birth control rules. It states that you are safe the evening of the fourth day after your Peak Day.

**Pergonal:** A powerful drug used to stimulate ovulation. It often triggers the release of more than one egg.

**Perimenopause:** The period of months or years preceding the menopause, during which time there may be emotional and physical changes, including irregularities in the menstrual cycle due to fluctuating hormone levels. Also called premenopause.

**Perineum:** The membrane between the vaginal opening and the anus.

**Periodic abstinence:** Various methods of family planning based on voluntarily abstaining from intercourse during the fertile phase of the cycle in order to avoid pregnancy.

**Pituitary gland:** The gland at the base of the brain that produces many important hormones, some of which trigger other glands into making their own hormones. The pituitary functions include hormonal control of the ovaries and testes.

**Polycystic ovaries:** A condition in which the ovaries are studded with many small cysts, which may prevent the woman from ovulating normally.

**Polyp:** A small, often teardrop-shaped growth, usually found in the cervix or endometrium. It is almost always benign.

**Postcoital contraception:** Emergency contraceptive measures in the form of high-dose pills or insertion of an IUD that must be implemented within 72 hours following unprotected intercourse.

**Postcoital test:** The examination of cervical fluid shortly after intercourse to determine whether sperm survive in it.

**Postovulatory phase:** See **Luteal phase.**

**Preejaculatory fluid:** A small amount of lubricating fluid that is emitted from the penis before ejaculation during sexual excitement. May contain sperm.

**Pregnancy test:** A blood or urine test designed to detect the presence of HCG, the pregnancy hormone emitted from the newly implanted embryo.

**Pregnancy wheel:** A calculating device used by doctors to determine a pregnant woman's due date. It is based on the assumption that ovulation occurs on Day 14, and is therefore often inaccurate.

**Pregnanediol:** A metabolite (breakdown product) of progesterone, excreted in the urine.

**Premenopause:** See **Perimenopause.**

**Preovulatory phase:** The variable-length phase of the cycle from the onset of menstruation to ovulation. See **Menstrual cycle.**

**Progesterone:** A hormone produced by the corpus luteum in the ovary following ovulation. It prepares the endometrium for a possible pregnancy. It is also responsible for the rise in waking temperature, and for the change in cervical fluid and cervical position in the postovulatory infertile phase.

**Prolactin:** A pituitary hormone that stimulates the production of breast milk and indirectly inhibits the ovarian production of estrogen.

**Prostaglandins:** A group of fatty acids that is believed to be responsible for severe menstrual cramps.

**Pubococcygeous:** See **PC muscles.**

**Reproductive endocrinologist:** A doctor who specializes in reproductive hormones.

**Rhythm method:** An unreliable method of family planning in which the fertile phase of the cycle is calculated according to the lengths of previous menstrual cycles. Because of its reliance on regular menstrual cycles and long periods of abstinence, it is neither effective nor widely accepted as a modern method of natural family planning.

**Rule of Thumb:** A guideline in which aberrant waking temperatures are discounted, particularly when calculating the coverline.

**Secondary fertility signs:** Physical and emotional changes that may provide supplementary evidence of the fertile phase. Secondary signs include *mittelschmerz* (ovulatory pain), spotting, breast tenderness, and mood changes.

**Secondary sex characteristics:** Features of masculinity or femininity that develop at puberty under hormonal control. In the male, this includes deepening voice in addition to the growth of beard and underarm and pubic hair. They are influenced by androgens. In the female, such characteristics include rounding of breasts, waist, and hips, as well as the growth of underarm and pubic hair. They are influenced by estrogens.

**Semen Emitting Technique (SETs):** The use of Kegel exercises (and tissue) in order to eliminate semen from the vagina.

**Seminal vesicle:** One of a pair of sacs that open into the top of the male urethra. Its secretions form part of the seminal fluid.

**Seminiferous tubules:** Microscopic tubes in the testes in which sperm are produced.

**Sexually transmitted diseases:** Any infection that is transmitted by sexual contact or intercourse.

**Slow-rise temperature shift pattern:** A type of thermal shift in which temperatures rise by merely one-tenth of a degree per day over several days.

**Speculum:** A two-bladed stainless steel or plastic instrument used to examine the inside of the vagina and the cervix.

**Sperm count:** A measure of a man's fertility which calculates the total number of sperm per ejaculate as well as that percentage of sperm that are both forwardly moving (motility) and of normal shape and size (morphology).

**Sperm washing:** The process by which the motility of the sperm is dramatically increased through mixing them in a culture media and then placing them in a centrifuge.

**Spinnbarkeit:** Fertile-quality cervical fluid that is generally stretchy, slippery, and clear.

**Spotting:** See **Midcycle spotting.**

**Stair-step temperature shift pattern:** A type of thermal shift in which an initial spurt of temperatures occurs over several days, followed by a higher pattern of temperatures usually resembling a bell curve.

**Sticky cervical fluid:** The type of cervical fluid that is often like the quality of library paste. It is usually the first type of cervical fluid that appears in a woman's cycle following menstruation. It is very difficult for sperm to survive in it.

**Subfertility:** A state of less than normal fertility.

**Sympto-thermal method (STM):** A natural method of family planning combining observation of the waking (basal body) temperature, cervical fluid, and cervical position, along with any other secondary fertility signs. The most comprehensive and effective natural method, and the one taught in this book.

**Temperature chart:** A graph showing variation in daily waking temperature recorded to detect ovulation. See **Biphasic** and **Monophasic temperature pattern.**

**Temperature method:** See **BBT method.**

**Temperature shift:** The rise in waking temperature that divides the preovulatory low temperatures from the later, postovulatory high temperatures on a biphasic chart. It usually results in temperatures that are at least two-tenths of a degree higher than those of the previous 6 days.

**Temperature Shift Rule:** One of the four natural birth control rules. It states that you are safe the evening of the third consecutive day your temperature is above the coverline.

**Testosterone:** A hormone produced by the testes, responsible for the development of male secondary sex characteristics and functioning of the male reproductive organs.

**Thermal shift:** See **Temperature shift.**

**Tubal ligation:** The surgical sterilization procedure that ties or cauterizes a woman's fallopian tubes to prevent the sperm and egg from uniting.

**Tubal pregnancy:** An ectopic pregnancy, in which the fertilized egg starts to implant in the fallopian tube rather than in the uterus.

**Ultrasound:** A diagnostic technique that uses sound waves, rather than X rays, to visualize internal body structures.

**Unchanging Day Rule:** One of the two natural birth control rules used during phases of anovulation. It states that if your 2-week Basic Infertile Pattern (BIP) is dry or the same-quality sticky cervical fluid day after day, you are safe for unprotected intercourse the evening of every dry or unchanging sticky day.

**Vaginismus:** A painful spasm of the vagina that prevents comfortable penetration of the penis.

**Vaginitis:** An inflammation of the vagina caused by an infection or other irritation.

**Varicocele:** A varicose-type vein in a man's scrotum that can impede his fertility by increasing the testicular temperature.

**Vas deferens:** One of a pair of tubes that carries the seminal fluid from the testis to the urethra.

**Vasectomy:** A male sterilization procedure in which each vas deferens is cut to prevent the passage of sperm.

**Waking temperature:** The temperature of the body at rest, taken immediately upon awakening, before any activity. Often referred to as basal body temperature (BBT).

**Withdrawal:** The act of removing the penis from the vagina before ejaculation occurs. Often used as a form of contraception.

**Withdrawal bleeding:** Vaginal bleeding resulting from a drop in the levels of estrogen necessary to maintain the uterine lining. It usually occurs during anovulatory cycles.

**ZIFT:** Zygote Intra-fallopian Transfer. A procedure in which a woman's egg is fertilized by her partner's sperm in a petri dish. The resulting zygote is then placed back in her fallopian tube.

**Zygote:** The fertilized ovum, a single fertilized cell resulting from fusion of the sperm and the egg. After further cell division the zygote is known as an embryo.

**Zygote Intra-fallopian Transfer:** See **ZIFT.**

# Bibliography

Many of the recommended books listed in Appendix N were also used as source material.

## AIDS

### Articles

Bylund, David J., M.D., Ulrike H. M. Ziegner, M.D., Ph.D., & Dennis G. Hooper, M.D., Ph.D. "Review of Testing for Human Immunodeficiency Virus," *Clinics in Laboratory Medicine* 12 ( June 1992): 305–333.

Sloand, Elaine M., M.D., et al. "HIV Testing: State of the Art," *Journal of the American Medical Association* 266 (November 27, 1991): 2861–2866.

### Books

Berer, Marge. *Women and HIV/AIDS: An International Resource Book.* San Francisco: HarperCollins, 1993.

Vargo, Marc E., M.S. *The HIV Test: What You Need to Know to Make an Informed Decision.* New York: Pocket Books, 1992.

## BREASTFEEDING

### Articles

Family Health International, Consensus Statement. "Breastfeeding as a Family Planning Method," *The Lancet* (November 19, 1988): 1204–1205.

Gray, Ronald H., Oona M. Campbell, Ruben Apelo, Susan S. Eslami, Howard Zacur, Rebecca M. Ramos, Judith C. Gehret, & Miriam H. Labbok. "Risk of Ovulation During Lactation," *The Lancet* 335 ( January 6, 1990): 25–29.

Howie, P. W., A. S. McNeilly, M. J. Houston, A. Cook, & H. Boyle. "Fertility After Childbirth: Post-Partum Ovulation and Menstruation in Bottle and Breast Feeding Mothers," *Clinical Endocrinology* 17 (October 1982): 323–332.

Kennedy, Kathy J., & Cynthia M. Visness. "Contraceptive Efficacy of Lactational Amenorrhoea," *The Lancet* 339 (January 25, 1992): 227–229.

Labbok, Miriam, Kristin Cooney, & Shirly Coly. *Guidelines: Breastfeeding, Family Planning, and the Lactational Amenorrhea Method—LAM.* Washington, DC: Institute for Reproductive Health, 1994.

Lewis, Patricia R., Ph.D., et al. "The Resumption of Ovulation and Menstruation in a Well-Nourished Population of Women Breastfeeding for an Extended Period of Time," *Fertility and Sterility* 55 (March 1991): 520–535.

Perez, Alfredo, Miriam H. Labbok, & John T. Queenan. "Clinical Study of the Lactational Amenorrhoea Method for Family Planning," *The Lancet* 339 (April 18, 1992): 968–970.

Tay, Clement C. K., MBChB, MRCOG. "Mechanisims Controlling Lactational Infertility," *Journal of Human Lactation* 7 (March 1991): 15–18.

### Books

Paranteau-Carreau, Suzanne, M.D., IFFLP, & Kristin A. Cooney, M.A., IRH. *Breastfeeding, Lactational Amenorrhea Method, and Natural Family Planning Interface: Teaching Guide,* 1–35. Washington, DC: Institute for Reproductive Health, 1994.

Riordan, Jan, Ed.D., R.N., IBCLC, & Kathleen G. Auerbach, Ph.D., IBCLC. *Breastfeeding and Human Lactation.* Boston and London: Jones and Bartlett Publishers, 1993.

## CONTRACEPTIVE EFFECTIVENESS

### Articles

Barbato, Michele, M.D., & Giancarlo Bertolotti, M.D. "Natural Methods for Fertility Control: A Prospective Study—First Part," *International Fertility Supplement* (1988): 48–51.

Flynn, Anna M., & John Bonnar. "Natural Family Planning." In *Contraception: Science and Practice,* edited by Marcus Filshie & John Guillebaud, pp. 203–205. London: Butterworth Press, 1989.

Frank-Herrmann, Petra, M.D., et al. "Effectiveness and Acceptability of the Symptothermal Method of Natural Family Planning in Germany," *American Journal of Obstetrics & Gynecology* 165 (December 1991): 2052–2054.

Ghosh, A.K., S. Saha, & G. Chattergee. "Symptothermia Vis à Vis Fertility Control," *Journal of Obstetrics and Gynecology of India* 32 (1982): 443–447.

Hume, K. "Fertility Awareness in the 1990s—The Billings Ovulation Method of Natural Family Planning, Its Scientific Basis, Practical Application and Effectiveness," *Advances in Contraception* 7 (June–Sept. 1991): 301–311.

Lethbridge, Dona J., R.N., Ph.D. "Coitus Interruptus: Consideration as a Method of Birth Control," *Journal of Obstetrics, Gynecologic and Neonatal Nursing* 20 (1991): 80–85.

Petotti, Diana B. "Statistical Aspects of the Evaluation of the Safety and Effectiveness of Fertility Control Methods." In *Fertility Control,* edited by Stephen L. Corson, Richard J. Derman, & Louise B. Tyrer, pp. 13–25. Boston: Little Brown, 1985.

Rice, Frank J., Ph.D., Claude A. Lanctôt, M.D., & Consuelo Farcia-DeVesa, Ph.D. "Effectiveness of the Sympto-Thermal Method of Natural Family Planning: An International Study," *International Journal of Fertility* 26 (1981): 222–230.

Royston, J. P. "Basal Body Temperature, Ovulation and the Risk of Conception, with Special Reference to the Lifetimes of Sperm and Egg," *Biometrics 38* (June 1982): 397–406.

Ryder, R. E. J. " 'Natural Family Planning': Effective Birth Control Supported by the Catholic Church," *British Medical Journal* 307 (September 18, 1993): 723–726.

Trussell, James, & Laurence Grummer-Strawn. "Contraceptive Failure of the Ovulation Method of Periodic Abstinence," *Family Planning Perspectives* 22 (March/April 1990): 65–75.

Trussell, James, & Kathryn Kost. "Contraceptive Failure in the United States: A Critical Review of the Literature," *Studies in Family Planning* 18 (September/October 1987): 237–283.

Trussell, James, Ph.D., et al. "A Guide to Interpreting Contraceptive Efficacy Studies," *Obstetrics & Gynecology* 76 (September 1990): 558–567.

Trussell, James, Ph.D., et al. "Contraceptive Failure in the United States: An Update," *Studies in Family Planning* 21 (January/February 1990): 51–54.

Wade, Maclyn E., M.D., et al. "A Randomized Prospective Study of the Use-Effectiveness of Two Methods of Natural Family Planning," *American Journal of Obstetrics & Gynecology* 141 (October 1981): 368–376.

Woolley, Robert J., M.D. "Contraception—A Look Forward, Part I: New Spermicides and Natural Family Planning," *Journal of the American Board of Family Practice* (January 1991): 33–44.

World Health Organization, Task Force. "A Prospective Multicentre Trial of the Ovulation Method of Natural Family Planning. II. The Effectiveness Phase," *Fertility and Sterility* 36 (November 1981): 591–598.

World Health Organization, Task Force. "A Prospective Multicentre Trial of the Ovulation Method of Natural Family Planning. III. Characteristics of the Menstrual Cycle and of the Fertile Phase," *Fertility and Sterility* 40 (December 1983): 773–778.

### Books

Hatcher, Robert A., M.D., MPH, et al. *Contraceptive Technology,* sixteenth revised edition. New York: Irvington Publishers, 1994.

## FERTILITY AND THE MENSTRUAL CYCLE

### Articles

Badwe, R. A., et al. "Timing of Surgery During Menstrual Cycle and Survival of Pre-menopausal Women with Operable Breast Cancer," *The Lancet* (May 25, 1991): 1261–1264.

Banks, A. Lawrence, M.D. "Does Adoption Affect Infertility?" *International Journal of Fertility* (1962): 23–28.

Barnes, Ann B., M.D. "Menstrual History and Fecundity of Women Exposed and Unexposed in Utero to Diethylstilbestrol," *Journal of Reproductive Medicine* 29 (September 1984): 651–655.

Barnes, Ann B., M.D. "Menstrual History of Young Women Exposed in Utero to Diethylstilbestrol," *Fertility and Sterility* 32 (August 1979): 148–153.

Brown, James B., D.Sc., Joanne Holmes, B.A., & Gillian Barker. "Use of the Home Ovarian Monitor in Pregnancy Avoidance," *American Journal of Obstetrics and Gynecology* 165 (December 1991): 2008–2011.

Burger, Henry G., M.D. "Neuroendocrine Control of Human Ovulation," *International Journal of Fertility* 26 (1981): 153–160.

Campbell, Doris M. "Aetiology of Twinning." In *Twinning and Twins*, edited by I. MacGillivray, D. M. Campbell, & B. Thompson, pp. 27–36. London: John Wiley & Sons, 1988.

Canfield, R. E., et al. "Development of an Assay for a Biomarker of Pregnancy and Early Fetal Loss," *Environmental Health Perspectives* 74 (October 1987): 57–66.

Chard, T. "Pregnancy Tests: A Review," *Human Reproduction* 7 (May 1992): 701–710.

Check, Jerome H., M.D., et al. "Comparison of Various Therapies for the Luteinized Unruptured Follicle Syndrome," *International Journal of Fertility* 37 (January/February 1992): 33–40.

Croxatto, H. B., et al. "Studies in the Duration of Egg Transport by the Human Oviduct. II. Ovum Location at Various Intervals Following Luteinized Hormone Peak," *American Journal of Obstetrics & Gynecology* 132 (November 15, 1978): 629–634.

Cunha, G. R., Ph.D., et al. "Teratogenic Effects of Clomiphene, Tamoxifen, and Diethylstilbestrol on the Developing Human Female Genetic Tract," *Human Pathology* 18 (November 1987): 1132–1143.

Daly, Douglas C., M.D., et al. "Ultrasonographic Assessment of Luteinized Unruptured Follicle Syndrome in Unexplained Infertility," *Fertility and Sterility* 43 (January 1985): 62–65.

Darland, Nancy Wilson, RNC, MSN. "Infertility Associated with Luteal Phase Defect," *Journal of Obstetric, Gynecologic and Neonatal Nursing* (May/June 1985): 212–217.

Daviaud, Joëlle, et al. "Reliability and Feasibility of Pregnancy Home-Use Tests: Laboratory Validation and Diagnostic Evaluation by 638 Volunteers," *Clinical Chemistry* 39 (January 1993): 53–59.

De Mouzon, Jacques, M.D., et al. "Time Relationships Between Basal Body Temperature and Ovulation or Plasma Progestins," *Fertility and Sterility* 41 (February 1984): 254–259.

DeVane, Gary W., M.D. "Prolactin Measurement: What Is Normal?" *Contemporary Ob/Gyn* (September 1989): 99–117.

Eggert-Kruse, W., I. Gerhard, W. Tilgen, & B. Runnebaum. "The Use of Hens' Egg White as a Substitute for Human Cervical Mucus in Assessing Human Infertility," *International Journal of Andrology* 13 (August 1990): 258–266.

Fehring, Richard J., R.N., DNSc. "Methods Used to Self-Predict Ovulation: A Comparative Study," *Journal of Obstetric, Gynecologic and Neonatal Nursing* 19 (May/June 1990): 233–237.

Field, Charles S., M.D. "Dysfunctional Uterine Bleeding," *Primary Care* 15 (September 1988): 561–573.

Filer, Robert B., M.D., & Chung H. Wu, M.D. "Coitus During Menses: Its Effect on Endometriosis and Pelvic Inflammatory Disease," *Journal of Reproductive Medicine* 34 (November 1989): 887–890.

Filicori, Marco, et al. "Evidence for a Specific Role of GnRH Pulse Frequency in the Control of the Human Menstrual Cycle," *American Journal of Physiology* 257 (December 1989): 930–936.

Fish, Lisa H., M.D., & Cary N. Mariash, M.D. "Hyperprolactinemia, Infertility, and Hypothyroidism," *Archives of Internal Medicine* 148 (March 1988): 709–711.

Flynn, Anna M., & John Bonnar. "Natural Family Planning." In *Contraception: Science and Practice,* edited by Marcus Filshie & John Guillebaud, pp. 203–205. London: Butterworth Press, 1989.

Fordney-Settlage, Diane, M.D., M.S. "A Review of Cervical Mucus and Sperm Interactions in Humans," *International Journal of Fertility* 26 (1981): 161–169.

France, John T., Ph.D. "Overview of the Biological Aspects of the Fertile Period," *International Journal of Fertility* 26 (1981): 143–152.

Freidson, Eliot, Ph.D. "The Professional Mind." In *The Sociology of Medicine, A Structural Approach,* pp. 130–131. New York: Dodd, Mead, 1968.

Gnant, Michael F. X., et al. "Breast Cancer and Timing of Surgery During Menstrual Cycle: A 5-Year Analysis of 385 Pre-Menopausal Women," *International Journal of Cancer* 52 (November 11, 1992): 707–712.

Goldenberg, Robert L., M.D., & Roberta White, R.N. "The Effect of Vaginal Lubricants on Sperm Motility in Vitro," *Fertility and Sterility* 26 (September 1975): 872–873.

Gondos, Bernard, M.D., & Daniel H. Riddick, M.D., Ph.D. "Cervical Mucus and Sperm Motility." In *Pathology of Infertility: Clinical Correlations in the Male and Female,* edited by Bernard Gondos & Daniel H. Riddick, pp. 337–351. New York: Thieme Medical Publishers, Inc., 1987.

Grodstein, Francine, et al. "Relation of Female Infertility to Consumption of Caffeinated Beverages," *American Journal of Epidemiology* 137 ( June 15, 1993): 1353–1359.

Guerrero, R., O. Rojas, & A. Cifuentes. "Natural Family Planning Methods." In *Human Ovulation,* edited by E. S. E. Hafez, pp. 477–479. Amsterdam and New York: Elsevier North-Holland Biomedical Press, 1979.

Guyton, Arthur C., M.D. "Endocrinology and Reproduction." In *Textbook of Medical Physiology,* 8th ed., edited by Arthur C. Guyton, p. 912. Philadelphia: W. B. Saunders Company, 1991.

Hamilton, Mark P. R., M.D., et al. "Luteal Cysts and Unexplained Infertility: Biochemical and Ultrasonic Evaluation," *Fertility and Sterility* 54 ( July 1990): 32–37.

Hibbard, Lester T., M.D. "Corpus Luteum Surgery," *American Journal of Obstetrics & Gynecology* 135 (November 1, 1979): 666–667.

Hilgers, Thomas W., Guy E. Abraham, & Ann M. Prebil. "The Length of the Luteal Phase," *International Review* (Spring/Summer 1989): 99–106.

Hilgers, Thomas W., M.D., & Alan J. Bailey, MSW, ACSW. "Natural Family Planning. II. Basal Body Temperature and Estimated Time of Ovulation," *Obstetrics & Gynecology* 55 (March 1980): 333–339.

Hilgers, Thomas W., M.D., FACOG, Guy E. Abraham, M.D., & Denis Cavanagh, M.D., FACOG. "Natural Family Planning: I. The Peak Symptom and Estimated Time of Ovulation," *The American College of Obstetricians and Gynecologists* 52 (November 1978): 575–582.

Howles, Colin M. "Follicle Growth and Luteinization." In *Encyclopedia of Human Biology,* Vol. 3, edited by Renalto Dulbecco, pp. 627–635. London: Academic Press, 1991.

Huggins, George R., M.D., & Vanessa E. Collins, M.D. "Fertility After Contraception or Abortion," *Fertility and Sterility* 54 (October 1990): 559–570.

Hull, M. G. R., et al. "Expectations of Assisted Conception for Fertility," *British Medical Journal* 304 ( June 6, 1992): 1465–1469.

Joesoef, M. Riduan, et al. "Are Caffeinated Beverages Risk Factors for Delayed Conception?" *The Lancet* (January 20, 1990): 136–137.

Jones, Ben Morgan, & Marilyn K. Jones. "Alcohol Effects in Women During the Menstrual Cycle," *Annals of the Academy of Sciences* 273 (1971): 1–664.

Jones, Howard W. Jr., M.D., & James P. Toner, M.D., Ph.D. "The Infertile Couple," *New England Journal of Medicine* 7 (December 2, 1993): 1710–1715.

Kerin, John F., M.D., FACOG, et al. "Incidence of the Luteinized Unruptured Follicle Phenomenon in Cycling Women," *Fertility and Sterility* 40 (November 1983): 620–626.

Knee, Gerald R., M.S., et al. "Detection of the Ovulatory Luteinizing Hormone (LH) Surge with a Semiquantitative Urinary LH Assay," *Fertility and Sterility* 44 (November 1985): 707–709.

Koninckx, P. R., & I. A. Brosens. "The Luteinized Unruptured Follicle Syndrome." In *The Inadequate Luteal Phase: Pathophysiology, Diagnostics, Therapy,* edited by H. D. Taubert & H. Kuhl, pp. 145–151. Lancaster: MTP Press, 1983.

Lamb, Emmet J., M.D., & Sue Luergans, Ph.D. "Does Adoption Affect Subsequent Fertility?" *American Journal of Obstetrics & Gynecology* 134 (May 15, 1979): 138–144.

Lambert, Hovey, Ph.D., et al. "Sperm Capacitation in the Human Female Reproductive Tract," *Fertility and Sterility* 43 (February 1985): 325–327.

Landy, Helain J., M.D., et al. "The 'Vanishing-Twin': Ultrasonographic Assessment of Fetal Disappearance in the First Trimester," *American Journal of Obstetrics & Gynecology* (July 1986): 14–19.

LeMaire, Gail Schoen, R.N., M.S.N. "The Luteinized Unruptured Follicle Syndrome: Anovulation in Disguise," *Journal of Obstetric, Gynecologic and Neonatal Nursing* (March/April 1987): 116–120.

Lenton, Elizabeth A., Britt-Marie Landgren, & Lynne Sexton. "Normal Variation in the Length of the Luteal Phase of the Menstrual Cycle: Identification of the Short Luteal Phase," *British Journal of Obstetrics and Gynecology* 91 (July 1984): 685–689.

Luciano, Anthony A., M.D., et al. "Temporal Relationship and Reliability of the Clinical, Hormonal, and Ultrasonographic Indices of Ovulation in Infertile Women," *Obstetrics & Gynecology* 75 (March 1990): 412–416.

MacGillivray, Ian, Mike Samphier, & Julian Little. "Factors Affecting Twinning." In *Twinning and Twins,* edited by I. MacGillivray, D. M. Campbell, & B. Thompson, pp. 67–92. London: John Wiley & Sons, 1988.

March, C. M. "Ovulation Induction," *Journal of Reproductive Medicine* 38 (May 1993): 335–346.

Marik, Jaroslav, M.D., & Jaroslav Hulka, M.D. "Luteinized Unruptured Follicle Syndrome: A Subtle Cause of Infertility," *Fertility and Sterility* 29 (March 1978): 270–274.

McCarthy, John J. Jr., M.D., & Howard E. Rockette, Ph.D. "A Comparison of Methods to Interpret the Basal Body Temperature Graph," *Fertility and Sterility* 39 (May 1983): 640–646.

Messinis, I. E., et al. "Changes in Pituitary Response to GnRH During the Luteal-Follicular Transition of the Human Menstrual Cycle," *Clinical Endocrinology* 38 (February 1993): 159–163.

Nesse, Robert E., M.D. "Abnormal Vaginal Bleeding in Perimenopausal Women," *American Family Physician* (July 1989): 185–189.

Nicholson, Roberto, M.D. "Vitality of Spermatozoa in the Endocervical Canal," *Fertility and Sterility* 16 (November/December 1965): 758–764.

O'Herlihy, C., MRCOG, MRCPI, & H. P. Robinson, M.D., MRCOG. "Mittelschmerz Is a Preovulatory Symptom," *British Medical Journal* 280 (April 1980): 986.

Olsen, Jorn. "Cigarette Smoking, Tea and Coffee Drinking, and Subfecundity," *American Journal of Epidemiology* 133(7) (April 1, 1991): 734–739.

Overstreet, James W., David F. Katz, & Ashley I. Yudin. "Cervical Mucus and Sperm Transport in Reproduction," *Seminars in Perinatology* 15 (April 1991): 149–155.

Padilla, Santiago L., M.D., & Kathryn S. Craft, RNC. "Anovulation: Etiology, Evaluation and Management," *Nurse Practitioner* 10(12) (December 1985): 28–44.

Pillet, M. Christine, M.D., et al. "Improved Prediction of Postovulatory Day Using Temperature Recording, Endometrial Biopsy, and Serum Progesterone," *Fertility and Sterility* 53 (April 1990): 614–619.

Pritchard, Jack P., Paul C. MacDonald, & Norman F. Gant. "Multifetal Pregnancy." In *Williams Obstetrics,* 17th ed., pp. 503–524. Norwalk, CT: Appleton-Century-Crofts, 1985.

Profet, Margie. "Menstruation as a Defense Against Pathogens Transported by Sperm," *The Quarterly Review of Biology* 68 (September 1993): 335–381.

Rebar, Robert W. "Premature Ovarian Failure." In *Treatment of the Post Menopausal Woman: Basic and Clinical Aspects,* edited by Rogerio A. Lobo, pp. 25–33. New York: Raven Press, 1994.

Ross, G. T. "HCG in Early Human Pregnancy." In *Maternal Recognition of Pregnancy,* edited by Julie Whelan, pp. 198–199. New York: Ciba Foundation Press, 1979.

Rossing, Mary Anne, D.V.M., Ph.D., et al. "Ovarian Tumors in a Cohort of Infertile Women," *The New England Journal of Medicine* 331(12) (September 22, 1994): 771–776.

Rousseau, Serge, M.D., et al. "The Expectancy of Pregnancy for 'Normal' Infertile Couples," *Fertility and Sterility* 40 (December 1983): 768–772.

Scholes, D., et al. "Vaginal Douching as a Risk Factor for Acute Pelvic Inflammatory Disease," *Obstetrics & Gynecology* 81 (April 1993): 601–606.

Simmer, Hans H. "Placental Hormones." In *Biology of Gestation,* edited by N. S. Assali, pp. 296–299. New York: Academic Press, 1968.

Smith, S. K., Elizabeth A. Lenton, & I. D. Cooke. "Plasma Gonadotropin and Ovarian Steroid Concentrations in Women with Menstrual Cycles with a Short Luteal Phase," *Journal of Reproduction and Fertility* 75 (November 1985): 363–368.

Smith, Stephen K., et al. "The Short Luteal Phase and Infertility," *British Journal of Obstetrics and Gynecology* 91 (November 1984): 1120–1122.

Souka, Abdel Razek, et al. "Effect of Aspirin on the Luteal Phase of Human Menstrual Cycle," *Contraception* 29 (February 1984): 181–188.

Thomas, R., M.D., & R. L. Reid, M.D. "Thyroid Disease and Reproductive Dysfunction: A Review," *Obstetrics & Gynecology* 70 (November 1987): 789–792.

Thrush, Parke, M.D., & Deborah Willard, M.D. "Pseudo-Ectopic Pregnancy: An Ovarian Cyst Mimicking Ectopic Pregnancy," *The West Virginia Medical Journal* 85 (November 1989): 488–489.

Tulandi, Togas, M.D., & Robert A. McInnes, M.D. "Vaginal Lubricants: Effect of Glycerin and Egg White on Sperm Motility and Progression in Vitro," *Fertility and Sterility* 41 (January 1984): 151–153.

Tulandi, Togas, M.D., Leo Plouffe, Jr., M.D. & Robert A. McInnes, M.D. "Effects of Saliva on Sperm Motility and Activity," *Fertility and Sterility* 38 (December 1982): 721–723.

Vermesh, Michael, M.D., et al. "Monitoring Techniques to Predict and Detect Ovulation," *Fertility and Sterility* 47 (February 1987): 259–264.

Veronesi, Umberto, et al. "Effect of Menstrual Phase on Surgical Treatment of Breast Cancer," *The Lancet* 343 ( June 18, 1994): 1545–1547.

Weir, William C., M.D., & David R. Weir, M.D. "Adoption and Subsequent Conceptions," *Fertility and Sterility* 17(2) (March/April 1966): 283–288.

Wilcox, Allen, Clarine Weinberg, & Donna Baird. "Caffeinated Beverages and Decreased Fertility," *The Lancet* (December 24–31, 1988): 1453–1455.

Wood, James W. "Fecundity and Natural Fertility in Humans." In *Oxford Reviews of Reproductive Biology,* Vol. 11, edited by S. R. Milligan, pp. 61–109. Oxford: Oxford University Press, 1989.

Worley, Richard J., M.D. "Dysfunctional Uterine Bleeding," *Postgraduate Medicine* 9 (February 15, 1986): 101–106.

Yong, Eu Leong, MRCOG, et al. "Simple Office Methods to Predict Ovulation: The Clinical Usefulness of a New Urine Luteinizing Hormone Kit Compared to Basal Body Temperature, Cervical Mucus and Ultrasound," *Australia and New Zealand Journal of Obstetrics & Gynecology* 29 (May 1989): 155–159.

Zacur, Howard A., M.D., Ph.D., & Machelle M. Seibel, M.D. "Steps in Diagnosing Prolactin-Related Disorders," *Contemporary Ob/Gyn* (September 1989): 84–96.

Zuspan, Kathryn J., & F. P. Zuspan. "Basal Body Temperature." In *Human Ovulation,* edited by E. S. E. Hafez, pp. 291–298. Amsterdam and New York: Elsevier North-Holland Biomedical Press, 1979.

**Books**

Biale, Rachel. *Women and Jewish Law: An Exploration of Women's Issues in Halakhic Sources.* New York: Schocken Books, 1984.

Bryan, Elizabeth M., M.D., MRCP, DCH. *The Nature and Nurture of Twins.* London: Baillière Tindall, 1983.

*Danforth's Obstetrics and Gynecology,* 6th ed. Philadelphia: J. B. Lippincott Company, 1990.

Edwards, Robert G. *Conception in the Human Female.* London: Academic Press/Harcourt Brace Jovanovich, 1980.

Gondos, Bernard, M.D., & Daniel H. Riddick, M.D., Ph.D., eds. *Pathology of Infertility: Clinical Correlations in the Male and Female.* New York: Thieme Medical Publishers, 1987.

Hafez, E. S. E., ed. *Human Reproduction: Conception and Contraception,* 2nd ed. New York: Harper & Row, 1980.

Herbst, Arthur L., M.D., & Howard A. Bern, Ph.D., eds. *Developmental Effects of Diethylstilbestrol (DES) in Pregnancy.* New York: Thieme-Stratton, 1981.

Kaplan, Abraham. *The Conduct of Inquiry: Methodology for Behavioral Science.* San Francisco: Chandler, 1964.

Mishell, Daniel R., Jr., M.D., & Val Davajan, M.D., eds. *Infertility, Contraception & Reproductive Endocrinology,* 2nd ed. Oradell, NJ: Medical Economics, 1986.

Older, Julia. *Endometriosis*. New York: Scribner's, 1984.

Sachs, Judith. *What Women Can Do About Chronic Endometriosis*. New York: Dell, 1991.

Taymor, Melvin L., M.D. *Infertility: A Clinician's Guide to Diagnosis and Treatment*. New York and London: Plenum, 1990.

## MALE FERTILITY

### Articles

Ahlgren, M., Kerstin Boström, & R. Malmqvist. "Sperm Transport and Survival in Women with Special Reference to the Fallopian Tube," *The Biology of Spermatozoa*, Institute National de la Santé et de la Recherche Medicale Int. Symp., Nouzilly, France (1973): 63–73.

Amelar, Richard D., M.D., Lawrence Dubin, M.D., & Cy Schoenfeld, Ph.D. "Sperm Motility," *Fertility and Sterility* 34 (September 1980): 197–215.

Austin, G. R. "Sperm Fertility, Viability and Persistence in the Female Tract," *Journal of Reproduction and Fertility,* Suppl. 22 (1975): 75–89.

Dawson, Earl B., William A. Harris, & Leslie C. Powell. "Relationship Between Ascorbic Acid and Male Fertility," *World Review of Nutrition and Diet* 62 (1990): 2–26.

Giblin, Paul T., Ph.D., et al. "Effects of Stress and Characteristic Adaptability on Semen Quality in Healthy Men," *Fertility and Sterility* 49 (January 1988): 127–132.

Harris, William A., A.A., Thaddeus E. Harden, B.S., & Earl B. Dawson, Ph.D. "Apparent Effect of Ascorbic Acid Medication on Semen Metal Levels," *Fertility and Sterility* 32 (October 1979): 455–459.

Jaszczak, S., & E. S. E. Hafez. "Physiopathology of Sperm Transport in the Human Female," *The Biology of Spermatozoa*, Institute National de la Santé et de la Recherche Medicale Int. Symp., Nouzilly, France (1973): 250–256.

Levin, Robert M., Ph.D., et al. "Correlation of Sperm Count with Frequency of Ejaculation," *Fertility and Sterility* 45 (May 1986): 732–734.

Makler, Amnon, M.D., et al. "Factors Affecting Sperm Motility. IX. Survival of Spermatozoa in Various Biological Media and Under Different Gaseous Compositions," *Fertility and Sterility* 41 (March 1984): 428–432.

Medical News. "Sperm Swim Singly after Vitamin C Therapy," *Journal of the American Medical Association* 249 (May 27, 1983): 2747–2751.

Megory, E., H. Zuckerman, Z. Shoham (Schwartz), & B. Lunenfeld. "Infections and Male Fertility," *Obstetrical and Gynecological Survey* 42 (1987): 283–290.

Schlegel, Peter N., M.D., Thomas S. K. Chang, Ph.D., & Gray F. Marshall, M.D. "Antibiotics: Potential Hazards to Male Fertility," *Fertility and Sterility* 55 (February 1991): 235–242.

Tulandi, Togas, M.D., Leo Plouffe, Jr., M.D., & Robert A. McInnes, M.D. "Effects of Saliva on Sperm Motility and Activity," *Fertility and Sterility* 38 (December 1982): 721–723.

Zinaman, Michael, et al. "The Physiology of Sperm Recovered from the Human Cervix:

Acrosomal Status and Response to Inducers of the Acrosome Reaction," *Biology of Reproduction* 41 (November 1989): 790–797.

### Books

Glover, T. D., C. L. R. Barratt, J. P. P. Tyler, & J. F. Hennessey. *Human Male Fertility and Semen Analysis.* London: Academic Press/Harcourt Brace Jovanovich, 1990.

Tanagho, Emil, & Jack W. McAninch. *Smith's General Urology,* 13th Edition. Norwalk, CT: Appleton and Lange, 1992.

## MENOPAUSE

### Articles

Cummings, D. C. "Menarche, Menses, and Menopause: A Brief Review," *Cleveland Clinical Journal of Medicine* 57 (March–April 1990): 169–175.

Flynn, Anna M., M.D., et al. "Sympto-Thermal and Hormonal Markers of Potential Fertility in Climacteric Women," *American Journal of Obstetrics and Gynecology* 165 (December 1991): 1987–1989.

Rosenberg, Leon E. "Endocrinology and Metabolism." In *Harrison's Principles of Internal Medicine,* edited by Jean D. Wilson et al., pp. 1780–1781. New York: McGraw-Hill, 1991.

Shideler, S. E., et al. "Ovarian-Pituitary Hormone Interactions During the Peri-Menopause," *Maturitas* 11 (December 1989): 331–339.

### Books

Utian, Wulf H. *Menopause in Modern Perspective: A Guide to Clinical Practice.* New York: Appleton-Century-Crofts, 1980.

## PMS

### Articles

Chakmakjian, Z. H., M.D., C. E. Higgins, B.S., & G. E. Abraham, M.D. "The Effects of a Nutritional Supplement, Optivite for Women, on Premenstrual Tension Syndromes," *Journal of Applied Nutrition* 37 (1985): 12–17.

Endicott, Jean. "The Menstrual Cycle and Mood Disorders," *Journal of Affective Disorders* 29 (October–November 1993): 193–200.

Faccinetti, Fabio, M.D., et al. "Premenstrual Fall of Plasma β-Endorphin in Patients with Premenstrual Syndrome," *Fertility and Sterility* 47 (April 1987): 570–573.

### Books

Severino, Sally K., M.D., & Margaret L. Moline, Ph.D. *Premenstrual Syndrome: A Clinician's Guide.* New York: Guilford Press, 1989.

# Index

Page numbers in *italics* refer to illustrations.